O9-ABE-632

APR 1 7 2003

RC
483
.L47
1991

WITHDRAWN

Lickey, Marvin E.,
1937-

Medicine and mental
illness.

$29.95

RC
483
.L47
1991

Lickey, Marvin
E., 1937-

Medicine and
mental illness.

$29.95

DEC 1 5 2004

DATE   BORROWER'S NAME

FEB 2 7 2002   CHECKED APR 0 9 2003

AUG 0 6 2002   DEC 1 8 2002

CHECKED AUG 0 5 2002

CHECKED JAN 0 6 2002

APR 1 7 2003

KVCC KALAMAZOO VALLEY
      COMMUNITY COLLEGE
      LIBRARY

BAKER & TAYLOR BOOKS

MEDICINE AND MENTAL ILLNESS

RC
483
.L47
1991

MEDICINE AND MENTAL ILLNESS

The Use of Drugs in Psychiatry

Marvin E. Lickey
and Barbara Gordon

Department of Psychology and Institute of Neuroscience
University of Oregon

W. H. FREEMAN & COMPANY · NEW YORK

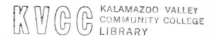
KALAMAZOO VALLEY
COMMUNITY COLLEGE
LIBRARY

MAR 0 5 1992

Library of Congress Cataloging-in-Publication Data

Lickey, Marvin E., 1937–
Medicine and mental illness : understanding drug treatment in
psychiatry / Marvin E. Lickey and Barbara Gordon.
p.   cm.
Rev. ed. of: Drugs for mental illness. c1983.
Includes bibliographical references and index.
ISBN 0-7167-2195-3 (hard). — ISBN 0-7167-2196-1 (soft)
1. Psychopharmacology.   2. Affective disorders—Chemotherapy.
3. Schizophrenia—Chemotherapy.   4. Anxiety—Chemotherapy.
I. Gordon, Barbara, 1942–   .   II. Lickey, Marvin E., 1937–   Drugs
for mental illness.   III. Title.
[DNLM: 1. Affective Disorders, Psychotic—drug therapy.
2. Anxiety Disorders—drug therapy.   3. Schizophrenia—drug therapy.
WM 402 L711d]
RC483.L47   1991
616.89′ 18z—dc20

DNLM/DLC   191-9562
for Library of Congress   CIP

Copyright © 1991 by W. H. Freeman and Company

No part of this book may be reproduced by any mechanical, photographic,
or electronic process, or in the form of a phonographic recording, nor may
it be stored in a retrieval system, transmitted, or otherwise copied for
public or private use, without written permission from the publisher.

Printed in the United States of America

1 2 3 4 5 6 7 8 9 0 VB 9 9 8 7 6 5 4 3 2 1

For our parents
Marjorie and Eugene Gordon
Veva Lickey

And in memory of
Harold Lickey

CONTENTS

——

PREFACE

—

Our desire to write about drugs for mental illness was kindled by two experiences. The first was connected with our work as professors in the Institute of Neuroscience and the Department of Psychology at the University of Oregon. Until the early 1970s we had not paid much attention in our research and teaching to the medical applications of neuroscience, supposing psychiatry a rather unscientific, not really medical profession whose responsibility was to look after helpless people who were not medically ill. In our effort to satisfy the rising demand of undergraduates for greater relevance in classroom studies, however, we found our aloofness unacceptable. Our students' desire for relevance was never greater than when we lectured about the actions of chemicals on brain cells. The youth drug culture was then in full flower; many of the students were taking psychoactive drugs recreationally, and they were curious to learn what neuroscience had to say about mind-altering drugs. Psychopharmacology thus became part of our course syllabus. To provide a balanced treatment, we began to teach about psychiatric drugs, as well as about recreational and illicit drugs, and of necessity we learned, too, about the practice of psychiatry.

Talking with students and friends, we found that the drug revolution in psychiatry was not widely understood. Most of our acquaintances believed, as we had before we studied the subject, that psychiatry's only legitimate tool was words; most were skeptical or disapproving of the use of drugs to treat mental illness. As our appreciation of contemporary psychiatric treatment grew, we became convinced that everyone should take some time to learn how the profession is practiced in the late twentieth century.

The second impetus for writing this book was a more personal event. At about the same time that we started teaching about psychoactive drugs, a colleague at another university suffered a severe episode of mental illness that seriously disrupted both his career and his personal life. After training at several famous universities and establishing himself as a competent researcher in neurophysiology, he experienced recurrent outbreaks of anger mixed with hopelessness and despair that brought his work to a halt. His ability to think and concentrate was lost because of mental turmoil. His relationships with his wife and children deteriorated. After nearly two years of floundering with ineffective therapies, misdiagnosis, and inappropriate drugs, our friend finally consulted a psychiatrist, who gave the correct diagnosis, an effective drug treatment, and effective psychotherapy. His recovery was so dramatic that in an earlier age it would have been called a miracle. There was nothing magical about his recovery, of course; on the contrary, proper treatment had constructively changed the physiological activity in his brain. And we intended to understand more deeply the reasons that his treatment and others like it produce such beneficial results.

Now it is about 20 years since we first started teaching about psychoactive drugs. Although the public is more broadly aware of the benefits and risks of drug treatments, there is still a need to continue exploring the nature of mental illness, its roots in brain activity, and its treatment with drugs and other therapies. Research moves rapidly: The number of drugs continually increases, and alternative psychotherapies are continually devised and tested. Moreover, since about 25 percent of the population will suffer an episode of mental illness at some point in life, everyone needs up-to-date information about available treatments.

Since 1982, when we finished writing the previous edition of this book, entitled *Drugs for Mental Illness*, there have been many developments. New drugs have been introduced. The *DSM-III* has been revised. Drug treatments have been developed for disorders that previously had not been treated with drugs. Scientific understanding of the biological bases of psychiatric disorders has increased. More is known about how psychiatric drugs affect the brain. Our concepts of the relationship between drug therapy and psychotherapy have become more sophisticated. These advances are reflected in this edition, which we have entitled *Medicine and Mental Illness: The Use of Drugs in Psychiatry*.

New drugs discussed include clozapine for previously intractable schizophrenia, fluoxetine, the most popular of the new antidepressants, and two new drugs for anxiety, alprazolam and buspirone. Several side effects of antipsychotics not discussed in the first edition are now included. The discussions of the mechanisms of action of antipsychotics, antidepressants, and lithium have been completely rewritten to reflect current research.

The discussion of the genetic basis of schizophrenia and bipolar disorder has been expanded to include modern molecular genetic studies. New results from brain imaging studies have been included in the discussions of relationships between brain structures and psychiatric disorders.

The chapters on diagnosis now explain the diagnostic categories in the *DSM-III-R* rather than the *DSM-III*. The sections on behavioral medicine have been strengthened with new material on cognitive and interpersonal therapy, the relation between stress and depression, and the cognitive side effects of antidepressants.

The largest change is the addition of two new chapters on drug therapy and psychotherapy for several anxiety disorders that were not mentioned in the first edition: panic disorder, phobias, and obsessive-compulsive disorder.

We thank Michael Powell for typing and bibliographic assistance. We also thank Dr. Charles Ksir, Lawrence H. Price, M.D., an anonymous reviewer, and Jonathan Cobb at W. H. Freeman for their penetrating and detailed reviews of the manuscript.

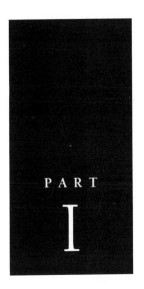

PART

I

BACKGROUND

1

DRUGS ENTER PSYCHIATRY

—

D uring the decade of the 1950s the introduction of several new drugs enabled psychiatrists to treat a variety of serious mental illnesses that had previously been intractable. The new drugs revolutionized psychiatry. Millions of psychiatric patients began receiving the new drug treatments. People who otherwise would have lived their entire lives in psychiatric hospitals became able to care for themselves, and some of the most dehumanizing symptoms of mental illness disappeared. Anguish was lifted from the families of the afflicted, and the cost of psychiatric hospitalization was radically reduced. Many psychiatrists place the psychiatric drugs introduced in the fifties among the great medical advances of the twentieth century, comparable in their impact to antibiotics and vaccines. In this chapter we describe some of the changes that occurred in the psychiatric environment as a result of the new drug treatments and we identify some of the controversies that were aroused by the new drugs as they were assimilated into psychiatric practice.

THE DRUG REVOLUTION IN PSYCHIATRY

The drug revolution in psychiatry began in 1949 when an Australian psychiatrist, John F. J. Cade, reported on some of his experiments with lithium. He had found that injections of lithium could produce tame behavior in otherwise defensive and fearful guinea pigs. In a great leap of overconfidence that would have left current medical researchers aghast (and would be illegal under present U.S. regulations governing the development of new drug therapies), Cade gave lithium to ten hospitalized manic and agitated psychiatric patients. The experimental treatment worked. The patients assumed emotional tones much closer to the normal range. One of the patients, who had been hospitalized for five years, almost continuously in a state of manic agitation, had failed to respond to many different types of treatment. After four weeks on lithium, however, he became so much calmer that he was able to leave the hospital, live at home, and resume his old job. A few years later, the French psychiatrists Jean Delay and Pierre Deniker successfully tested the drug chlorpromazine (brand name, Thorazine) for calming psychotic agitation. In the late 1950s, drugs for the effective treatment of depression became available.[1]

The new drugs were revolutionary because they worked. Before 1950, effective treatments for severely debilitated, hospitalized mental patients had been virtually unknown. Psychiatrists had searched for treatments since early in the nineteenth century,but with the exception of electroconvulsive shock treatment for depression, their search had been unsuccessful. In desperation psychiatrists had prescribed treatments like insulin shock and hydrotherapy. They had tried psychological therapies, including psychoanalysis. But convincing evidence that these treatments worked had always been scarce. By contrast, the new drugs were demonstrably effective in the majority of patients who received them.

Since about 1975, much progress has also been made in improving the effectiveness of psychotherapy. There are now nonpharmacologic procedures to help prevent relapses in schizophrenia and to relieve depression, phobias, and obsessive-compulsive disorder. The advances in psychotherapy, like the advances in drug therapy, have been brought about through careful collection of evidence about the success rate of particular forms of treatment. Thus new drug treatments have developed hand in hand with new psychotherapies. Although we concentrate on drug treatments in this book, we also point out situations in which both drugs and psychotherapy are used to treat the same mental disorder, and we try to explain how the two types of treatment supplement and complement each other.

The new psychiatric drugs were revolutionary because they made psychiatry more accessible to people in need. Psychoanalysis, the main type of psychotherapy that was available before 1960, was very time-consuming and expensive. In many cases it required sessions with a psychiatrist more than once a week for several years. Moreover, qualified psychiatrists were available only in major population centers. Such treatment was therefore logistically and financially impossible for most people. Hospitalized patients usually received no psychotherapy because there were not enough psychotherapists on hospital staffs. By comparison, psychiatrists and nurses could be more easily trained to administer the new psychotherapies. There was no longer a need for extended weekly conversations between patients and highly trained therapists. In many cases, psychotherapists interact with several patients at once in weekly meetings. In other cases, a substantial part of the therapy may be done as "homework." The new psychotherapies are clearly cheaper and easier to administer than those that prevailed before 1960.

The impact of the drug revolution on mental health care can be illustrated by examining the number of patients residing in state and county mental hospitals between 1905 and 1986 (Figure 1–1). During the first half of the twentieth century, the number of patients steadily increased from 150,000 to about 550,000. In the period just following World War II, there were so many hospitalized mental patients that it became a common joke that the sane and the insane would soon have to exchange housing. In 1956, the year the new drugs were introduced in the United States, the upward trend reversed, and by 1975 the number of hospitalized patients declined to 200,000. By 1986 the number dropped to 111,000. The decline in the number of hospitalized patients was not the result of a decrease in the rate of new hospital admissions. Rather, the new drugs made it

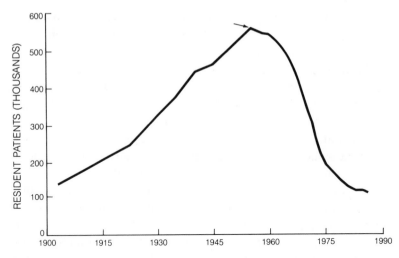

FIGURE 1-1   Resident patients in state and county mental hospitals. Arrow indicates year in which chlorpromazine was first used.

possible for patients to leave the hospital after a much briefer stay. Before 1956 patients often spent their entire lives in the hospital. In 1986 the average length of stay was only about two weeks.[2]

Current treatment for severe mental illness typically consists of an initial hospital stay during which the patient is medically and psychologically evaluated. If drug therapy is appropriate and if the patient has no medical problems that would make drug side effects too risky, an initial drug trial is carried out under close medical supervision. If the treatment is successful and without harmful side effects, the patient is released and the drug therapy continued outside the hospital. Outpatient psychotherapy may be called for in conjunction with drugs, depending on the needs of the particular patient. Careful attention to individual needs is an important part of any treatment.

The depopulation of mental hospitals in the late twentieth century, referred to as the deinstitutionalization of the mentally ill, has brought a new set of problems that we, as a society, are not dealing with effectively. As shown in Chapter 6, drug treatments for some of the most disabling disorders are only partially effective in some patients. The drugs may bring about significant improvement but fail to restore full normality. Partially recovered patients are usually able to live outside the hospital if they receive some guidance and protection in the community, but they may not be well enough to live independently. Unfortunately, the taxpayers and their governmental representatives have usually not provided for the needed guidance and protection of partially recovered patients. Instead, the drug revolution has been exploited as a way to cut public spending for mental health care. As a result some patients released from the hospital in fairly good mental health are subsequently unable to maintain their improved condition in the community.[3]

Psychiatric drugs dramatically improved the quality of life inside mental hospitals. Before 1956 the hospital environment was dismal. The quarters were typically overcrowded. Hallucinating patients talked to their "voices." Stuporous catatonic patients sat in one place, in one posture, for days, developing pressure sores. Withdrawn patients did not speak to anyone. Manic patients paced the floor purposelessly for days until exhausted, and those who were violent were physically restrained. Physicians and other hospital personnel, unable to find more effective ways to relieve the symptoms, desperately applied procedures like insulin shock, warm baths, and strapping patients in wet sheets to calm psychotic agitation. Often, patients were put in straitjackets, isolated in padded rooms, or given debilitating sedative drugs. Therapeutic success was usually only temporary, and physicians were mainly supervisors of custodial care. The new drugs have transformed the hospital environment into one that is free of bizarre psychotic symptoms. Many patients can now enjoy sports, handicrafts, music, entertainment, and even gainful employment.[4] The principal complaint is that patients suffer excessively from drug side effects.

CONTROVERSIES ABOUT DRUG TREATMENT

Like all revolutions, the drug revolution in psychiatry provoked controversy and criticism. Some of the controversy has been laid to rest, but some, revolving around four main issues, persists:

1. Is mental illness primarily biological or psychological?
2. Is psychotherapy or drug therapy better?

3. Does drug treatment violate patients' legal rights?
4. Are the side effects of the drugs worse than the mental illness itself?

These issues are introduced here and discussed further in Chapter 19.

Is Mental Illness Primarily Biological or Psychological?

In the United States and elsewhere there is a philosophical and semantic custom of distinguishing the mind from the body. In our everyday conversation, we habitually speak of psychological problems as if they were different from biological, medical illnesses. Depression, anxiety, and paranoia seem to be in the mind, not in the body. In colleges and universities, the psychology department is often isolated from the biology department. Biology majors are required to study physics and organic chemistry as a foundation for their major subject, but natural sciences are seldom seen as fundamental to the study of psychology.

Although the customary distinction between mind and body provides a practical method for referring to two different aspects of human existence, it also leads people to believe—mistakenly, in our opinion—that the mind and the body are fundamentally different. Because of this perceived difference, many people are uncomfortable with the fundamental assumption underlying biological treatments in psychiatry, the assumption that mental disorders are brain disorders. In the following chapters of this book, mental illness is discussed as if the mind and the brain are inextricably intertwined. It is often (perhaps always) impossible to say whether mental illness is primarily biological or psychological.

Is Psychotherapy or Drug Therapy Better?

Another source of resistance to biological psychiatry has been the vigorous tradition of psychoanalysis and other forms of psychotherapy in which the activities of the therapist are directed toward giving patients insight into the psychological causes of their distress. In the first half of the twentieth century, following the theories of Sigmund Freud, it became first fashionable and then customary to think of mental illnesses as being caused by psychological conflict. Freud thought that patients do not understand or are unaware of the conflicts causing their distress. He proposed that insight into these underlying conflicts was needed for a cure. Patients would have to laboriously recollect the critical experiences that created their conflicts and, with the help of a therapist, learn how those conflicts were causing their distress.

Although Freud's outlook was biological in the sense that he thought the mind obeyed the animal instinctual drives for reproduction and bodily security, he did not theorize about possible brain mechanisms. Knowledge of brain biology was irrelevant to the psychiatric treatment he recommended. At the time of his seminal work, about 1895, knowledge of the brain was rudimentary; early neuroscientists did not even know about synapses or chemical transmitters (discussed in Chapter 2). It would have been hopelessly impractical to base treatment for mental illness on theories of brain physiology, so Freud formulated his theories in the language of psychology. He had to hope, for the sake of his patients, that knowledge of brain physiology would not be necessary for the development of effective treatments.

Freud's influence has been very great. To the U.S. public and to many mental health workers, it has seemed both sensible and correct to conceptualize mental illnesses as unfavorable psychological reactions to overwhelming conflicts. The physiology of the brain has been largely ignored. For example, in a conversation with a New York psychoanalyst whom we first knew as an Oregon graduate student, we were told, "The man [Freud] was amazing. He said it all! His insights are a wholly sufficient explanation for how we act and think. Others merely rediscover what he saw clearly fifty years ago." Another psychotherapist, in a conversation about drug treatments for depression, declared, "Yes, it could well be that some depressions result from a biochemical imbalance, but I've found that in ninety percent of the cases, when you really probe in therapy, when you really dig deep, you always find hostility."

Proponents of psychoanalysis and other talk therapies commonly allege that drug therapy provides only superficial relief of symptoms. The charge is not that drugs are ineffective but that their benefits are of lesser value than the benefits of psychological insight. The fact that drugs get patients out of the hospital is discounted by the observation that modern mental hospitals have revolving doors — patients leave only to return a few months later. The implication is that patients would stay out of the hospital if they were treated properly with psychotherapy.

Another common opinion is that psychiatric drugs, including those used for schizophrenia, turn mental patients into "zombies," so sedated they cannot participate productively in the psychotherapy they need. (We heard a neuroanatomy professor at an Ivy League university express this opinion.) The fact that some psychiatric drugs are called tranquilizers encourages the idea that they are merely powerful sleeping pills or, worse, chemical straitjackets.

Opponents of drug therapy sometimes charge that medication subverts mental patients by tempting them with a cheap and easy escape from the hard work of gaining psychological insight. We knew a young woman in New York who had been seeing her analyst four times a week for four years. During this time, she had made a great deal of progress, but she needed more analysis. When we suggested to her boyfriend that drug treatment might be appropriate, he told us, "Well, maybe, but then she might leave therapy before she completes the work she is going to have to do." Advocates of drug treatment have sarcastically referred to this attitude as psychiatric Calvinism—the harder the patient works, the better the cure.

We believe that the effectiveness of drug therapies and talk therapies can be compared only by evaluating the results of properly conducted research. One must demand *evidence* that a particular therapy is the most effective way to provide relief from a particular illness. Are drugs better for some disorders, while talk therapies are better for others? Maybe, unlikely as it seems, psychotherapy and drug therapy are about equally effective for certain illnesses. What are the undesirable side effects of the various forms of treatment? What are the social and economic costs? Such questions will be settled only by data, not by polemics or appealing to a tradition.

Does Drug Treatment Violate Patients' Legal Rights?

The custom of segregating the mentally ill in special institutions (madhouses, asylums, hospitals) began about 300 years ago. A recurrent problem associated with this practice is the difficulty of judging whether a particular patient should be placed in the hospital or allowed to remain free in the community. Often patients do not want to go to the hospital; they prefer to stay in the community, no matter how much danger they present to themselves and others. Traditionally it has been possible to forcibly place the gravely debilitated in a hospital where they can be given the necessities of life in safety. Those making the decision to force hospitalization on unwilling patients have traditionally been physicians and members of the patients' immediate family. Decisions about the kind of treatment for hospitalized patients have traditionally been made by the hospital staff.

Opposition to these traditions has recently surfaced. For example, in 1988 the American Civil Liberties Union of Oregon filed a suit against the Oregon State Hospital seeking to force personnel to stop compelling patients to accept drug treatments. The ACLU maintained that the patients did not want the drug treatment, they were adults and capable of making up their own minds, and the state had no authority to coerce them to take drugs against their will. This is not an isolated incident. Since the mid-1970s, many similar suits have been filed in many states. In the Oregon case, an out-of-court settlement was achieved when the hospital agreed to a substantial limitation on hospital authority to force patients to take drugs. We will have more to say on this issue in Chapter 19 after we have discussed the various treatments that are at the center of contention in civil liberties cases like these. Here, we simply state the two sides of the issue.[5]

The civil liberties argument has been made forcefully by Thomas Szasz, a psychiatrist and radical libertarian. In his books, including *The Myth of Mental Illness*, Szasz argues that psychiatric patients are not ill, just non-conformists. Since, in most cases, these non-conformists have committed no crimes, their forced hospitalization is equivalent to imprisonment without charge and without due process of law. Forcing them to take drugs against their will is a violation of their body (battery) and a cruel and unusual punishment. Thus, psychiatric patients, like slaves, are stripped of their constitutional rights, psychiatrists are like slave masters, and enslavement is justified by calling it medical treatment.[6]

The view that psychiatric hospitalization is punishment, not treatment, is also expressed by Ken Kesey in *One Flew over the Cuckoo's Nest*.[7] In this novel a hospitalized "mental patient" is given pills to control his offensive behavior. His offense is that he is mischievous and a nuisance: He uses naughty language and creates a commotion, gambling and passing smutty cards. When the authorities fail to control him with drugs, they try electroconvulsive shock. When that, too, fails, the villainous physicians perform a lobotomy!

Psychiatrists and the families of mental patients have a different view. They are often less impressed with the necessity of protecting a patient's civil rights than with the need to provide therapeutic help. From their perspective, it seems obvious that patients are sometimes in deteriorating health, incapable of taking care of themselves, and a danger to themselves and others. For example, when a suicidally depressed patient refuses to take antidepressant drugs, wanting instead to die and believing that he or she does not deserve to get better, the psychiatrist and the patient's family are likely to think treatment should be forced on the patient.

A conflict exists between freedom and benevolence. How should this conflict be resolved?

Are the Side Effects of the Drugs Worse Than the Mental Illness Itself?

Some people object to drug treatment out of fear that the drug side effects may be worse than the mental illness being treated. This is a realistic concern. Many anxiety-relieving drugs can lead to addiction and dependence (discussed in Chapter 17). Some drugs used for schizophrenia, for example, can cause a debilitating movement disorder called tardive dyskinesia that is sometimes incurable (see Chapter 8).

The problem of adverse side effects is not unique to psychiatry, of course. Practitioners of general medicine face the same problem. For example, some people become gravely ill or even die from an allergic response to penicillin. Nonetheless, penicillin is a beneficial drug because the number of lives its saves is thousands of times greater than the number it takes. The judgment of whether a psychiatric drug is likely to be beneficial requires thorough knowledge of the drugs actions and the potential harms of the illness. In the following chapters we try to convey this information with respect to the most commonly used psychiatric drugs and the illnesses they are designed to treat.

The decision about the use of drugs for mental illness should not, in our opinion, be dictated by intuition regarding the source of a disorder, that is, whether it is biological or psychological. It should not hinge on what authorities thought before 1960 about biological

treatments. We do not think the existence of effective psychotherapies for some disorders precludes the use of drugs in mental health
care, and we do not think that the possibility of the unjust use of
drugs for social control means they are always used unjustly. We
think there are two important questions to ask about treatment,
regardless of whether it is pharmacological or psychological: (1) Is
there evidence that the treatment works, and (2) do the probable
benefits outweigh the risks and costs?

2

HOW DRUGS WORK ON
THE BRAIN

—

Many misconceptions surround the use of drugs to treat psychiatric illnesses. A number of these ideas can be dispelled through an understanding of how such drugs affect the brain. This chapter describes the fundamental workings of the nervous system and then provides an overview of the various ways in which psychiatric drugs can alter transmission of information in the brain, making treatment of certain mental illnesses possible.

The most important assumption underlying our contention that drugs can be used effectively to treat mental illness is that the thoughts, emotions, and behaviors of animals, including humans, result from the activity of nerve cells in the brain and spinal cord (see Figure 2–1).[1] The activity of nerve cells depends, in turn, on a complex system of chemical reactions and movements of molecules. We believe that, without these chemical reactions and molecular

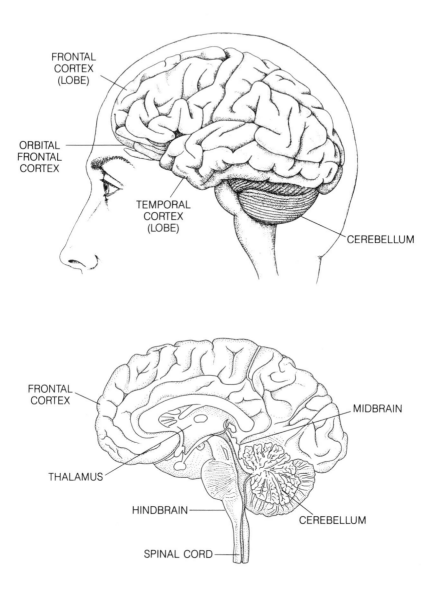

FIGURE 2–1 Top: Human brain in the skull. The outer surface of the brain is visible. Bottom: The cut surface of the human brain is now visible. The brain has been cut down the middle dividing it into left and right halves. (Top from ''The Brain'' by David H. Hubel, Copyright 1979 by Scientific American, Inc. Bottom from *Brain, Mind, and Behavior* by F. E. Bloom et al., W. H. Freeman and Co. New York, 1985.)

movements, thoughts, emotions, and behavior could not exist; indeed, mental phenomena are the result of a very highly organized collection of molecular activities carried out by the nerve cells of the brain. Though these assumptions are unprovable, they have become our credo because they are the foundation for the progress that neuroscience has made in understanding the brain.

A change in behavior signifies a change in brain chemistry. This change in brain chemistry is usually not drug induced; it results from ordinary everyday experiences. Although many people know that changes in brain chemistry cause changes in behavior like falling asleep and making love, they may not appreciate their role in more subtle alterations in behavior. Chemical reactions in the brain are responsible for the ability to balance on a bicycle and the desire for orange juice in the morning. One stands in awe of a sunset in the mountains because the scene initiates chemical reactions in one's brain. The brain is the ultimate provider of "better living through chemistry."

A person develops a mental illness when the brain chemistry changes in a way that affects his or her ability to function well. The goal of treatment is to modify the brain's chemical reactions in a way that produces good health, and taking drugs is one way to alter brain chemistry. When drugs reach the brain, they alter ongoing chemical reactions. A drug is an effective treatment if it alters brain chemistry so that the symptoms of mental illness are relieved.

Drugs are not the only way to improve a malfunctioning brain; psychotherapy can also alter the brain chemistry. As the sunset caused chemical reactions in the brain, so can the advice of a psychotherapist. Effective psychotherapy initiates chemical reactions that decrease the symptoms of the illness.

Although neuroscientists know more about how drugs work than about how psychotherapy works, they do not know the fine details of how either alters brain chemistry to alleviate mental illness. They understand many of the immediate effects of drugs on nerve cells, but these effects are only the first in a cascade of drug-initiated chemical changes, many of which are not yet well understood.

Better judgments about the role of chemical treatment in mental illness will be made if one understands the effects of drug molecules on brain chemistry. Aware that the brain is a complex and delicate mechanism, many people are reluctant to tamper with it. When the brain is working well, this reluctance is appropriate. Even though the brain may not be functioning perfectly, "Leave well enough alone" may be the best advice because chemical intervention may do more harm than good. But when serious mental illness strikes, the situation is quite different. Then the brain is no longer "well enough." At this point, some intervention, perhaps drug treatment, is justified. Of course, all treatments have risks as well as benefits. Both the risks and the benefits result from the effects of these substances on brain chemistry. Drug treatment will seem more acceptable and less capricious if these effects are understood.

Gaining knowledge of how drugs influence brain activity can also help dispel certain misconceptions about psychiatric drugs. One common misconception is that these drugs are chemical straitjackets or chemical scalpels wielded against socially undesirable behavior. A second misconception is that psychiatric drugs are all the same. (Proponents of this view usually refer to all psychiatric drugs as tranquilizers.)

A third misconception is that a drug ought to cure the disease it treats; that medication ought not continue indefinitely. This idea has taken hold because of the successful treatment of bacterial infections with antibiotics. However, most medical illnesses — diabetes, arthritis, heart disease, for example — are managed rather than cured. They cannot be cured because the basic abnormality, usually a chemical one, remains. For example, physicians cannot correct the abnormality that prevents a diabetic's pancreas from making insulin; they can only supply the insulin that the pancreas fails to make. As we will see, psychiatric drugs can compensate for chemical abnormalities in the brain, but they cannot cure them.

Understanding the action of drugs on the brain requires some knowledge about the normal brain. One needs to know what brain cells look like and how they work. One needs to know how the brain is organized and what regions are affected by mental disorders. Finally, one needs specific information about the effects of psychiatric drugs upon the molecules and the chemical reactions in the brain.

The brain has three basic functions: (1) It collects information from the outside world, (2) it uses this information to decide on a course of action, and (3) it implements the decision by commanding muscles to move and glands to secrete. A brain and spinal cord seen with the naked eye give no indication about the ways these functions are performed. They present the appearance of a squishy pink material squeezed tightly into a skull. Only the microscopic examination of small pieces of brain tissue will lead to an understanding of the structure of the brain, showing that the brain is composed of individual elements, the nerve cells, or neurons. These are the specialized cells that exchange information in the vast communications network of brain activity. A current popular analogy compares the workings of these billions of organic elements with the interaction of the electronic components of a digital computer.

BRAIN AND COMPUTER: SIMILARITIES AND DIFFERENCES

The analogy between brain and computer illuminates the function and complexity of the brain but it must not be carried too far. Nerve cells are fundamentally different from computer components: A computer cannot be repaired with drugs, and a brain cannot be repaired with electronic chips. That being said, we will note analogies between the brain's and the computer's modes of dealing with information.

The computer receives information from the outside world via a keyboard, a magnetic disk, or a scanning device. Similarly, the brain receives its information from sense organs. This information travels to the brain over specialized parts of nerve cells called *axons*, which are long, thin, extensions of neurons.

The computer's central processing unit, made up of integrated circuits, combines information and makes decisions. The decision rules reside in the computer's program. The brain is the central processing unit of the nervous system. The connections among the nerve cells create the rules for making decisions. One of the major goals of neuroscientists is to discover these decision-making rules.

The computer produces output via a video terminal or printer. The brain uses the muscles and glands to express the results of information processing. Again, the information is transmitted along the axons of nerve cells from the brain to the muscles or glands.

Each message that the brain or the computer sends to an output device is the result of thousands of small decisions. The brain and the computer use radically different hardware to make these decisions, of course. The computer performs its logic linearly by means of integrated circuits. The brain uses a multitude of simultaneous synapses, the junctions between nerve cells, to make decisions. Although each output from the computer to the printer is the net result of decisions made by many individual electronic devices, the printer receives only the final decision. Likewise, each output from the nervous system to the muscles is the result of decisions at thousands of synapses, but the muscles receive only the final commands. The muscles are ignorant of how the nervous system arrived at that command.

INNATE AND LEARNED PROGRAMS

The brain and computer differ not only in the hardware they use to process information but also in the way they are programmed. A modern general-purpose computer is truly like John Locke's *tabula rasa*, the presumed blank slate of a newborn's mind. It comes off the assembly line without a program. The programmer determines the programs to be run on the computer and hence decides all the computer's functions. In contrast, the brain of the newborn infant is not 'in fact' a *tabula rasa*. At birth, it is already elaborately programmed. Some of the innate programs, such as those controlling breathing and suckling, are necessary for survival. Others limit the abilities of the adult that the infant will become. For example, innate programs may dictate that a person will be left-handed or will have exceptional skill at composing music.

Of course, the brain of the infant does not contain all the programs that will eventually reside in the brain of the adult. New programs are developed as the child matures; this development is called learning. Learning results from interactions between the brain and the environment. The environment influences brain function in yet another way: Environmental inputs are often required to run inborn programs. The amount of carbon dioxide in the blood, for example, determines how the breathing program runs.

Differences in behavior reflect differences in brains. Species-specific behaviors present dramatic examples of such differences. For instance, humans find it difficult to make a nest out of twigs and straw, whereas robins can do it easily. On the other hand, no amount of training will teach robins to talk, whereas humans learn spontaneously, without special instruction. Robin behavior and human behavior are different because robin brains and human brains are different.

Although behavioral variations among individual humans are less dramatic, these variations also reflect biological differences in individual human brains. Some humans are mentally ill because their brains possess abnormalities. Intervention from the social environment may effectively treat some abnormalities, but in other cases, this intervention is not successful; then drugs or some other physical intervention may be desirable.

NERVE CELLS

A clear understanding of how the brain functions requires an understanding of individual nerve cells. Nerve cells in different parts of the brain have different functions and look different from one another under a microscope. Nevertheless, all nerve cells have basic similarities in structure, as illustrated in Figure 2–2.

A *cell membrane* separates the contents of each cell from the fluid that surrounds it. Just as skin is the boundary between what is inside the body and what is outside, the cell membrane is the boundary between the inside and the outside of the cell. The membrane also controls the chemical contents of the cell. Because the membrane is primarily fatty material, water and water-soluble molecules cannot pass through it unless special gates or channels are opened.

The metabolic center of the nerve cell is called the *cell body*. It ranges in size from about 0.005 to about 0.1 mm in diameter, depending on the type of cell. The cell body contains the nucleus and the chemical machinery needed to keep the cell alive. Many thin extensions diverge from the cell body. Most nerve cells have numerous short extensions called *dendrites* and a single longer one called the *axon*. The dendrites and the cell body are the parts of the nerve cell that usually receive signals from other neurons. The dendrites range from 0.01 to 2.0 mm in length, and they usually branch profusely, giving the cell a bristly appearance when seen under the microscope.

The axon is the part of the cell that sends signals from the region of the cell body to regions of the nervous system a considerable distance away. Axons are often much longer than dendrites and do not branch except very near their ends. The axon illustrated in Figure 2–2 is folded like an accordion so that it fits within the diagram; in the brain it would be straighter. If the cell were involved

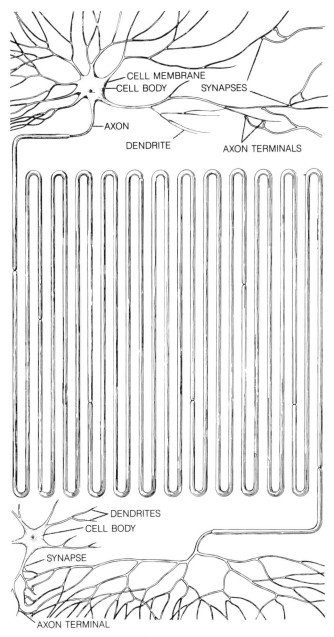

FIGURE 2–2 Diagram of typical nerve cells. Cell bodies for axon terminals at the top are beyond the edge of the diagram. Axon of cell body at lower left runs off diagram. Most of the axon terminal branches extend beyond the edge of the diagram, and their synapses are not shown. (From "The Neuron" by Charles F. Stevens. Copyright © 1979 by Scientific American, Inc. All rights reserved.)

in controlling the feet of a tall man, its axon might reach from the top of the brain to the end of the spinal cord. It would be about a meter long, though only about 0.01 mm in diameter. By contrast, if the cell communicated only with neighboring cells in the brain, its axon might be only 0.1 mm long and less than 0.001 mm in diameter.

At the tips of the small branches at the end of the axon are small bulblike swellings called *axon terminals*. Axon terminals are almost always found close to a dendrite or cell body of another nerve cell. The junction between an axon terminal of one nerve cell and a dendrite or cell body of another nerve cell is called a *synapse*.

The vast majority of nerve cells are completely confined to the central nervous system. Of course, the input and output cells must have axons that reach beyond the central nervous system to the sense organs and muscles. Many of the nerve cells involved in sensory input have their cell bodies located in clumps just outside the spinal cord.

THE TRANSMISSION OF INFORMATION

Each nerve cell must perform many of the same tasks that are performed by the brain as a whole. The cell must receive information, usually at its cell body and its dendrites. It must use that input to make decisions; this is usually the job of the cell body. The decision must be communicated to other nerve cells, usually by sending a signal down the axon. Because most psychiatric drugs do not affect the transmission of information from the cell body down the axon to the axon terminals, we will discuss this aspect of nerve cell function only briefly.

Nerve Impulses

To send a signal to the spinal cord, a nerve cell in the brain generates a *nerve impulse*. The nerve impulse is a momentary change in the electrical conductivity of the axon membrane. This change lasts only about 0.001 seconds. Signaling with nerve impulses is like signaling with a Morse code that has only dots and no dashes; the message that travels down the axon is conveyed by the rate of nerve impulses. Nerve cells can generate as many as 200 impulses per second. A nerve impulse travels rapidly down the axon from the cell body to the axon terminal. It never travels in the reverse direction. The speed of the nerve impulse is different in different types of nerve cells. It can be as fast as 100 meters per second or as slow as one-tenth of a meter per second. A fast-conducting axon would send a message from its cell body in the brain to synapses in the tail of the spinal cord in only 0.01 seconds.

Synapses

A neuron generates impulses under the control of signals it receives at synapses from other neurons. Psychiatric drugs modify synaptic signals in specific ways. The effects of drugs on synapses are similar in both ill and normal brains. Understanding drug action requires a fairly detailed understanding of transmission across synapses. Figure 2–3 shows the detailed structure of a typical synapse as it looks under an electron microscope. A synapse is so small that examina-

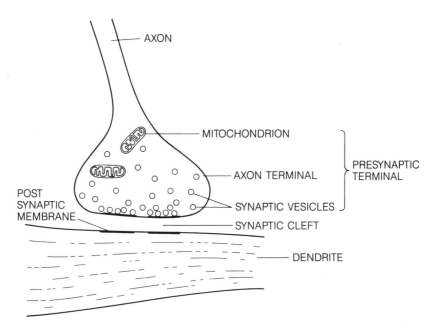

FIGURE 2-3 Diagram of a synapse as seen with an electron microscope. The synaptic vesicles contain transmitter. The mitochondria supply the energy needed for synthesis and release of transmitter.

tion of the detailed structure requires a magnification about 100 times greater than the magnification of the cells in Figure 2–2.

The axon terminal of the neuron sending a message is called the *presynaptic terminal* (*pre*-meaning "before," "in front of"). *Synaptic vesicles* are clustered close to the membrane. They are approximately spherical in shape and look like circles in the presynaptic terminal. These vesicles contain molecules of *transmitter*, the chemical that carries the message to the postsynaptic cell. Depending on the type of transmitter used by the presynaptic cell, the vesicles may appear clear or they may appear to be filled with dense material. The receiving portion of the synapse is called the *postsynaptic membrane* (*post*-meaning "behind," "after"). The postsynaptic membrane is a patch of membrane on the cell body or dendrite of the receiving, or postsynaptic, cell. The presynaptic and postsynaptic regions of the membrane appear slightly thicker and darker than the neighboring regions because they have special proteins inserted into the fatty material of the membrane. Notice that the presynaptic and postsynaptic membranes are very close to each other but do not quite touch. The space between them, the *synaptic cleft*, is about 20 millionths of a millimeter wide.

It is important to realize that the terms *presynaptic* and *postsynaptic* do not refer to entire nerve cells but only to their roles at a particular synapse. At a particular synapse between a brain cell and a spinal cord cell, the brain cell may be presynaptic, and the spinal cord cell, receiving information, postsynaptic. But when that spinal cord cell transmits information to another spinal cord cell or to a muscle, it is presynaptic.

Transmitters

How do signals cross the cleft between the presynaptic terminal and the postsynaptic membrane? A nerve impulse cannot cross the cleft because nerve impulses travel only in membrane and no membrane spans the synaptic cleft. Instead, the signals are carried across the cleft by chemical transmitters that are released from vesicles in the presynaptic terminals. The transmitter diffuses across the cleft and attaches to special protein molecules, called *receptors*, embedded in the postsynaptic membrane. This process of attachment is called *binding.* The binding of transmitters to receptors constitutes the signal that triggers a change of activity in the postsynaptic nerve cell. Many drugs affect brain function by altering the binding of transmitters to receptors.

To understand the many ways that drugs can affect synaptic transmission, it is useful to follow the path of the transmitter molecules moving from a presynaptic terminal to the postsynaptic receptors. In the absence of a nerve impulse in the presynaptic neuron, the transmitter is stored in the synaptic vesicles. When a nerve impulse arrives at the presynaptic terminal, some of the vesicles fuse with the presynaptic membrane and rupture at the point of fusion, releasing their contents into the synaptic cleft (Figure 2–4). Less than 0.0005 seconds elapses between the arrival of the nerve impulse at the presynaptic terminal and the receipt of the message by the postsynaptic receptors.

What happens to the postsynaptic cell when a transmitter binds to a receptor? The binding of the transmitter activates chemical changes in the postsynaptic membrane. At some synapses the

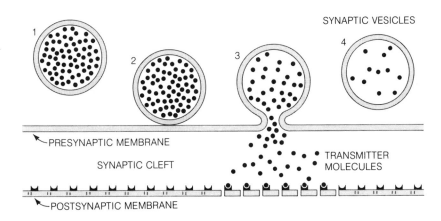

FIGURE 2–4   Diagram of the rupturing of synaptic vesicles and release of transmitter into the cleft. The transmitter diffuses across the cleft and attaches to the receptor. The vesicle membrane is reclaimed by the presynaptic terminal. (From "The Neuron" by Charles F. Stevens. Copyright © 1979 by Scientific American, Inc. All rights reserved.)

change in the postsynaptic membrane encourages the production of nerve impulses in the postsynaptic axon; at other synapses the changes induced by binding discourage the production of nerve impulses. When the binding of a transmitter to a receptor encourages the production of nerve impulses, the process is called *synaptic excitation*. Without synaptic excitation, information cannot travel through the nervous system. When the binding discourages the production of nerve impulses, the process is called *synaptic inhibition*. Inhibition prevents inappropriate production of nerve impulses; for example, it prevents two muscles that pull in opposite directions from contracting vigorously at the same time, which would tear the tendons off the bones.

Different nerve cells use different molecules as transmitters, but a given nerve cell probably releases the same few chemical transmitters at each of its presynaptic terminals. The predominant chemical is called the *transmitter* for that nerve cell. At many synapses, other molecules, called *cotransmitters*, are released along with the predominant transmitter. Some of these other molecules may be as important as the predominant transmitter, but since they have been discovered only recently, comparatively little is known about their function.

Although a particular transmitter is often described as excitatory while another is described as inhibitory, a single transmitter does not always produce the same effect on all its postsynaptic cells. Whether a given transmitter is excitatory or inhibitory is not determined by the transmitter alone. It depends on the postsynaptic machinery that the receptor controls. For example, acetylcholine, the transmitter released by axons onto muscles controlling the arms and legs, excites these muscles, causing them to contract. But acetylcholine is also released by axons controlling the heart. This transmitter inhibits the heart muscle, causing the heartbeat to slow down.

We do not know how many different kinds of chemicals are used as transmitters in the central nervous system. At present, there is good evidence for about 40 different kinds, but there may be many more. The psychiatric drugs affect mainly synapses that use one of five different transmitters: norepinephrine, dopamine, serotonin (also called 5-HT), acetylcholine, and gamma-aminobutyric acid (GABA). But we must always keep in mind that even the drugs we understand best might have actions we are unaware of at synapses using transmitters as yet unknown to us.

The Binding of Transmitters and Receptors

Usually the dendrites and cell body are studded with synapses (Figure 2–5). Each postsynaptic cell receives input from many different presynaptic cells, perhaps 20, perhaps several hundred. Collectively, these presynaptic cells release several different kinds of transmitter, but each kind of receptor molecule is specialized for binding to one particular transmitter. Some other transmitters will bind to the receptor, but the attachment is weak. Still others will not bind at all. Therefore, a single postsynaptic cell must have several different kinds of receptors to match the several different transmitters it

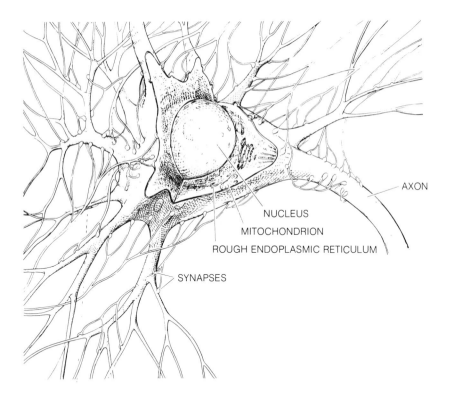

AXON

NUCLEUS
MITOCHONDRION
ROUGH ENDOPLASMIC RETICULUM

SYNAPSES

FIGURE 2–5 Nerve cell covered with synapses. The nucleus contains the genetic material of the cell. The rough endoplasmic reticulum is part of the protein-synthesizing machinery. Cell bodies of the presynaptic cells are off the diagram. (From "The Neuron" by Charles F. Stevens. Copyright © 1979 by Scientific American, Inc. All rights reserved.)

receives. Each kind of receptor is located where it will receive the proper transmitter, that is, across the synaptic cleft from a presynaptic terminal releasing that transmitter. A few thousandths of a millimeter away, another kind of receptor, located across from another presynaptic terminal, will respond to a different kind of transmitter.

As a result of this structure, every cell receives a continuously fluctuating barrage of excitatory and inhibitory synaptic signals. Each nerve cell must evaluate all its inputs on a moment-to-moment basis and decide whether there is enough net excitation to generate a nerve impulse. At one moment, excitation may be greater than inhibition, and the cell will send nerve impulses down its axon. A few hundredths of a second later, the opposite may be true, and the cell will stop sending impulses. This seems complex enough, but now imagine a human brain consisting of 100 billion nerve cells. At every moment, each cell is deciding whether to produce an output while depending on thousands of other cells for help in making its decision. No computer or social organization can rival this complexity.

Some kinds of transmitter—for example, dopamine, norepinephrine, and serotonin—have another kind of effect on postsynaptic cells: They change the cells' biochemistry. When these transmitters bind to receptors, they activate one or more enzymes that cause biochemical changes inside the cell, usually the synthesis of specific chemicals. Altering biochemical reactions can alter the cell's ability to send out impulses for several minutes or hours. In contrast, excitation or inhibition that is not mediated by biochemical reactions lasts only a few thousandths of a second.

The Removal of Transmitter

A receptor cannot respond to a second nerve impulse until the transmitter released by the first impulse is removed from both the receptor and the cleft. Fortunately, the union between receptor and transmitter is reversible. Transmitter molecules easily become unattached from a receptor. No special mechanism is required because all molecules in solution move continuously. They vibrate even when attached to a receptor. By chance, some of these vibrations have enough force to pull the transmitter off the receptor.

Once the transmitter has left the receptor, it is removed from the cleft in one of two ways. First, some types of transmitters are split into two smaller molecules by an enzyme in the synaptic membrane. Any transmitter molecule that happens to hit the enzyme is split. Neither of the two molecules formed by this split can function as a transmitter. Second, other types of transmitters leave the cleft by reentering the presynaptic terminal. The membrane of the presynaptic terminal, as well as the membrane of the postsynaptic terminal, has receptors for the transmitter. When a transmitter molecule binds to a presynaptic receptor, the transmitter is taken inside the terminal. This process is called *reuptake*, even though the implied preceding "uptake" is nonexistent. After reuptake, the transmitter either reenters a vesicle so that it can be released again or is destroyed by an enzyme inside the presynaptic terminal.

THE ORGANIZATION OF THE BRAIN

So far we have described how nerve cells communicate with one another but have said nothing about how nerve cells are organized to make a brain. The brain is not a random network of nerve cells; rather, each brain region has special functions. Just like individual nerve cells, each region receives information from other regions, processes that information, and sends the results of its processing to still other regions. Some regions of the brain consist of clumps of cells called nuclei (not to be confused with the nuclei of individual cells). These nuclei are usually visible in the microscope as dense clusters of cell bodies surrounded by regions that have fewer cell bodies and more axons. Many nuclei have fairly well understood functions; for example, the nuclei called the basal ganglia are important in the control of movement.

Complexity of function usually increases as we move up the nervous system from bottom to top. The basic regions of the brain are indicated in Figure 2–1. In our overview of brain organization, our description of each region will be a gross oversimplification, of course.

The *spinal cord* is the lowest region of the central nervous system. Its main functions are to receive sensory information and to issue commands to muscles. The spinal cord contains circuits that help coordinate the movements of walking and other basic reflexes. Like any other region of the brain, the spinal cord does not act independently; it uses information from the rest of the brain when it directs muscles to contract. For this purpose the spinal cord has large bundles of axons that send information to and receive it from the brain.

The *hindbrain* is instrumental in controlling vegetative functions like respiration, vomiting, heart rate, and sleep. It also contains clusters of neurons that manufacture serotonin. The axons of these cells secrete serotonin in many distant parts of the nervous system. Some of these serotonin cells help control the experience of pain. Drugs that help relieve depression and obsessive compulsive disorder act on serotonin-secreting neurons like these in the hindbrain and others in the midbrain.

The *cerebellum* sits on top of the hindbrain. It is primarily involved in motor coordination and its role in mental illness appears to be small.

The top of the *midbrain* is involved in vision and hearing. The bottom of the midbrain collaborates with the hindbrain in the control of sleep, alertness, and pain. Like the hindbrain, it contains nuclei of cells that manufacture serotonin. It also contains a group of nuclei that manufacture norepinephrine; in fact, the norepinephrine in all brain regions originates from the widespread axons of these midbrain cells. The activity of these norepinephrine-secreting cells makes an important contribution to the mental states of alertness, vigilance, and fear. These norepinephrine-secreting cells, as well as the serotonin-secreting cells, are important targets for drugs used to treat depression. The bottom part of the midbrain also contains a group of nuclei whose cells secrete dopamine. These cells are an important target for drugs that relieve schizophrenia.

Much of the *thalamus* is involved in processing sensory information. The functions of its nonsensory regions are poorly understood. These are important regions of the brain, but they do not have an important role in our study of psychiatric drugs.

The *forebrain* is an important region for psychiatry. Its largest and most visible part is the *cerebral cortex*, a mantle of neurons that covers up the midbrain and thalamus. Beneath the surface of the cerebral cortex lie the basal ganglia, which are involved in the control of voluntary movement, and the amygdala, which is important in the control of emotions. The forebrain probably controls all the higher mental functions including perception, imagery, language, abstract thought, some types of memory, and social responsibility. Different cortical regions have different functions. Malfunctions of the frontal and temporal areas of the cortex, as well as of the basal ganglia and amygdala, are probably involved in the psychiatric illnesses considered in this book.

A SUMMARY OF BRAIN FUNCTION

1. The brain must receive information from sense organs, use this information to make decisions, and instruct muscles and glands to implement its decisions.
2. The decisions depend both on the information received from sense organs and on the brain's programs. Some of these programs are learned or refined from experience; others are inborn.
3. Communication between nerve cells occurs at synapses. A synapse consists of an axon terminal (the presynaptic terminal), a postsynaptic receptor (located in a patch of postsynaptic membrane), and an intervening synaptic cleft.
4. A nerve impulse in the presynaptic terminal causes synaptic vesicles to fuse with the terminal membrane and release their transmitter into the cleft.
5. The transmitter binds to postsynaptic receptors, and the postsynaptic membrane responds with either excitation or inhibition.
6. A nerve cell produces nerve impulses on the basis of moment-to-moment evaluations of the excitation and inhibition it is receiving from its synapses.
7. The binding of transmitter to receptor can also alter the biochemistry of the postsynaptic cell.
8. Before the synapse can be used again, the transmitter must be removed from the cleft in one of two ways: Either an enzyme splits the transmitter, or the transmitter is taken up inside the presynaptic terminal.
9. The brain is organized into discrete regions, each with its own function. The frontal and temporal regions of the cortex, the basal ganglia, the amygdala, and the midbrain are probably the regions most crucially involved in psychiatric disorders.

HOW DRUGS AFFECT THE TRANSMISSION OF INFORMATION

Drugs are known that can alter virtually every step in synaptic transmission. For example, they can prevent the synthesis of a transmitter; they can increase or decrease transmitter release; they can bind to the postsynaptic receptor and thus prevent the normal transmitter from binding. Drugs can alter the shape of the receptor so that it becomes more or less difficult for the transmitter to bind; they can increase or decrease the number of receptors manufactured, inactivate enzymes that destroy transmitters, and prevent reuptake. Most of the drugs used to treat mental illness affect transmitter–receptor binding, reuptake of transmitters, and the manufacture of receptors. In later chapters, we will discuss in more detail how specific psychiatric drugs affect synapses. Here we present a brief preview.

Drugs used to treat schizophrenia block receptors for the transmitter dopamine which is secreted by cells in the midbrain that send their axons to the basal ganglia and frontal lobe. Dopamine usually causes inhibition of nerve impulses, but the drugs used for schizophrenia bind to dopamine receptors without causing inhibition. As long as a drug molecule occupies a receptor, dopamine cannot bind to it; thus, the receptor is blocked. A drug that blocks dopamine receptors is called a *dopamine antagonist*. Other drugs bind to dopamine receptors but do not block them. These drugs mimic the effects of dopamine by producing inhibition and by causing the biochemical changes normally caused by dopamine. The dopamine-mimicking drugs are called *dopamine agonists*. The primary use of dopamine agonists is in research, but they are also used experimentally for a few psychiatric disorders.

Drugs used to treat depression alter norepinephrine and serotonin synapses, preventing the reuptake of both transmitters. They also decrease the sensitivity of some postsynaptic receptors for norepinephrine and serotonin. These effects are complex, and their relation to relief of depression is not yet well understood.

Finally, drugs used in the treatment of anxiety interact with receptors for the transmitter GABA. Antianxiety drugs bind to the GABA receptor. When bound, the antianxiety drug changes the shape of the GABA receptor and causes the postsynaptic cell to respond more readily to GABA.

Each particular psychiatric drug acts primarily on synapses using a particular transmitter. For example, the transmitters dopamine and norepinephrine are very similar chemically, but a drug that affects dopamine synapses usually has much less effect on norepinephrine synapses, and vice versa. Dopamine receptor blockers bind only weakly to norepinephrine receptors, and blockers of norepinephrine reuptake have almost no effect on dopamine reuptake. The specificity is not absolute, however. Sometimes, the lack of specificity is important clinically. For example, dopamine antagonists also block certain acetylcholine receptors. The blocking of acetylcholine receptors causes some of the side effects of the dopamine antagonists used to treat schizophrenia.

The ability of psychiatric drugs to affect specific synapses indicates that they are not generalized poisons that merely prevent mental illness by turning the brain off or, worse, by destroying large parts of it. It is also clear that psychiatric drugs are not all the same. Different drugs act on different kinds of synapses and have different effects on behavior and mental life.

Finally, this overview suggests that taking a drug might compensate for a biochemical abnormality in the brain. Suppose a person has nerve cells that manufacture too many dopamine receptors. Because of the excess receptors, this person has excessive synaptic action at synapses using dopamine as a transmitter. In the proper dose, a drug that blocks dopamine receptors could compensate for the abnormality by preventing dopamine from binding with the extra receptors, thus restoring brain function to normal. In later chapters, we provide more evidence for both the therapeutic and the biochemical specificity of psychiatric drugs.

3

DIAGNOSING MENTAL ILLNESS

—

W hen we do not feel well, we go to the doctor to find out whether we have a recognized illness, what kind of illness it is, and how it can be treated. To provide answers, the doctor must have a valid system of diagnosis, that is, a method of naming illnesses. The doctor arrives at a diagnosis by classifying our symptoms according to their similarity to symptoms in other cases. Classification allows physicians and patients to communicate, physicians to prescribe treatments that control or cure diseases, and researchers to study the causes of diseases and to invent more effective treatments.[1]

To appreciate the importance of communication, imagine how uninformed you would be if you simply learned that an aunt had had a nervous breakdown or had become emotionally disturbed. You would not know her symptoms; you would have no idea whether treatment was available or desirable; you would know nothing about the seriousness of her condition. About the only thing you would know would be that something was wrong. The words *emotionally disturbed* and *nervous breakdown* fail to convey much information because they do not name a mental illness that has a distinct set of symptoms. Everyone defines the terms differently. People use the words *nervous breakdown* and *emotionally disturbed* because they lack more precise terms. By contrast, if you heard that the same relative had rheumatoid arthritis or mumps, you would be well informed about the nature of the illness. You would know something about the symptoms, something about the seriousness of the disease, whether effective treatments were available, and whether the prognosis was good or bad. A reliable system of diagnosis allows people to agree about definitions of diseases.

A reliable system of psychiatric diagnosis is required before researchers can study mental illnesses, discover their causes, and invent treatments. Suppose that two psychiatric researchers, Drs. Nader and Watt, each decided to investigate whether "nervous breakdowns" are related to unburned hydrocarbons emitted in the exhaust of automobiles. Using well-established methods, each would measure the level of unburned hydrocarbons in the air over various population centers and later sample the same populations to determine the rate of "nervous breakdowns." At that point, they might begin to disagree. Lacking an established definition, they would be free to define "nervous breakdown" idiosyncratically to suit their separate objectives. Dr. Nader, whose work is sponsored by the Political Action Coalition for Cleaner Air, would probably find that hydrocarbons are indeed associated with a high incidence of "nervous breakdowns," while Dr. Watt, whose work is sponsored by the International Consortium of Gasoline Refiners, would find that hydrocarbons have no relationship to "nervous breakdowns."

Contrast these results with the likely outcome of research by the same two doctors on the relation between unburned hydrocarbons and the birth rate and death rate in the exposed populations. In this study, they would agree about what was being measured, and although they might disagree on the implications of their results for public policy, they would probably agree on the degree of correlation between birth and death rates and the levels of specified chemicals.

Effective treatment, as well as valid research, requires a reliable system of diagnosis. When there are several kinds of illness and several kinds of treatment, diagnosis is required to obtain the optimal match between treatment and illness. If there were only one kind of treatment or if all treatments were ineffective, then diagnosis would lack therapeutic significance and would be of interest only to researchers and academicians.

THE FUNCTION OF DIAGNOSIS

Psychiatry and clinical psychology are just emerging from an era when only one treatment was used for nearly all mental disorders — and when there was no effective treatment for most disorders. During the twentieth century, until about 1960, any disorder — a nervous breakdown, an emotional disturbance, an inferiority complex, an Oedipal conflict, a neurosis, . . . —was treated with psychotherapy. The therapist tried to help by talking with the patient; usually, the therapist tried to discover how the mental problems were derived from the patient's personal development. Most talk therapies were based on the theories of authorities like Freud, Jung, and Sullivan and owed little to empirical research. No one tried to collect statistics on whether a treatment was having the desired effect. Therapists relied on personal insight to validate their therapeutic practices.

Recently, this tradition has been challenged by the advent of psychotherapeutic drugs and developments in clinical psychology. Drug laws in the United States demanded that a new psychiatric drug be proved both safe and effective for a particular disorder before being marketed. Similarly, clinical psychologists demanded that the effectiveness of psychotherapy be proved. These demands required objective evidence for treatment effectiveness. Only if researchers carefully created diagnostic categories and precisely described treatment methods could they determine the treatment that was effective for a particular disorder. As a result of these developments, mental health workers today pay a great deal of attention to diagnosis and to matching particular treatments to particular illnesses.

CONTEMPORARY DIAGNOSIS

Although diagnostic practice has greatly improved since 1960, scientific knowledge is still rudimentary and diagnostic concepts continue to change rapidly under the influence of new research. A reliable, valid, and generally accepted diagnostic system for mental disorders remains a goal, not an accomplishment.

Jill is an example of a patient whose illness was incorrectly diagnosed. Though Jill wanted desperately to be an efficient housewife and a loving mother, each day her good intentions were somehow overwhelmed by forces beyond her control. There were times lasting several weeks when, day after day, she refused to get breakfast, lunch, or dinner. She said she was "just not up to it." Sometimes, out of an unsubstantiated fear that her family would become poverty stricken, she refused to give her children lunch money. At such times, she was frightened and weepy. She had to be comforted even though nothing threatening or sad had happened. When she repented of her stinginess and passivity, she went to the opposite extreme, insisting that the whole family eat in expensive restaurants that they could not afford. At these times, she was too busy and impatient to cook.

At her husband's insistence, Jill visited a psychiatrist, who diagnosed her illness as a personality disorder. He prescribed an anxiety-relieving drug (Valium) and insight psychotherapy. Jill's failures and unhappiness continued. Two years later, her husband insisted that she consult another psychiatrist. Neither Jill nor her husband ever found out what her diagnosis was, but this psychiatrist prescribed a phenothiazine, a drug usually prescribed for schizophrenia, along with more insight psychotherapy. Though Jill wept less often, she still had trouble. A year later, in desperation, Jill went to a third psychiatrist, who diagnosed Jill as having unipolar depression and prescribed an antidepressant drug and rational emotive psychotherapy. Jill improved somewhat, but some of her symptoms remained. After six months the same psychiatrist changed the diagnosis, this time to bipolar disorder, and prescribed the mood-stabilizing drug lithium. The lithium worked, and Jill improved dramatically. She said to her husband, "I feel normal for the first time in years."

Only four classes of drugs are commonly used in psychiatry today: antianxiety drugs, antipsychotics, antidepressants, and mood stabilizers. It is an embarrassment to the art of psychiatric diagnosis that Jill received the drug of the correct class only after drugs from all three of the other classes had been incorrectly prescribed and had failed.

On March 30, 1981, John Hinkley shot and injured President Ronald Reagan and three other members of the president's party as they were leaving the Washington Hilton Hotel.[2] In the subsequent trial it was necessary for the jury to determine the state of Hinkley's mental health at the time of the shooting because Hinkley's plea was not guilty by reason of insanity. The courtroom attempt to evaluate Hinkley's mental health exemplifies the imprecision of diagnostic techniques in psychiatry. Psychiatrists for the defense testified that Hinkley had schizophrenia and, because of the illness, had not been rational when he shot President Reagan. They said that Hinkley was driven to shoot by the delusion that killing the president would win him the love of actress Jodie Foster. Psychiatrists for the prosecution disagreed. They testified that Hinkley did not have schizophrenia and that he could rationally control his behavior. They said that he planned the shooting in order to become famous without having to work hard. The jury was convinced by the psychiatrists for the defense, but that does not mean that the psychiatrists for the prosecution were "wrong." As expressed by Tom Wicker of the New York Times, these flagrant disagreements created two impressions: "One was that these doctors are little better able to agree than any two laymen might be on who's sane or insane; the other was that the opinions of some psychiatrists, at least, may be for sale.[3]"

In view of episodes like these, it is hardly surprising that many people regard psychiatry as unscientific or even fraudulent. Imagine the low regard you would have for nonpsychiatric medical doctors if they routinely disagreed about the appropriate name for your illness and even argued about whether or not you were sick. At the very least, psychiatry needs a uniform system of nomenclature so that professionals will agree on the meaning of terms like *neurosis, psychosis, insanity, schizophrenia, depression*, and *mental illness*. Moreover, a psychiatrist should not assign a name to a particular patient's illness when there is no broad professional agreement on that name. Sometimes the psychiatrist should say, "I don't know what to call your illness. I don't even know whether you're ill or not." The patient may not be comforted, but this kind of honesty is vastly superior to assigning names that will be misunderstood.[4]

Unfortunately, psychiatrists have used the same name to represent different kinds of illnesses. Gerald Klerman and several associates from the National Institute of Mental Health recently reviewed the use of the term *neurotic depression* in the psychiatric research literature. They found that psychiatric researchers used the term to represent six different kinds of psychological disorders. Some psychiatrists, for example, used *neurotic depression* to mean depression that is a reaction to a sad environmental event, such as a death in the family or a divorce. Other psychiatrists used the same term to mean mild depression, distinguishing it from psychotic depression, which is more severe.[5]

Conversely, psychiatrists have sometimes called the same illness by different names. In 1971 R. E. Kendall, J. E. Cooper, and several other psychiatrists from the United Kingdom and the eastern United States reported the outcome of an important study comparing the diagnostic practices of U.S. and British psychiatrists. They had shown videotapes of diagnostic interviews with patients to large groups of psychiatrists on both sides of the Atlantic. After viewing the same tapes, the British psychiatrists diagnosed manic depression and personality disorder much more often than the Americans, and the Americans diagnosed schizophrenia much more often than the British. After observing one of the taped diagnostic interviews, 92 percent of the Americans diagnosed schizophrenia, while only 2 percent of the British did so; 72 percent of the British psychiatrists diagnosed personality disorder, while only 8 percent of the Americans did so.[6]

Calling the same disorder by different names also creates problems for researchers. It may be necessary to find out if a particular drug—let's call it Mindclear—is effective in treating, say, schizophrenia. Researchers may find that, according to British psychiatrists, Mindclear works for 90 percent of the cases, whereas U.S. psychiatrists report success in only 30 percent of the cases. It could take decades to figure out the cause of such a discrepancy.

Different psychiatrists use different procedures for obtaining diagnostic information. Psychiatrists of Freudian persuasion may use free association to help patients uncover repressed, threatening memories. Psychiatrists impressed by modern statistical methods may give patients a written test designed to identify certain personality traits. Some psychiatrists may simply ask questions about a patient's mental state currently and in the recent past. Still others may use a structured psychiatric interview with a fixed sequence of questions to identify a patient's symptoms. These procedures yield different kinds of information that, in turn, yield different diagnoses.[7]

A reliable system of diagnosis will achieve at least two elementary goals. First, it will clearly define each disorder by describing its symptoms. Second, it will specify the methods for determining whether a patient has the symptoms. Only after these goals have been achieved will psychiatrists be able to agree in naming a patient's disorder.[8] If various psychiatrists and psychologists can agree with one another about naming of disorders, then the diagnostic system is said to have the property of reliability.

Beyond clear definitions and reliability (agreement), the third, and highest, goal of diagnosis is *validity*. A valid diagnosis is an accurate directory to knowledge about the causes of the disorder, the risk factors for contracting it, the course of the disorder, and its response to various types of treatment. The difference between reliability and validity can be shown by an analogy, using the problem of classifying animals. A reliable but invalid rule for naming giraffes would be to call an animal a giraffe if its neck is as long as its hind leg. This would be a reliable definition, since all people could agree on whether a particular animal's neck was as long as its leg. It would not be valid, however, since it would lead us to call geese and swans giraffes.

The goal of validity seems easy to achieve in the classification of animals because people have been studying animals for thousands of years. Validity has not yet been achieved for classifications in the relatively young disciplines of psychiatry and psychology. Proof that diagnostic categories in psychiatry are valid or invalid requires more research into differences and similarities among disorders. For most psychiatric diagnoses, validity is lacking or only partially present. Among the diagnoses discussed in this book, the ones with the highest degree of validity are schizophrenia, bipolar affective disorder, and obsessive compulsive disorder. The diagnosis whose validity is most suspect is probably generalized anxiety disorder.

DISTINGUISHING ILLNESS FROM HEALTH

To promote mental health, it is essential to have a concept of how mental health can be distinguished from mental illness. This is not easy to attain. Indeed, it is difficult to define what is meant by good health in general medicine. Does good health require a clear complexion, a slim waist, becoming pregnant, avoiding pregnancy? This is a matter that physicians deal with routinely.

Thomas Szasz proposed that mental illness exists only when the mental condition is caused by an anatomical defect in the brain.[9] He would also accept physiological or biochemical defects. If there is no such defect, he said, "illness" is a misnomer (in his words, a "myth"). Unfortunately, given the present state of knowledge, Szasz's definition provides no help to those who must decide whether they have a mental illness and need mental health care.

The first problem with Szasz's definition is that we do not have the biochemical, physiological, and anatomical knowledge to apply it. Many types of brain defects are as yet unknown, and knowledge of all brain defects will not be possible for many decades, if ever. At present, too, many known types of brain defect cannot be detected directly in living people, but are apparent only at autopsy. An example is Alzheimer's disease, one of a number of physiological conditions that cause loss of mental function during the later years of life.

A second problem is that every brain, like every kidney, is different from all others. In the case of the brain, this uniqueness produces individual talents, personality, and mental life. Distinguishing defects from normal variations cannot be done decisively on physiological grounds. The presence of a measurable brain defect is not yet a practical basis for defining mental illness.

Third, it is inhumane to withhold care from a sufferer on the grounds that we do not know the biological cause of the suffering. For example, a patient with lower back pain may have a legitimate reason to receive treatment with pain killing drugs even though the cause of the pain is not understood. Ignorance of the cause of pain does not mean that the pain is fake or that the patient is malingering. In fairness to Szasz, he does not recommend withholding treatment from suffering patients. He does claim, however, that most conditions we recognize as mental disorders, including schizophrenia, do not involve suffering but are instead cases of benign nonconformity.

In this book we adopt the distress and disability definition of mental disorders. According to this definition people are said to have a disorder when (1) they feel distressed by their condition and (2) the condition impairs their ability to pursue their life. We have been persuaded by Thomas Jefferson and others that people have "unalienable Rights [to] Life, Liberty and the pursuit of Happiness." When a person's ability to exercise these rights is impaired by a condition of his or her own mind, and when the mental condition causes suffering, we say that the person has a mental disorder.

The brief stresses and strains of daily living usually do not require treatment. These brief episodes of distress usually go away by themselves, the way a cold goes away. To receive treatment for them would be worse in most cases than the original distress. It would be a waste of time to seek treatment for the distress of being turned down for a date, for example, or of getting a C rather than a B on a college assignment.

Of course, when the distress is severe and long lasting, and when the disability is incapacitating, there is no uncertainty about the need for treatment. For example, Charlotte, now in her forties, was healthy throughout childhood, but when she was about 18, she began to have mental health problems. She sits or stands for hours at a time frozen rigidly in an uncomfortable posture and refuses to speak. Raymond, who is 20 years old, did well during his freshman year of college, but he had to leave school as a sophomore because he began spending several hours a day making faces in the mirror and talking incoherently, sometimes to imaginary companions. No elaborate diagnostic procedure is required to determine that Charlotte and Raymond are ill. They need care and treatment.

More commonly, the disability is less than completely incapacitating, and the symptoms are less bizarre than Charlotte's and Raymond's. How much sadness indicates the illness of depression? How much suspicion indicates paranoia? How much self-confidence indicates mania? Such quantitative questions make the definition of illness difficult. If a disability is not severe enough to keep a person off the job or to disrupt his or her family life, and if the distress is not painful enough to make a person cry for help, there will be uncertainty about whether mental disorder exists. This uncertainty is at present unavoidable.

Robert L. Spitzer, in summarizing the problem of defining "clinically significant mental illness," suggests that a psychiatric condition should be called illness only if almost everyone, including the patient, agrees that there is both distress and disability.[10] Thus, Charlotte and Raymond would be called mentally ill. Patients may not recognize their need for treatment while in the midst of an acute crisis of illness, but afterward, when the crisis has passed, they should agree that they were suffering and disabled. In these clear-cut cases, treatment is indicated even though it may involve some risk, expense, and interference with the patient's established pattern of living.

Spitzer recommends that the term *illness* not be applied to cases in which there is significant disagreement about whether the person is distressed and disabled. For instance, some people who are heterosexually oriented regard homosexuality as a distressing disability. On the other hand, many homosexually oriented people feel neither impaired nor distressed. Because of this disagreement, we would not call homosexuality an illness.

Mental illnesses are not simply rare qualities of mind that set an individual apart from the average person. As Spitzer points out, unusual behavior is often admired and rewarded. Intellectual and artistic geniuses are not considered ill simply because they are not average. Einstein was neither distressed nor disabled by his scientific intelligence, nor was Mozart by his musical ability. Van Gogh was considered mad, not because of his unusual artistic talent (which was neither distressing nor disabling), but because of his depressions, rages, self-mutilation, and suicide. In fact, the existence of healthy nonconformity helps defend the mental health profession against the charge of surreptitiously enforcing conventional standards of conduct by branding nonconformists as ill and coercively suppressing them with drugs and brainwashing.

Although Spitzer defines only those conditions that unambiguously cause distress and disability as illnesses, he does not imply that one should seek mental health care only if one has a well-defined illness. On the contrary, professional mental health services may be appropriate for a wide spectrum of problems in which the presence of distress and disability is ambiguous. Each prospective patient must personally decide whether to seek treatment for such conditions. The prospective patient may want professional advice about the probable benefits, risks, and expense of treatment. Therapists, whether psychologists or psychiatrists, should honestly explain what would be gained and lost by treatment, but they should not diagnose ambiguous cases as illness.[11]

Like physicians practicing general medicine, most psychologists and psychiatrists see their mission as broader than merely treating the ill; they also want to help those in need. When a woman goes to the doctor to obtain the means for birth control, for example, her doctor can help solve her personal problem without considering her to be ill. Similarly, a psychiatrist or psychologist, need not, and usually will not, refuse assistance just because a person's condition does not fit Spitzer's definition of illness.

Some people think that bearing hardship and pain in silence is admirable. The stoic has little sympathy for complainers and certainly would not consider asking a psychiatrist for help with a mere problem of daily living. Such a person turns to personal resources to "straighten up and fly right," seeking only "self-control." Secretly (or not so secretly), the stoic takes pride in not needing a psychiatrist. The first meeting with a psychiatrist, if it ever occurs, is likely to be in an emergency situation, when a small "problem of living" has become a crisis.

There are other people who are always worried that life is not just right. They may seek psychiatric help to assuage even minor unhappiness. "Why doesn't the baby sleep through the night?" "Why does my two-year-old get into everything?" "Why does my husband look at other women?" "Where did I go wrong, doctor?" If professional care can help such a person, then help should be given. Perhaps the request is reason enough for help. Furthermore, in such a person there may be substantial distress and disability, even though the same problems are dismissed with a chuckle by most people.

STANDARDIZING DIAGNOSTIC TECHNIQUES

When it is agreed that illness exists and treatment is desirable, how does a psychiatrist or a psychologist determine what kind of illness that patient has? It would be nice if mental health workers could order a laboratory test like the one used to diagnose strep throat. The laboratory personnel would wipe some bacteria off the patient's throat with a cotton swab and grow them in a dish until the colonies were large enough to see. Then the colonies would be identified as "schizophrenococcus," "depressococcus," or "neurotococcus" organisms by their particular visible characteristics. If mental illness were due to infection, the same diagnostic tests could be used each time, and the results would always be valid provided the tests were performed according to the recipe. Also, the same method of interpreting the results would be used each time, no matter who evaluated them. In fact, mental health workers would not have to make diagnoses at all; they could just certify the diagnoses made by laboratory personnel.

The idea of diagnosing mental illnesses by a throat culture is facetious, of course, but the suggestion of using a laboratory test is not farfetched. Tests are currently being developed. The dexamethasone suppression test measures the response of a patient's hormone system to the drug dexamethasone. In some people who have depression, the hormone system fails to respond normally to this drug. This failure to respond can be measured as an abnormality in the amount of hormone in the blood following ingestion of dexamethasone; thus, the hormonal abnormality can be considered a symptom of the mental disorder. However, the problem with the dexamethasone suppression test, and the reason it remains experimental, is its lack of sufficient validity. About 50 percent of the people with depression do not have abnormal responses to dexamethasone, and there are circumstances in which people who have no mental illness show abnormal responses to dexamethasone. Thus, at present, the dexamethasone suppression test is merely a research clue, not a clinically useful diagnostic procedure.[12]

Unlike strep throat, in which a few invariant symptoms suffice to establish a diagnosis, psychiatric illnesses are everchanging, complex sets of behaviors that are somewhat different in each individual. No set of simple observations and no single symptom differentiates one psychiatric illness from another. In many mental illnesses there is not even a single symptom that all patients express. For example, not all people with depression attempt suicide, just as they do not all have an abnormal hormone response to dexamethasone. Not all people with mania spend money profligately. Not all people with schizophrenia believe they can read others' minds.

Psychologists and psychiatrists must try to recognize a pattern of symptoms that corresponds to an illness, even though many possible symptoms may be absent from the pattern in a particular case. Often the mental health professional must use information about the development of the illness over the months or years prior to the episode at hand. Another technique is to use exclusion criteria. An exclusion criterion is a circumstance or symptom that excludes a particular diagnosis. Sometimes, however, the professional will be unable to classify an illness although the patient is obviously ill.[13]

Since the brain is the organ that is functioning improperly, we expect, solely on biological grounds, that the symptoms of mental illness will be highly variable from one patient to another. The social and psychological functions of the brain are determined by the details of communication in its vast network of synaptic connections, the construction and maintenance of which are in turn dependent both on heredity and on environment. Except for identical twins, everyone is born with a unique set of genes and hence a functionally unique set of brain circuits. Everyone grows up in a unique environment that further individualizes the details of his or her circuitry. Indeed, it has recently become possible, using microscopes and electronic recording instruments, to observe functionally significant environmental and hereditary effects on the synaptic connections of brain cells. Of course, other organs are also individualized by genetic and environmental history. One's cardiopulmonary system will be unusually efficient if one's biological parents passed along genes for a strong heart and lungs and if one jogs regularly. One's skin will be darker if one's parents passed along genes for heavier skin pigmentation and if one regularly spends time outdoors in the sun. However, in comparison to the other organs, the brain has a more significant impact on behavior. In the brain, the effects of heredity and environment individualize one's mental life, one's social and behavioral functioning.

Because each brain is unique, we expect the same type of mental illness to be expressed differently in different people. Suppose, for instance, that two people — one religious, the other not — have the symptom of bizarre delusions. The religious person may believe that the devil is speaking to him or her directly, ordering him or her to disobey the laws of his or her religion, to stay away from church, and to conduct an occult mass; the nonreligious person may believe that the leader of an extraterrestrial society is ordering him or her to prepare a site for invaders from outer space. In another example, take two people suffering from depression. One may be overcome with the mistaken belief that he or she is penniless and cannot afford the expense of simple pleasures like buying an ice cream cone or going to the movies; the other may lie in bed sobbing, day after day, obsessed with the idea that he or she is incompetent at work and worthless to others. Psychiatric diagnosis is difficult, not because mental illness is a myth, not because mental illness is nonbiological, and not because psychiatry is unscientific, but because the same underlying problem is not always expressed in the same way by individuals who are unique.

THE DIAGNOSTIC AND STATISTICAL MANUAL

In 1980 the American Psychiatric Association published *The Diagnostic and Statistical Manual, Third Edition* (the *DSM-III*), a book that brought about a significant advance in the art and science of psychiatric diagnosis. In 1987 a revision of the *DSM-III* was issued, the *DSM-III-R*.[14] (A new edition, the *DSM-IV*, is due in 1992.) The *DSM-III-R* defines 313 distinct mental disorders. Mental health professionals can use these definitions to make standard diagnoses of the cases they encounter in their practice. Each disorder is defined by a set of descriptive criteria that refer to patients' objectively observable behavior or to statements made in response to the examiner's questions. Some criteria describe symptoms that are often present in the disorder; others describe symptoms or conditions that preclude a given diagnosis. Often a criterion does not require a particular symptom but rather the expression of one or more symptoms from a long list of possibilities. The criteria do not depend on the professional's opinion about the cause of the illness, such as events during the patient's childhood, or on the professional's inferences about the patient's thoughts.

The purpose of the *DSM-III-R* is to establish reliability of diagnosis, that is, to reduce confusion by encouraging everyone to use the same name for the same condition. Its criteria are chosen to give each diagnostic category as much validity as possible based on the current state of knowledge. Thus, the *DSM-III-R* represents a summary of widely agreed-upon knowledge about mental illness.[15]

The *DSM-III* and *DSM-III-R* are products of committee work. In 1974 the American Psychiatric Association appointed a group of prominent psychiatrists, under the leadership of Robert L. Spitzer, to prepare a new diagnostic manual that would reflect scientific advances since the publication of the *DSM-II*, in 1968.[16] These psychiatrists, with other invited experts, formed committees specializing in particular families of mental disorders. The committee members debated whether given conditions should be considered disorders, determined the symptoms for diagnosis and decided on a name for each disorder. They also consulted with representatives of other professional organizations, such as the American Psychological Association and the American Psychoanalytic Association. At a special convention about a hundred experts in psychiatric diagnosis presented research data and debated the issues. Material in preliminary drafts of the manual was also tested extensively in field trials for practicality and reliability in typical clinical settings. Over 12,000 patients, 550 clinical psychiatrists, and 212 psychiatric facilities were involved in testing the criteria in the drafts of the *DSM-III*.[17]

At many times during the project, the committee work was more like a treaty negotiation than a scientific deliberation. The experts represented many different orientations, from Freudian to behaviorist. Mental health workers protect and defend their theories as valiantly as monarchs defending their territories. Difficult compromises had to be hammered out. For example, in an early draft of the *DSM-III*, mental conditions were defined as "medical disorders." Objections from the American Psychological Association led the task force to change the phrasing to "psychological disorders." The word *neurosis* was not used in early drafts because it was considered too ambiguous, but objections from the psychoanalytic lobby restored this esteemed word to the final draft, though it was placed in parentheses.

The inclusion of diagnostic criteria in the *DSM-III* was a pioneering departure from earlier diagnostic manuals and diagnostic practices. Although diagnostic criteria had been used in research as early as 1972,[18] their clinical use had never before been advocated by an official body of clinical psychologists or psychiatrists. The recommendation that psychiatrists make their diagnoses by referring to explicit, published criteria rather than by relying on professional judgment, insight, and empathy moved psychiatry closer to other branches of medicine.

Even with the use of criteria, the *DSM-III-R* leaves considerable latitude for judgment. Moreover, a large amount of information must be collected about a patient before the criteria can be applied, and the procedures for collecting it are complicated and not fully described. Opportunities for disagreement remain, and indeed psychiatrists do sometimes disagree about the diagnosis when applying criteria to the same cases.[19]

To further standardize diagnostic decisions, research psychiatrists have recently begun using a procedure called the structured interview, which is a standard set of questions the diagnostician asks the patient. The questions are organized so that all the information required by the criteria will be obtained efficiently and in the same way for every patient regardless of who is conducting the interview.[20]

One objection to structured interviews is that they are too impersonal. Many mental health professionals are uncomfortable asking every patient exactly the same questions. They feel they cannot be sensitive to the patient's unique needs when constrained by a rigid protocol. A possible solution is to have a trained diagnostician conduct the standardized interview, much as laboratory personnel perform throat cultures for the family physician. The psychologist or psychiatrist can then confirm the results of the interview through follow-up questions and deal with aspects of treatment that require individualized attention and interpersonal sensitivity. One should never lose sight of the fact that individualized attention and interpersonal sensitivity are essential features of all treatments.

The *DSM-III-R* is not a final statement about diagnosis. It is merely the current "still frame in the ongoing process of attempting to better understand mental disorders."[21] Many of the definitions and criteria are based only on the collective opinion of the task force members in 1986. Collective professional opinion is better than individual professional or nonprofessional opinion, of course, but it is no substitute for knowledge based on well-designed, well-replicated research. For a proper classification of mental disorders, their causes and course of development must be known. The causes of most mental illnesses, however, are not known in detail, so research must proceed, and as it does, *The Diagnostic and Statistical Manual* will have to be repeatedly revised.

In Chapter 4 we take a close look at the *DSM-III-R* criteria for schizophrenia, in Chapter 9 we examine the criteria for mania and depression, and in Chapter 15 we look at the criteria for anxiety disorders. We selected these disorders for three reasons. First, they are clinically significant in that they are both prevalent and debilitating. Second, diagnosis of these disorders is supported by a considerable amount of research. Finally, schizophrenia, mania, depression, and anxiety disorders are the categories of mental illness that are frequently and successfully treated with drugs.

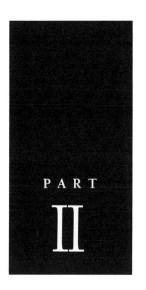

SCHIZOPHRENIA

4

DIAGNOSING SCHIZOPHRENIA

—

I n this chapter we describe schizophrenia and explain its diagnosis according to criteria listed in the *DSM-III-R*. Examples are given to indicate how the criteria apply to individual cases. Special attention is paid to situations in which the symptoms of schizophrenia can be confused with symptoms of other mental disorders.

Schizophrenia is a seriously debilitating mental illness in which the victim is afflicted with bizarre delusions and prominent hallucinations. The delusions are profoundly invalid beliefs, and the hallucinations are equally invalid perceptions. There is also a disordering of the reasoning process, disordered emotional expression, and loss of motivation for work and social living. Typically, the illness starts in adolescence or early adulthood and, if untreated, usually worsens with age.

This grim description of schizophrenia was first set forth by the German psychiatrist Emil Kraepelin in 1896. It was not until 1952 that Kraepelin's discouraging picture was leavened with a dash of hope. In that year the drug chlorpromazine was found to provide substantial relief from several of the most debilitating symptoms of schizophrenia. As a result, the quality of life experienced by schizophrenia patients has improved considerably in the past four decades. There remains, however, a large gap between the treatment that is presently available and a treatment that is completely effective for schizophrenia.

Schizophrenia is best conceived of as a family of related disorders. The symptoms, the way the illness develops, and the response to treatment may vary from case to case. This variation no doubt reflects underlying variation in the biological and social causes of the illness. At present, however, we lack agreement on the number of distinct varieties, the ways to distinguish among them, and the proper name for each. We face this problem of defining, counting, and naming whenever we categorize. For example, ornithologists classifying the varieties of warbler would ask: Does this warbler look and act different enough from all others to represent a separate species? The more they know about the birds, the better their position to answer that question. Similarly, we need to know more about schizophrenia before we can be secure in defining its subtypes. In this chapter we concentrate on the features, as spelled out in the *DSM-III-R*, that define the whole family of schizophrenic disorders. A discussion of subtyping can be found in more advanced works and in the *DSM-III-R* itself.[1] In Chapter 6 we discuss the treatment of schizophrenia with drugs and psychotherapy, and in Chapter 7 we discuss its known biology.

The delusions of schizophrenia are not commonly held mistakes or superstitions; the schizophrenic does not learn them from other people. Rather, the afflicted individual invents personal delusions and hallucinations. The delusions have a distinct, bizarre quality. They often concern the mind itself, focusing on mind reading, occult or supernatural experience and knowledge, and magic power. A patient may believe, for example, that others can read his or her mind (thought-broadcasting delusion), that an alien power is inserting thoughts into his or her mind (thought insertion), or that trivial events are actually signs of colossal significance (delusions of reference). Non-schizophrenics are usually amazed that anyone in our culture could believe such things. But the patient does believe and holds the beliefs with such conviction that reasoned argument is powerless to dissuade. When asked how he or she knows about mental intrusions or occult significances, a patient may typically assert, "I just know."

The hallucinations of schizophrenia usually consist of hearing voices that give orders, criticize, warn of disaster, maintain a running commentary on the patient's activities, or plot against the patient. The patient may pay more attention to the voices than to anything else, believing that the voices convey messages that have profoundly greater significance than the trivial affairs of everyday life.

We can illustrate schizophrenia most easily by describing a fictionalized patient who exhibits typical features of the illness. Judy, a 23-year-old college graduate, was brought to the hospital by her parents because she had developed a severe mental illness. About eight months earlier, she had quit her job as a proofreader and become unusually withdrawn and uncommunicative. This behavior was astonishing because Judy had never before been particularly shy or anxious.

When Judy quit her job, she knew that something was happening to her, but she did not understand what it was. She became more and more preoccupied with her thoughts. She ruminated on the meaning of existence and religious matters. Her personal appearance deteriorated. She stopped taking care of her hair, using cosmetics, and keeping her clothes clean. Then, a few weeks before she was brought to the hospital, she became convinced that her mission was to save the United States from cataclysmic destruction. According to Judy, no one else knew about the imminent threat or appreciated the need for action. Although vague about how the destruction was to be brought about, Judy knew it was inevitable because the information had been supernaturally implanted in her mind.

She remembered the exact moment when she had been called to assume her mission. One morning she had awakened early. She had stood in her room, looking out at the early light of dawn. An unusually bright planet had been visible near the eastern horizon. As she had watched, the top edge of the sun had broken over the horizon, and she had seen a ray of orange light reach from the sun to the planet. The planet had disappeared, and a dog had barked. She had known then that she had been chosen. Recently, Judy had received many new proofs of her role in the cosmic struggle. She knew that certain events, which others thought to be meaningless, were really signs. For example, just before she entered the hospital, a fly had landed on the television and started cleaning its wings while the newscaster reported on satellite pictures from the planet Neptune. It was a sign that little time was left.

Her enemies knew, too, that she had been chosen, and they tried to thwart her. They could read her mind; every time she thought of a plan to overcome them, they stole the plan from her mind. She tried to occupy herself with trivia to prevent their clairvoyant espionage, and she started wearing a black hat to hide her thoughts. She frequently heard the voices of her enemies talking among themselves about her, swearing at her, and plotting to stop her. Sometimes Judy talked back to them. The enemies did not stop at merely manipulating her mind. They placed coiling snakes in her abdomen and slipped poison into the medicine that she refused to take in the hospital.

Judy made it clear that she had important information about an upcoming disaster and that she was being opposed by magic enemies, but some schizophrenics communicate less well or not at all. Their grammar and pronunciation are fine, but there is no information in what they say or write. They jump from one idea to another without making anything clear. They may use made-up words whose meaning others can only guess about. In extremely ill patients, speech may deteriorate into a hash of random words. Such patients may show no awareness that they are not being understood; in fact, they may believe their ideas are profound. Psychiatrists use the term *formal thought disorder* for this garbled thinking. Formal thought disorder has been regarded as a prominent feature of schizophrenia ever since the illness was first described by Kraepelin a hundred years ago.

Heinz E. Lehmann described a schizophrenia patient who was well enough to retain a part-time job as a secretary. She was generally preoccupied with ideas about religion, invisible forces, radiation, psychology, and other esoterica. One day she typed the following memo:

> Mental health is the Blessed Trinity, and as man cannot be without God, it is futile to deny His Son. For the Creation understands germ-any in Voice New Order, not lie of chained reaction, spawning mark in temple Cain with Babel grave'n image to wanton V day "Israel."

Lucifer fell Jew prostitute and Labeth walks by roam to sex ritual, in Bible six million of the Babylon woman, inferno salvation.

Lehmann presented another example of schizophrenic writing that is even more difficult to decode:

The seabeach gathering homestead building upon the site of the bear mountains. Time placed of the dunce to the recovery of the setting sun, upon the stream, poling paddleboat, Mickey, Rooney, Bill. Proceeded of, to the enlivenment. Placed upon the assiduous laboriousness of keeping aloof, yet alive to the forest stream. Haunting the distance of the held possession, requiring means of liberty to sociability.[2]

Another symptom that Judy did not experience is *catatonia*, the practice of making bizarre movements, adopting weird postures, and acting in disorganized and purposeless ways. A well-known catatonic sign is remaining motionless in a fixed, uncomfortable posture for a long time. A patient may stand for hours with one arm raised or sit rigidly in one position day after day, developing pressure sores. During these postural episodes the patient seems stuporous, unresponsive, staring, and silent. The injection of a small dose of barbiturate, a drug that causes relaxation and sleep in normal people, will often release the catatonic patient from his or her statue-like pose. Another catatonic symptom is the so-called waxy flexibility, in which patients hold any posture they are put into. For example, if the hospital attendant raises the patient's arm, the patient will hold the arm up indefinitely; if the attendant turns the patient's head to the right, the patient continues looking to the right. In a third version, excited catatonia, the patient emits excessive, purposeless, disorganized movements. Patients with excited catatonia can become so hyperactive and uncontrolled that they become dangerous to themselves and others.

Catatonia is seldom seen in hospitals today because modern drug treatments are quite effective in relieving it. No discussion of schizophrenia would be complete, however, without a description of catatonia in the absence of treatment.

Catatonic behavior may reflect a profoundly disturbed emotional life. Of course, since we cannot read minds, we cannot speak with complete confidence about another's emotions, but we can draw hints from observation of a person's movements: There is a close relation between motion and emotion. In schizophrenia, facial, bodily, and verbal expressions of emotion are often disturbed or paralyzed. Psychiatrists call this deficit *flat and inappropriate affect*. The patient may stand too close while talking to another. He or she may show inappropriate emotions, laughing while telling of a child's death or becoming enraged when greeted with "How are you?" In some patients, the face is as inexpressive as a mask; showing no external sign of pleasure, amusement, anger, sadness or other feelings within the normal emotional range. Other examples of bizarre behavior associated with schizophrenia include grimacing in front of a mirror for hours, failing to wash or use the toilet, eating feces, dressing outlandishly, and inappropriately displaying nudity. The schizophrenic commonly retreats into a private world of fantasies and hallucinations, ignoring work, family, and body. In a journalistic account of a schizophrenic patient, Susan Sheehan described Sylvia Frumkin, who adorned herself by knotting silverware into her hair and tying a T-shirt around her neck and periodically wearing it around her head like a headband. When she was not hospitalized, Sylvia would often appear on the street dressed in her underwear, giving away phonograph records.[3]

Schizophrenia rarely occurs in childhood. Usually it first appears in adolescence or young adulthood. With the benefit of hindsight, it can often be recognized that the patient had strange, eccentric ways even before the first episode of the debilitating illness. The disease usually lasts for the patient's lifetime, but there may be alternating periods of improvement and worsening.

Schizophrenia is not rare. About 1 percent of Americans suffer from schizophrenia at some point in their lives, and about the same prevalence has been observed in other countries. The illness appears to be slightly more common in women than in men.[4] If you have not done so already, you will probably come into contact with several people suffering from schizophrenia during your lifetime.

DIAGNOSTIC CRITERIA

Criteria for a disorder are listed in the *DSM-III-R* to enable a reliable diagnosis. The description of all aspects of an illness is a secondary objective. Therefore, the criteria focus on those aspects of an illness that are easy to describe objectively and easy to recognize; features that are not useful diagnostically are not emphasized. Six criteria, labeled A through F, must be satisfied for a diagnosis of schizophrenia. For clarity we have paraphrased parts of the criteria below. Direct quotes are indicated.

Criterion A

One or more of the following subcriteria have been satisfied for a period of at least one week.

1. **two of the following symptoms:**
   a. delusions
   b. prominent hallucinations (throughout the day for several days or several times a week for several weeks, each hallucinatory experience not being limited to a few brief moments).
   c. incoherence or marked loosening of associations
   d. catatonic behavior
   e. flat or grossly inappropriate affect
2. **bizarre delusions (i.e., involving a phenomenon that the persons' culture would regard as totally implausible, e.g., thought broadcasting, being controlled by a dead person)**
3. **prominent hallucinations [as defined in 1.b, above] of a voice with content having no apparent relation to depression or elation, or a voice keeping up a running commentary on the person's behavior or thoughts, or two or more voices conversing with each other.**

Criterion A defines the psychotic symptoms that must occur if the illness is to be called schizophrenia. These are the *sine qua non* of schizophrenia. The criterion will be satisfied if the person either has bizarre delusions that cannot possibly be true (item 2) or repeatedly hears voices talking extensively about him or her (item 3). It is not necessary that the patient have both hallucinations and delusions. However, the delusions and hallucinations must be of the particular type that is common to schizophrenia. Under circumstances described in item (1), it is possible to diagnose schizophrenia when the hallucinations and delusions are too mild to satisfy items 2 and 3.

Judy's illness satisfies item 2 of criterion A. Some of Judy's delusions are magical and utterly impossible. In psychiatry, delusions like these are called bizarre. Judy's bizarre delusions include her beliefs that thoughts have been placed directly into her mind by telepathic communication (thought insertion delusion), that others can read her mind (thought broadcasting), that thoughts have been removed from her mind (thought withdrawal), that her behavior and thinking are controlled by an outside power (delusion of being controlled), that meaningless events are profoundly significant (delusion of reference), and that she has snakes in her abdomen (a somatic delusion).

Delusions do not always satisfy item 2; that is, they are not always bizarre. For example, if a woman falsely believes that she is engaged to an heir to the Spanish throne, item 2 would not be satisfied. This delusion could conceivably be true. Judy has some nonbizarre delusions. These include her beliefs that her medicine has been poisoned (persecutory delusion), that her enemies are persecuting her in other ways, and that she has an important role to play in preventing a large disaster (grandiose delusion).

Judy's illness also satisfies item 3. She hears voices. To satisfy item 3, the voices must speak more than just a few words; that is, the hallucinations must be "prominent." There may alternatively be many voices that talk to each other about the patient or a single voice that talks extensively to the patient. Voices that are heard only briefly when the person is emotionally very depressed or very elated do not qualify. The voices must continue speaking even, and especially, when the patient is in a thoughtful mood.

Hearing a single voice that says only a few words can occur in illnesses that are not schizophrenia. In depression, for example, a hallucinated voice may deprecate the patient during periods of intense emotional despair. The voice might say, "You fool!" or "You're despicable!" In the case of mania, a voice might speak during times of emotional elation, in which case the message would be laudatory. The voice might say, "Congratulations, Roger!" But in neither depression nor mania are the voices talkative, and they don't speak unless the person is overcome with intense emotion.

Hallucinations other than voices may occur in schizophrenia, but they are much less common. Only rarely do people with schizophrenia see things. Visual or tactile hallucinations are common in other illnesses and impairments, for example, in various types of drug intoxication and during delirium tremens, the alcoholic withdrawal illness. In obsessive compulsive disorder the person may experience distressing visual images, such as the vision of pushing his or her child off a bridge. In depression, the person may experience visual images of his or her own violent death during periods of intense emotion. However, hallucinations like these do not satisfy item 2 of criterion A.

Item 1 of criterion A can be satisfied when the delusions are less bizarre or the hallucinations are less prominent than those required to satisfy items 2 and 3, but the patient must have two symptoms, rather than just one. If the patient mistakenly believes that she is engaged to the Spanish heir and on two occasions has heard a lady-in-waiting say, "Yes, your highness," item 1 would be satisfied. But item 1 would not be satisfied by either the delusion or the hallucination alone. Item 1 can also be satisfied in the absence of any hallucinations or delusions if the person has two of symptoms c, d, and e.

Symptom 1c, incoherence or loosening of associations, refers to the formal thought disorder described above. "Loosening of associations" means that the patient skips from one idea to the next without clarifying any single idea. Symptom 1d, catatonic behavior, refers to disordered patterns of movement and posture. Symptom 1e, flat or grossly inappropriate affect, refers to abnormalities in the expression of emotion. Judy did not express symptoms c, d, or e.

Criterion B

During the course of the disturbance, functioning in such areas as work, social relations, and self-care is markedly below the highest level achieved before the onset of the disturbance (or, when the onset is in childhood or adolescence, failure to achieve expected level of social development).

As in Judy's case, the onset of schizophrenia is indicated by clear-cut changes from previously established patterns of behavior, thought, and emotional expression. Thus the patient's family and friends may remark, "Judy has changed," or "Judy didn't used to be this way." Patients may alienate or lose interest in their friends.

Employed patients may lose their jobs or be transferred to positions of lesser responsibility. Students may lose interest in their studies, stop going to class, and experience a drop in grades. Married patients may have new difficulties with their spouses. Of course, some people exhibit eccentric behavior almost from birth. Some never learn to speak coherently. Some are passive, shy, or withdrawn. Such lifelong traits, distressing though they may be, are not symptoms of schizophrenia according to the *DSM-III-R*. Personality traits and lifelong illnesses that have no clear time of onset are excluded from the category.

If the illness begins in childhood, the failure of the child to develop as expected can satisfy criterion B. In the *DSM-III Case Book*, Robert L. Spitzer and colleagues describe a schoolgirl of 15 who, though not mentally retarded, has only fifth-grade reading skills and third-grade arithmetic skills. The problem seems to be that the girl is profoundly uninterested in school. Rather, she is preoccupied with drawing pictures of robots, spaceships, and futuristic inventions. She talks to herself in odd voices and makes up bizarre stories involving magic and the future. She believes that she is a supergenius and that other people simply fail to appreciate her ability to hear things that they cannot hear and to communicate with a creature from another planet.[5]

Criterion C

Schizoaffective Disorder and Mood Disorder with Psychotic Features have been ruled out, i.e., if a Major Depressive or Manic Syndrome has ever been present during an active phase of the disturbance, the total duration of all episodes of a mood syndrome has been brief relative to the total duration of the active and residual phase of the disturbance.

The purpose of this criterion is to deal with complications arising from the fact that some patients with the psychotic symptoms of criterion A also suffer from symptoms of mania or depression. For medical and scientific reasons it is important not to confuse these patients with those who suffer more exclusively from the symptoms in criterion A. If a patient suffers from mania or depression as much as or nearly as much as he or she suffers from the symptoms of criterion A, then the condition is not called schizophrenia; rather it is called either schizoaffective disorder or mood disorder with psychotic features. The criteria for diagnosing schizoaffective disorder and mood disorder with psychotic features are given in other sections of the *DSM-III-R*. The symptoms of mania and depression are described in other sections of the *DSM-III-R* and are discussed in Chapter 9.

Criterion D

Continuous signs of the disturbance for at least six months. The six-month period must include an active phase (of at least one week, or less if symptoms have been successfully treated) during which there were psychotic symptoms characteristic of Schizophrenia (symptoms in A), with or without a prodromal or residual phase, as defined below.

Prodromal phase: A clear deterioration in functioning before the active phase of the disturbance that is not due to a disturbance in mood or to a Psychoactive Substance Use Disorder and that involves at least two of the symptoms listed below.

Residual phase: Following the active phase of the disturbance, persistence of at least two of the symptoms noted below, these not being due to a disturbance in mood or to a Psychoactive Substance Use Disorder.

Prodromal or Residual Symptoms:

1. Marked social isolation or withdrawal
2. marked impairment in role functioning as wage-earner, student, or homemaker
3. markedly peculiar behavior (e.g., collecting garbage, talking to self in pubic, hoarding food)
4. marked impairment in personal hygiene and grooming
5. blunted or inappropriate affect
6. digressive, vague, overelaborate, or circumstantial speech, or poverty of speech, or poverty of content of speech
7. odd beliefs or magical thinking, influencing behavior and inconsistent with cultural norms, superstitiousness, belief in clairvoyance, telepathy, "sixth sense," "others can feel my feelings," overvalued ideas, ideas of reference

8. **unusual perceptual experiences (e.g., recurrent illusions, sensing the presence of a force or person not actually present)**
9. **marked lack of initiative, interest, or energy**

Examples: Six months of prodromal symptoms with one week of symptoms from A; no prodromal symptoms with six months of symptoms from A; no prodromal symptoms with one week of symptoms from A and six months of residual symptoms.

The main purpose of this criterion is to ensure that the name *schizophrenia* is not applied to brief psychotic episodes. In order to be called schizophrenia the illness must last at least six months. Symptoms as severe as those specified in criterion A, however, do not have to be present continuously for six months. Schizophrenia waxes and wanes in severity. The time spent in the severe phase (criterion A) plus the time in less severe phases must total at least six months.

A *prodromal phase* is a period of lesser severity that precedes the outbreak of an intense episode of criterion A symptoms. A *residual phase* is a period of less intense illness that follows an intense episode. Symptoms 1–9 in criterion D are mild symptoms that, by themselves, do not justify the diagnosis of schizophrenia. But they can be used to satisfy the six-month duration requirement when they are combined with at least one week of symptoms in criterion A.

Symptoms 1–9 of criterion D refer to the same underlying mental and emotional malfunctions referred to in criterion A. Impairment in everyday living (criterion B) is represented in symptoms 1, 2, 4, and 9. Mild catatonia is reflected in symptoms 3 and 4. Symptoms 3, 4, 5, and 9 reflect loss of emotional responsiveness and flat affect. Symptom 6 is impairment in meaningfulness of verbal communication. A tendency toward delusional beliefs is suggested by symptoms 3 and 7. Symptom 8 indicates mild hallucinations. Judy had a prodromal phase that preceded the outbreak of frank delusions and hallucinations. During this phase, she quit her work (symptom 2), became socially withdrawn (symptom 1), and let her personal appearance deteriorate (symptom 4). She also became preoccupied with thoughts about the meaning of existence and other religious matters (perhaps symptom 7).

Criterion E

It cannot be established that an organic factor initiated and maintained the disturbance.

Here the *DSM-III-R* committee is warning psychiatrists and psychologists against being misled by known brain defects that can cause, at least temporarily, symptoms satisfying criterion A. It is fairly common to find people among the elderly who are victimized by paranoid delusions. They may believe that family members are trying to steal their money or forcibly kidnap them from their homes. They may hide their money or physically assault relatives who are trying to help them. These delusions of persecution are unleashed by the death of neurons in the brain. Such degeneration can be caused by neural diseases such as Alzheimer's or failure of the brain's blood vessels (stroke). These degenerative diseases can easily be distinguished from schizophrenia by concomitant neurological symptoms, such as loss of memory or specific deficits in movement (shakiness, weakness in arms or legs). As mentioned above, drug intoxications (for example, with cocaine, amphetamines, PCP) and alcoholic withdrawal can give rise to hallucinations and delusions, especially of the paranoid type.

Other nonschizophrenic illnesses that can produce schizophrenia-like symptoms include cerebral tumors, traumatic injuries to the brain, epilepsy, multiple sclerosis, carbon monoxide poisoning, thallium poisoning, and vitamin B_{12} deficiency. If one of these nonpsychiatric illnesses is misdiagnosed as schizophrenia, effective treatment will be delayed or prevented, and the patient will have to endure unnecessary suffering.[6]

Even though some symptoms of schizophrenia are similar to symptoms of neural degeneration, the two classes of disease do not appear to have the same biological causes. Schizophrenia does not involve the large-scale loss of neural tissue that occurs in Alzheimer's disease or follows strokes. On the other hand, schizophrenia may be associated with subtle changes in brain anatomy and may arise from biochemical deterioration that is not visible in the microscope.

Criterion F

If there is a history of Autistic Disorder, the additional diagnosis of Schizophrenia is made only if prominent delusions or hallucinations are also present.

Autistic disorder is a rare, lifelong deficit in social interaction and emotional expression that afflicts about three times as many males as females. Both in childhood and adulthood, the afflicted person fails to become involved in the normal panoply of human activity. The afflicted child typically fails to show normal affectionate response to parents, siblings, and potential playmates. Normal imaginative activity is lacking; the child will not play make-believe games with other children. Rather, the child may adopt obsessional behaviors, such as becoming fascinated with rotating objects (e.g., fans), or become compulsively involved with repetitive activities, such as making faces, lining up a string of toys the same way over and over again, or repeating the same phrase.

The lack of emotional responsivity in autism may be confused with the flat affect of schizophrenia. The repetitive behaviors, odd mannerisms, or staring at moving objects may be confused with catatonia. The meaningless speech may suggest the incoherence of schizophrenia. Thus autistic disorder may seem to satisfy criterion A, symptoms 1.c, d, and e, as well as criteria B (failure of normal development), C (mood disorder does not predominate), D (lasts six months), and E (no known organic factor). Autistic disorder, however, does not have delusions and hallucinations of the type that are specified in criterion A, items 2 and 3. Also, schizophrenia is seldom present in young children.

CONCLUSION

In closing this chapter it is appropriate to emphasize that the criteria in the *DSM-III-R* do not take all the guesswork out of diagnosing schizophrenia. The criteria only hint at the nature of schizophrenia. They contain many weakly defined terms that allow psychiatrists to disagree about whether a particular patient suffers from schizophrenia. For example, it is stated in criterion A 1.b that hallucinations must be "prominent." "How prominent?" we may ask. How do we draw the line that separates prominent from mild hallucinations? The same problem exists in criterion A 2 where it is stated that the delusions must be bizarre. We are not told how to determine whether a delusion is weird enough to be called bizarre; the individual mental health professional must make judgment for each patient. Thus, though the criteria in the *DSM-III-R* may help significantly in producing agreement among different diagnosticians, diagnosis is not yet a fully objective procedure. Research is needed to clarify the term *schizophrenia*.

5

CAUSES OF SCHIZOPHRENIA

—

T hree different types of evidence support the conclusion that schizophrenia is the behavioral manifestation of an abnormal brain. First, the anatomy and activity of the schizophrenic brain are often abnormal. Second, a predisposition to schizophrenia is inherited. Third, drug treatments that alter brain biochemistry often cause a dramatic improvement in schizophrenic symptoms. We present a detailed discussion of drug treatments in Chapters 6 and 7. In this chapter we discuss the first two points, the brain abnormalities and the genetics of schizophrenia, in detail and consider other theories of the origins of schizophrenia.

RESEARCH ON BRAIN STRUCTURE AND FUNCTION

If the biology of schizophrenia were really understood, we would be able to describe precisely how the brain of a person with schizophrenia differs from the brain of a healthy person. From the discussion of the biology of the brain in Chapter 2, we can imagine many ways in which the function of a healthy brain might be disrupted. For example, the neurons in a schizophrenic brain might fail to produce a particular transmitter, they might produce too much or too little transmitter, or they might make the wrong transmitter. As another possibility, a particular class of receptors might not function normally. There are, of course, many other possible causes of mental illness.

Although neuroscientists do not yet know what causes schizophrenia, they are fairly certain that both the structure and the activity of schizophrenic brains are abnormal. This conclusion is based primarily on studies using recently developed techniques to create images of the living brain.

The ability to study the living human brain permits scientists to relate brain anatomy and function to behavior in the living patient. For several reasons, studies using live patients can provide more reliable information than postmortem studies about abnormalities in the schizophrenic brain. First, most schizophrenia patients receive medication that changes the brain; only by studying live patients before they receive medication can scientists be certain that brain abnormalities have resulted from disease and not from medication. Second, the brain may change rapidly after death; apparent abnormalities seen in postmortem studies may be the result of postmortem changes rather than disease. Third, in order to study the relationship between changes in the brain and particular symptoms or behaviors, the scientist must observe the brain and the behavior at the same time.

Computed tomography (CT) is one way to obtain an image of a living brain. This technique uses a series of x-ray images combined by a computer to create an image of a particular region of the living brain. Researchers can use the image to measure the size of brain structures in healthy people and in schizophrenic people. Although no large structures are missing from them schizophrenic brains are, on the average, abnormal.[1] In many schizophrenia patients, for example, the fluid-filled spaces in the brain, called ventricles, are enlarged. The enlargements are slight, difficult to see by eye, but detectable with careful measurements and statistical analysis. There is also a subtle abnormality in the pattern of cortical folds in the frontal and prefrontal regions of the brain, regions that scientists think are particularly involved in complex reasoning (see Figure 2–1). Other brain structures adjacent to the enlarged ventricles are abnormally small. Perhaps brain deterioration has left behind an enlarged ventricular space.

There has been some controversy over the significance of these findings. First, enlarged ventricles are not specific to schizophrenia. They accompany many neurological diseases. Second, ventricular size varies greatly among individuals whether or not they have schizophrenia, so in many individuals with schizophrenia, ventricular size falls within the normal range. Nevertheless, the preponderance of the evidence is that ventricular size is abnormally large in many schizophrenia patients. In order to decrease the uncertainty that biological variability introduces into these studies, scientists have compared ventricular size in identical twins, where one member of the pair has schizophrenia and the other does not. The ventricles are almost always larger in the ill twin.[2]

Perhaps some studies have failed to find ventricular enlargement because the enlargement occurs only in certain types of schizophrenia. Schizophrenia is probably not a single disease; certainly the symptoms are not identical in all patients. Several investigators have found that patients with predominantly negative symptoms, such as social withdrawal and flattened affect, are more likely to have enlarged ventricles than are patients with positive symptoms, such as hallucinations and delusions.[3] Perhaps these two types of symptoms have different biological bases. At present, we do not know.

Other studies suggest that people with schizophrenia may have damage to the temporal lobe of the brain (see Figure 2–1). Through postmortem measurements, E. C. Crow and his colleagues have found that the ventricles in this region were enlarged in people with schizophrenia.[4] Again, the increase in ventricular size implies that the brain tissue has shrunken. In studies of the temporal lobes, Daniel Weinberger and his colleagues provide support for this hypothesis. Using another new imaging technique, magnetic resonance imaging (MRI), they found that the gray matter of the temporal lobe was smaller in schizophrenia patients than in healthy controls.[5] It is not surprising that schizophrenia often involves a defect in the temporal cortex, which is involved in hearing, because people with schizophrenia often have auditory hallucinations.

More remarkable than the ability to study the structure of the living brain is the ability to study the living human brain at work. Measurements of blood flow in the brain have shown that brains of people with schizophrenia function differently from brains of normal people. In these experiments, the subject inhales a radioactive gas that enters the blood rapidly. The radioactivity in particular regions of the brain in detected by sensors around the patient's head. The greater the blood flow through a particular region of the brain, the more rapidly the radioactivity leaves that region. Increased blood flow means increased neural activity.

Daniel Weinberger and Karen Faith Berman and their colleagues at the National Institute of Mental Health (NIMH) have used this technique to study the relation between schizophrenia and brain activity during problem solving.[6] They focused on a task requiring abstract reasoning; the patient had to figure out whether a set of cards should be sorted by color, number, or shape. They found that regional blood flow, and presumably neural activity, increased in the prefrontal cortex of normal people performing this task. Schizophrenia patients performed much more poorly on the task and did not show an increase in prefrontal blood flow. Weinberger and Berman do not think that this finding was the result of medication since the results were similar for patients who had not received medication for at least four weeks.

Another research group at the NIMH has obtained similar results using a more complex method of brain imaging called positron emission tomography (PET). In PET scanning the scientist measures particles called positrons that are emitted from a radioactive chemical injected into the patient. A computer makes images of brain "slices," and the amount of positron emission from each region of the brain is indicated on these images. The scientist can use the rate of positron emission to evaluate the metabolic rate of nerve cells in particular regions of the brain. Robert Cohen and his colleagues used PET scanning to measure differences between the brains of normal people and the brains of schizophrenia patients. They asked subjects to discriminate between two different auditory signals. While doing this task, patients with schizophrenia had abnormally low metabolism in the prefrontal cortex.[7] Perhaps the attention abnormalities that accompany schizophrenia are reflected in decreases in metabolism that occur when patients are performing specific tasks.

Scientists at Washington University in St. Louis have discovered a different abnormality in the PET scans of schizophrenia patients who were resting quietly rather than doing a specific task during their scans. In these patients one portion of the basal ganglia on the left side of the brain showed abnormally high blood flow.[8] This is particularly interesting because schizophrenia patients seem to neglect the portion of the environment perceived by the left side of the brain.[9]

The conclusion that schizophrenia patients often have anatomical and functional brain defects has been confirmed by at least four imaging techniques: CT, MRI, regional blood flow, and PET. As time goes on, schizophrenia looks less and less like a myth.

INFLUENCE OF HEREDITY AND ENVIRONMENT ON DISEASE

Among diseases that affect the brain and behavior, all degrees of genetic transmission and environmental causality exist. For example, Huntington's chorea is a neurological disease of purely genetic origin.[10] Patients carrying the gene for Huntington's disease usually seem healthy until they are between 30 and 50 years old. About this time the first symptoms, involuntary jerky movements, appear. Mental deterioration and death follow. Physicians know that the disease is inherited because they understand its mechanism of transmission. Half the children of an affected parent will develop the disease. At the other extreme is deprivation dwarfism, a brain disease with proven environmental causes. In this syndrome, children who receive little love, cuddling, or attention actually stop growing normally and are therefore extremely small for their age.[11] The release of the hormones responsible for growth is controlled by the brain, and lack of normal social stimulation prevents the child's brain from producing the proper amounts of these hormones.

The relative influences of heredity and environment in schizophrenia have been more difficult to distinguish. Schizophrenia is neither purely hereditary like Huntington's chorea nor purely environmental like deprivation dwarfism. Researchers have not yet succeeded in discovering either the mechanism of genetic transmission or the environmental factors that precipitate the disease. Nevertheless, scientists do know that both heredity and environment are involved in its development.

The fact that schizophrenic parents frequently have schizophrenic children suggests, but does not prove, that schizophrenia is genetically transmitted. A family shares its environment as well as its genes, so either the shared environment or the shared genes might cause the disease to run in families. As the well-known psychiatrist Seymour Kety pointed out, the vitamin-deficiency disease pellagra exemplifies the importance of a shared environment in the development of disease within a family: It runs in families not because it is inherited, but because all family members eat the same food.[12]

To show that schizophrenia is heritable, one must distinguish the effects of genes from the effects of environment. The simplest approach to this problem is to compare the rate of schizophrenia in identical and fraternal twins. Identical twins originate from a single egg that splits after fertilization; therefore, both twins have identical genes. Fraternal twins, on the other hand, come from two different eggs and are no more genetically alike than are ordinary brothers and sisters. Presumably the members of a pair of twins share a similar environment regardless of whether they are identical or fraternal. (That is a reasonable assumption, but, it cannot be proved with certainty.)

We say a pair of twins is concordant for schizophrenia if both members have the disease. The pair is discordant if only one member is afflicted. If a predisposition to schizophrenia is genetically transmitted, the concordance for identical twins should be substantially greater than the concordance for fraternal twins. And in fact, it is. The concordance for schizophrenia is about 50 percent for identical twins but only about 6 percent for fraternal twins.[13]

Studies of identical twins provide another kind of evidence for the heritability of schizophrenia. The children of the normal twin and the children of the schizophrenic twin have approximately the same prevalence of schizophrenia,[14] and this prevalence is much higher than the prevalence of schizophrenia in the general population. The normal twin clearly carries the schizophrenia genes because he or she transmits them to his or her children.

The effects of heredity and environment can also be separated by studying adopted children. Adopted children receive their genes from their biological parents but their environment from their adoptive parents. Therefore, if the biological parents but not the adoptive parents of schizophrenic adopted children have an abnormally high incidence of schizophrenia, we can conclude that schizophrenia is heritable. (As mentioned in Chapter 4, the prevalence of schizophrenia in the general population is about 1 percent.) This sort of study can be done only in countries, such as Denmark, where adoption records are not sealed by the courts.

The best known and most conclusive studies on the heritability of schizophrenia were conducted in Denmark by the U.S. psychiatrist Seymour Kety, who compared healthy and schizophrenic adopted "children" (in fact, most were grown up by the time the study was done). The two groups were as similar as possible in age, sex, socioeconomic class of adoptive family, time spent with biological relatives before adoption, and time spent in institutions or foster homes. After locating the adoptive and genetic relatives of each adopted child, Kety's team interviewed each relative. Then, from these interviews, psychiatrists diagnosed each person as healthy, suffering from schizophrenia, or having a nonschizophrenic psychiatric illness. They found that about 6.4 percent of the genetic relatives of the schizophrenic adopted children had suffered from schizophrenia. In contrast, only 1.4 percent of the adoptive relatives had the disease. Both genetic and adoptive relatives of the normal adopted children had a low prevalence of schizophrenia—less than 2 percent.[15]

How do these statistics translate into the probability that schizophrenia will occur in any one family? If a genetic family of a schizophrenic child includes two parents and two additional siblings, there is a 25 percent chance that at least one member of this family will suffer from schizophrenia. On the other hand, in an adoptive family that includes two adoptive parents and their two genetic children, there is only a 6 percent chance that at least one of these relatives will also suffer from schizophrenia.

Clearly, a person with schizophrenic genetic relatives is at risk for schizophrenia even though raised in a family that is free from schizophrenia. Kety's results provide excellent evidence that a predisposition to schizophrenia is genetically transmitted.

Before Kety's conclusions can be accepted, however, a number of interpretations of the data must be ruled out. First, the hypothesis that schizophrenic parents are more likely than healthy parents to give their children up for adoption could explain, without recourse to genetics, Kety's finding that schizophrenia is prevalent in the genetic relatives of adopted schizophrenic children. Nevertheless, this hypothesis is probably wrong because it makes another prediction that is false: It predicts that many healthy adopted children will have schizophrenic genetic parents, whereas Kety's group found that the genetic relatives of healthy adopted children do not have an abnormally high prevalence of schizophrenia.

Second, Kety's data might be explained by the hypothesis that schizophrenia is transmitted by the biological mother, but not genetically. Perhaps the environment inside the uterus is responsible for the disease, or perhaps the mother's behavior toward her baby during the first few weeks of life, before adoption, causes schizophrenia. To eliminate such possible causes of schizophrenia, Kety searched for paternal half-siblings of the schizophrenic adopted children — half-siblings who had the same genetic father but not the same genetic mother. These children not only developed in a different uterus from the schizophrenic children but also lived with a different mother immediately after birth. However, the schizophrenic adopted children and their paternal half-siblings inherited genes from the same father, and the paternal half-siblings, like the schizophrenic adopted children, had a high prevalence of schizophrenia. Clearly, the uterine environment and the environment of the first few weeks after birth are not the sole causes of schizophrenia.

Third, biased diagnostic procedures could explain the results. Maybe the interviewers were more lenient in diagnosing schizophrenia when they interviewed relatives of a schizophrenic adopted child than when they interviewed relatives of a healthy adopted child. However, Kety's experimental design took great care to avoid such bias. First, his interviewers did not know whether they were interviewing a relative of a healthy child or a relative of a schizophrenic child. Next, transcripts of the interviews were carefully edited to remove any inadvertent hints about the relation of the interviewed relative to a particular adopted child. Finally, three psychiatrists who had never seen the relatives or read the unedited transcripts each provided diagnoses from the interviewees' transcripts.

A fourth explanation for the data is that, though unbiased, Kety's diagnostic procedures were inadequate; clearly, he was measuring some genetically transmitted behavior, but it might not have been schizophrenia. After all, Kety conducted his research several years before the *DSM-III* was published; his diagnostic criteria were less precise than those used today. However, an independent team of psychiatrists that rediagnosed all the relatives from the transcripts of Kety's interviews, using *DSM-III* criteria, confirmed Kety's conclusion: The genetic relatives of the schizophrenic adoptive children were more likely than any of the other groups to suffer from either schizophrenia or a less severe variant called schizotypal personality disorder.[16] (Again, the diagnoses were blind; the psychiatrists did not know whether or not a person interviewed was a genetic relative of a schizophrenic or healthy adopted child.)

The best way to show that schizophrenia is inherited is to locate the gene or genes responsible for it and to show these genes are abnormal in people with the disease. To locate the relevant genes, geneticists find a large family with a high incidence of schizophrenia, examine the DNA of family members, and search for a short sequence of DNA that is different in schizophrenic and in normal family members. If family members with a particular DNA sequence at a particular location on the chromosome frequently have schizophrenia, but family members with a different sequence at that location never have the disease, then that DNA sequence is either part of the disease-causing gene or very close to it on the chromosome.[17]

In November 1988 Robin Sherrington and colleagues at the University of Miami School of Medicine proposed in the journal *Nature* that a particular DNA sequence located on a particular chromosome occurred primarily in schizophrenic members of several large Icelandic and British families. However, the same journal also published two other studies that failed to find a link between this DNA sequence and schizophrenia.[18] Even so, this discrepancy might not be fatal to Sherrington's proposal. Although three groups used similar techniques, they studied different families. Because schizophrenia is probably not a single disease, the schizophrenia gene or genes identified in one family may not be the cause of the disease in another family.

Kety's adoption studies, the high concordance of schizophrenia in identical twins, and recent successes in locating genes possibly responsible for schizophrenia all argue that genetics is important. Schizophrenia is not just "a special strategy that a person invents in order to live in an unlivable situation," in the words of the prominent British psychiatrist R. D. Laing.[19] Laing's view implies that for each patient there is at least one guilty party who causes the illness by making the patient's situation unlivable. It also implies that the mind of the newborn baby is a blank slate and that all thoughts can reside equally easily in all brains; that is, no brains are predisposed to schizophrenic thought. This tacit assumption does not holdup, of course, in light of recent observation. Using Kety's data, we can also argue against Thomas Szasz's idea that schizophrenia is just a myth. In Kety's words, "If schizophrenia is a myth, it is a myth with a strong genetic component."[20]

Someone who has schizophrenia in his or her family should be sobered but not panicked by this information when considering having children. Assessing the risk of schizophrenia in any particular family is complex; the risk depends on exactly how many normal and how many ill relatives there are and their precise relationship to you. The prospective parent would be wise to assess the risk realistically by seeking the advice of one of the genetic counselors listed in the *International Directory of Genetic Services*.[21]

The future possibility of genetic testing for schizophrenia and other psychiatric disorders raises a host of ethical and public policy issues.[22] Who should be tested? If I want to know my vulnerability but my brother or, worse, my identical twin does not want to know, should the test be done? Should employers or insurance companies be allowed to mandate testing? Furthermore, interpreting the test to nonscientists may be difficult: Everyone who carries the gene will not get the disorder, but anyone who tests positive will be frightened. Might we cause one psychiatric disorder by testing for another? When genetic knowledge becomes available, as it surely will, scientists, physicians, and the public will have to think hard about its humane use.

ENVIRONMENTAL FACTORS

The fact that identical twins are 50 percent concordant for schizophrenia is evidence that genetics contribute to the development of the illness, but the fact that the concordance is not 100 percent is evidence that other factors are also important. If schizophrenia were determined solely by genetics, we would expect that either both twins or neither twin would be schizophrenic. The fact that the children of the normal twin have a high incidence of schizophrenia[23] is further evidence that expression of the gene requires a nongenetic trigger. Presumably, both the normal twin and his or her schizophrenic children have the required gene or genes. The normal twin does not express these genes, but some of his or her children do.

The nongenetic factors, like the genetic ones, must involve the brain. The brain gathers information from the environment, information that can change behavior and cause sanity or madness. Yet scientists have not been able to determine what features of the environment are critical for the development of schizophrenia. Studies of the families and societies of schizophrenia patients have not provided good clues.

Psychiatrists have come up with many conflicting theories about the characteristics of families that produce schizophrenic children. For example, mothers who allegedly produce schizophrenic children have been accused of being dominating by some and passive by others.[24] The role of the parents' personalities is particularly doubtful when one twin develops schizophrenia and the other remains healthy; both children after all have the same parents and very similar family environments.

In any event, studies of the behavior of parents of schizophrenic children cannot elucidate the effects of the environment if only genetic parents are examined. Abnormal behavior in both the child and the parents may be derived from common genes. Only an adoption study can separate genetic and environmental effects.

To study the effects of a schizophrenic environment, Kety's team compared the prevalence of schizophrenia in three groups of adopted children: those with a schizophrenic genetic parent, those who had a schizophrenic adoptive parent, and those who had healthy genetic and adoptive parents.[25] The researchers found that only children with a schizophrenic genetic parent had a high prevalence of schizophrenia. Children with a schizophrenic adopted parent or with healthy parents had the usual 1 percent rate of schizophrenia.

The organization of Israeli society provides another opportunity to study the effect of schizophrenic parents on their children. On the one hand, some families live on kibbutzim, where parents are not directly responsible for rearing their children. On the other hand, in towns children live in nuclear families and are reared by their parents. Yet children of schizophrenic parents have a similar prevalence of schizophrenia regardless of whether they come from kibbutz families or from town families.[26]

In summary, most studies show that heredity is substantially more important than environment as a cause of schizophrenia.[27] The disorder is less frequent when there is no genetic susceptibility. Nevertheless, nongenetic factors must play a role in the genesis of the disorder. The best evidence for this conclusion is that the concordance for schizophrenia in identical twins is only about 50 percent. For two reasons, we do not think family interactions are a primary environmental cause: First, rearing by a schizophrenic parent does not cause schizophrenia; second, discordant identical twins have usually been raised in the same family environment. In any event, the nature of the nongenetic event is unknown. It need not be an observable environmental event like a failure experience; it may be something uncontrollable like exposure to a virus or a toxin as a fetus or infant.

Perhaps this information can allay some of the guilt that often burdens the parents of a child who has schizophrenia. Parents often ask what they have done wrong. Sometimes, mental health professionals are all too eager to tell them. But parents probably cannot cause schizophrenia in a child who is not genetically susceptible. Furthermore, psychiatrists do not know any way to prevent the disease in a susceptible child. Genes determine susceptibility, and we are not responsible for our genes. We received them from our ancestors at the moment we were conceived, and we pass along half our genes to each of our children at the moment of conception.

THE LABELING AND OPPRESSION THEORIES OF SCHIZOPHRENIA

There are two versions of the notion that society causes schizophrenia. The labeling theory claims that labeling deviant people mentally ill creates a self-fulfilling prophecy; that is, because of the label, deviant people are encouraged to behave in an even more deviant manner.[28] The oppression theory admits that mental illness is real but contends that it is not caused by a genetic defect in the brain but by social and/or economic oppression.

These theories are not satisfactory. If the labels do not describe preexisting phenomena but rather create patterns of deviant behavior, similar patterns of behavior labeled mental illness would not exist in widely different cultures. However, both the Eskimos and the

Yoruba, a rural African culture, have words for a cluster of symptoms that bears an uncanny resemblance to our European-American description of schizophrenia.[29] The Eskimo word *nuthkavihak*, for example, describes people who scream at someone who does not exist, refuse to talk, refuse to eat, make strange grimaces, and hide in strange places. The content of the symptomatic delusions is culturally determined, of course. For example, a *nuthkavihak* Eskimo might believe that a fox lives insider her, whereas an American with schizophrenia might believe that he is possessed by a powerful electromagnetic force. Eskimos and Yorubas also recognize as sick those people with symptoms that U.S. pyschiatrists call severe anxiety and depression, even though these two cultures do not have a label for these symptoms.

In fact, studies conducted by the World Health Organization (WHO) comparing schizophrenia in the United States, Europe, Asia, and Africa have found that patients from a wide diversity of cultures use similar language to describe their symptoms. They describe hearing voices talking about them in the third person. They describe having their thoughts read or "broadcast" by some outside force.[30]

The response of society to these symptoms is also similar in different cultures. Eskimos and Yorubas both consider schizophrenia to be an illness to be treated by healers. Furthermore, neither Eskimos nor Yorubas consider all deviants to be ill. There are evil deviants, who are "witches," and good deviants, who are faith healers, and they have no difficulty distinguishing between a person with schizophrenia and either a witch or faith healer. The fact that these very diverse cultures believe that very similar behaviors are symptoms of illness suggests that the illness existed before the label, not vice versa. We do not know whether mental illness is ever created by labeling, but we are quite sure that it is not always created by labeling.

If schizophrenia were a product of social oppression in Western society, it ought not to exist in non-Western societies. But in fact all societies that have been studied in Asia, Africa, Europe, and the Americas have a prevalence of schizophrenia between 0.2 and 1.0 percent. Non-Western societies have approximately as much schizophrenia as do Western societies.[31]

We do not think that industrialization and its associated psychological stress have increased the incidence of schizophrenia. The rate of first hospital admissions for young and middle-aged psychotics in

Massachusetts, for example, did not increase from 1840 to 1940.[32] Industrialization may, however, have affected the long-term outcome of schizophrenia. The WHO found that in developing countries about half the patients recovered from their initial episode and had no continuing disability, whereas such a favorable outcome was rare in developed countries.[33] We do not have any plausible speculations about the reason for this difference.

Oppression theorists usually point out that schizophrenia is more common in the lower than in the higher socioeconomic classes. Socioeconomic class is measured by education and occupation, so people in lower classes tend to have little education and unskilled jobs. According to oppression theory, poverty causes schizophrenia. An alternative, intuitively reasonable explanation is that schizophrenia causes poverty. After all, many patients leaving the hospital have residual symptoms. Many are young adults, and their residual symptoms may prevent them from completing their education. Their illness may also rob them of the subtle social skills that are required for success in a high-paying career.

A study examining the social class of schizophrenia patients and their parents supports the notion that schizophrenia causes downward social mobility. In families without schizophrenia, the children's social class is similar to the parents' social class, but schizophrenia patients tend to have a much lower social class than their parents. This downward mobility is a specific effect of schizophrenia, not a general effect of psychiatric illness or hospitalization. The social class of schizophrenia patients is much lower than the social class of other hospitalized psychiatric patients, yet the social class of the parents of schizophrenia patients does not differ from the social class of parents of patients with other psychiatric illnesses.[34]

Psychiatrists know that both heredity and environment are important in the genesis of schizophrenia, but they do not know precisely how either acts on the brain to encourage or retard the development of the disease. They do not know how to change the environment to reduce the incidence of schizophrenia. Schizophrenia is a chronic illness; it cannot be cured. But it can be treated. To work, the treatment must change the patient's brain chemistry.

TREATMENT OF
SCHIZOPHRENIA

—

W̲e begin this chapter with the early history of antipsychotic drugs. We then provide descriptions of drugs effects in acutely schizophrenic patients, including case studies as well as the results of research demonstrating effectiveness. After a discussion of the use of antipsychotics for recovering patients, we deal with the misuse of antipsychotics. Finally, we briefly discuss psychotherapy in the treatment of schizophrenia.

THE DISCOVERY AND ACCEPTANCE
OF PHENOTHIAZINES

The first effective drug used to treat schizophrenia was chlorpromazine (brand name, Thorazine). It belongs to the category of drugs called phenothiazines. Phenothiazines were not discovered through research designed to find a treatment for schizophrenia. On the contrary, the history of phenothiazines reads like a story of a drug in search of a disease. The molecule on which the modern drugs are based, the phenothiazine nucleus, was first synthesized by the German dye industry in 1883. All phenothiazines currently in use are chemical modifications of this parent compound. No one thought that this molecule might have important medical uses until 1944, when several phenothiazine variants were tested as antimalarial agents, both in France and in the United States, because some chemically related dyes were known to have antimalarial value. Phenothiazines failed as a treatment for malaria, but the researchers discovered their potential value as sedatives and antihistamines.

Rhone-Poulenc, the French pharmaceutical firm that had synthesized the compounds, became interested in developing a phenothiazine that was an effective antihistamine but had minimal sedative effects. Chemists at Rhone-Poulenc synthesized several variants of the phenothiazine nucleus and tested their effects on rats. The chemists looked for effective antihistamines that would not make the rats sleepy or impair their muscular coordination.

In 1949, while Rhone-Poulenc was testing phenothiazines for antihistaminic properties, the French surgeon Henri Laborit was working on the theory that antihistamines would prevent surgical shock. To test this theory, he began giving phenothiazines to surgical patients. Although his theories about shock turned out to be wrong, Laborit described dramatic effects of the drug on the central nervous system. Like the Rhone-Poulenc scientists, he found that most phenothiazines had sedative effects. Because he was working with people rather than rats, Laborit also had the opportunity to observe another effect of phenothiazines: In low doses the drugs calmed anxious surgical patients without making them fall asleep.

Probably it was Laborit's work in conjunction with their own animal research that made the scientists at Rhone-Poulenc do an abrupt about-face and start searching for a phenothiazine variant with maximal rather than minimal effects on the central nervous system. In December 1950 these researchers synthesized chlorpromazine, and tests on animals suggested that it had considerable clinical potential. But it is not clear that the Rhone-Poulenc scientists could have answered the question, potential for what?

Rhone-Poulenc began testing chlorpromazine on patients in March 1951, only three months after the drug had been synthesized. (This quick transfer from the chemistry laboratory to the hospital would be impossible today. Extensive animal trials showing both efficacy and safety are required before a new drug can be tested on humans.) At first, chlorpromazine was used in conjunction with barbiturates in both surgical anesthesia and in psychiatric treatment. (For want of any better treatment, barbiturates were often used to sedate violent and uncontrollable mental patients.) Until chlorpromazine was used alone, its antipsychotic properties—that is, its ability to suppress psychotic thoughts and behaviors—were not obvious. In 1951 two French psychiatrists, Jean Delay and Pierre Deniker, used chlorpromazine alone to treat six manic patients. Shortly afterward, they published the first paper on the antipsychotic properties of chlorpromazine, claiming that chlorpromazine caused rapid improvement in their patients. Yet several years passed before the physicians in the French psychiatric hospitals made any substantial use of the drug. Their reluctance to use chlorpromazine may have resulted from the low scientific standards of psychiatric research in the 1940s. Although French psychiatrists had a tradition of faith in physical and chemical treatments for mental illness, they had been assailed too many times by worthless drugs touted as cures. The drug companies had cried "salvation" too often.

Chlorpromazine with first introduced to the United States when Rhone-Poulenc asked the Smith, Klein, and French Corporation, a large U.S. drug company, if it would be interested in a licensing agreement to market the drug in the United States. Smith, Klein, and French was very interested. The company performed laboratory tests and clinical trials for two years and in May 1954 began to market chlorpromazine under the trade name Thorazine.[1]

The development of other antipsychotic drugs followed rapidly. Some, like chlorpromazine, were members of the phenothiazine family; others, such as haloperidol (trade name, Haldol), were chemically unrelated to chlorpromazine. Sixteen effective antipsychotics are currently described in a standard pharmacology text, and that list includes only a small fraction of all the drugs with antipsychotic effects (see the Appendix).[2]

As Deniker has pointed out, the source of the initial U.S. resistance to chlorpromazine was quite different from that in France. In the United States the psychoanalytic tradition originating with Freud led many psychiatrists to believe that psychotherapy was the only proper treatment for mental illness. Although Freud himself never claimed that psychoanalysis could cure schizophrenia, many of his disciples in the United States believed that it would, and they resisted the use of drugs. Nevertheless, by 1955 antipsychotics were commonly used to treat schizophrenia in U.S. mental hospitals, and consequently the population of these hospitals began to decrease.

BEHAVIORAL CHANGES PRODUCED BY ANTIPSYCHOTICS

Antipsychotics are so effective in treating schizophrenia that many patients in mental hospitals appear quite healthy. A visitor to a psychiatric hospital, particularly one providing primarily short-term care, might wonder why many of the patients were hospitalized at all. It might appear that psychiatrists cannot tell the sane from the insane. David L. Rosenhan, a psychologist at Stanford University, expressed this opinion in an article in *Science* entitled "On Being Sane in Insane Places."[3] Rosenhan and some of his colleagues gained admittance to a psychiatric hospital by claiming that they were having hallucinations and hearing voices. After admission, they reported that their symptoms disappeared; however, they were not released. The pseudopatients claimed that the staff assumed that all patients were "crazy" and refused to recognize any evidence to the contrary.

Rosenhan and his associates did not consider the possibility that antipsychotic drugs were helping many schizophrenia patients to behave normally much of the time. Rather, they interpreted their experience as evidence of psychiatrists' incompetence. However, experienced professionals know that the absence of florid psychotic behavior does not mean that a patient is cured and ready to leave the hospital.

During their first few weeks in the hospital, floridly schizophrenic patients show dramatic changes in behavior. Upon entering the hospital, they excitedly converse with their voices, broadcast their thoughts to the president, or proclaim that enemy forces are poisoning their food. The first doses of antipsychotic will probably make them somewhat sleepy, but the sedative effects of the drug wear off after a few weeks. These sedative effects may be somewhat useful in the case of violent or excited patients, but sedation is neither the main effect of antipsychotics nor the reason for their effectiveness in treating schizophrenia. After a week or two, the patients' symptoms begin to improve.

As treatment progresses, patients stop conversing with their voices. They are no longer harassed by voices' commands to harm themselves or others. "External forces" no longer instruct them to be hostile and belligerent, so these behaviors, too, decrease. As paranoia and suspiciousness fade, patients no longer accuse the hospital staff of trying to harm them. If patients were incoherent, their speech becomes connected and comprehensible.

Not only do symptoms of illness decrease, but symptoms of health return. Patients become emotionally more responsive. They begin to listen and respond to the staff and fellow patients, perhaps because they are no longer completely absorbed by the demands of their hallucinations. They begin to care for themselves. Those who rarely spoke may now engage in conversations, their sentences becoming more grammatical and complex. Those who rarely moved now begin to walk around and participate in activities. Catatonic patients no longer stand or sit in their fixed positions; their pressure sores begin to heal.[4]

Mental health workers have vividly described the changes brought about by antipsychotics in hospitalized psychiatric patients:

> The opinion seems to be almost unanimous that patients who exhibit psychomotor activity, assaultiveness, hostility, and negativism show a reduction in their motor output [movements] with the administration of the drug. They are less restless, are quite ready to sit quietly, are less assaultive and destructive, are orderly and well-behaved. Subjectively, they exhibit a marked reduction in anxiety. They are clear mentally, in good contact with their surroundings, and are able to discuss their hallucinations and delusions calmly and with a considerable degree of objectivity.[5]

In another report a hospital official said: "It is a distinct pleasure to think of the patients . . . who formerly paced about more like caged animals than any group of patients that I have ever seen, now going to the general dining room and eating with silverware."[6] Such changes in the patients' behavior have caused dramatic changes in the hospital environment. Hospitals can now provide more recreational and therapeutic programs, and the patients can take advantage of them. Patients, no longer catatonic, violent, or incoherent, can learn social and occupational skills.

CASE STUDIES

In *The Eden Express* Mark Vonnegut poignantly documented his own recovery from mental illness.[7] Vonnegut's diagnosis of schizophrenia was made before the publication of the *DSM-III*, so we cannot be certain that it was correct. Nevertheless, he clearly had schizophrenic symptoms. His case is a good example of the ability of antipsychotics to alleviate these symptoms and to restore rational thought.

When Vonnegut became ill, he was living on a communal farm in British Columbia, trying hard to be a "good hippie" during the peak of the counterculture period (1969–1970). Even his hippie friends, admiring as they were of deviant behavior, recognized that he was ill. Vonnegut vividly described the hallucinations and delusions of his schizophrenic episodes. But his descriptions of schizophrenic thought, though culled from his own memory, cannot quite capture the aberrant quality of schizophrenic thought that is so obvious in a direct quote from a schizophrenia patient (see Chapter 4).

Vonnegut's recovery, like that of most patients, took several weeks. The first sign of improvement was that he began to notice his surroundings. Vonnegut explains:

> I was all taken up with voices, visions and all. I vaguely knew I was in a mental hospital, but it wasn't any different from being anywhere else. Where I was was beside the point. Little by little with the help of massive doses of Thorazine in the ass and in my milkshakes (which was all they could get me to eat), little by little it started mattering to me where I was and what was going on.[8]

Though Vonnegut does not like Thorazine, he admits that he needed it.

Vonnegut's first episode was not his only one. He was rehospitalized twice before he enjoyed a lasting recovery. After he recovered, he wrote, studied biochemistry, and applied to medical school. He says that he "got more and more disgustingly healthy." Interestingly, the healthier he got, the more convinced he became that schizophrenia is a biochemical disease. Mark Vonnegut was fortunate; he seems to have recovered fully and permanently. His compelling and elegant book is in itself evidence of his recovery.

There are other literary accounts of schizophrenia (*I Never Promised You a Rose Garden*, for example) that describe recovery rather than chronic illness and psychiatric deterioration. However most of these accounts diagnosed their protagonists without the benefit of the *DSM-III* or the *DSM-III-R*, and we cannot know whether these patients would have satisfied modern criteria for schizophrenia. In fact, researchers who analyzed the symptoms described in several such narratives concluded, in a 1981 article in the *Archives of General Psychiatry*, that none of the protagonists actually suffered from schizophrenia. Of particular interest, they proposed that Vonnegut had bipolar affective disorder. (Unless Vonnegut relapses, we will never be certain what his diagnosis would have been under *DSM-III-R* criteria.) Furthermore, they suggested that these literary accounts gave the public an unrealistically optimistic view of the prognosis for schizophrenia patients.[9]

Another patient, Paul, also recovered from schizophrenia, but his recovery was less complete than Vonnegut's. As a child, Paul spent a lot of time with his parents but little with friends his own age. His adolescence was uneventful, although a skilled observer would have noticed that his emotional development was not normal. He never went out with girls, for example. Moreover, at the age of 17 he often told, with great relish and amusement, foolish stories and jokes appropriate to a six-year-old, unresponsive to the obvious boredom of his listeners (this unresponsiveness is called blunted affect). However, he worked hard at school and was a brilliant student. He went to a prestigious college, and although he was somewhat demoralized by the competition, he continued to do well academically. Nonetheless, he still showed no signs of maturing emotionally.

After college, he went to graduate school, studying biology for a year. During this year, be became discouraged with academic work and increasingly religious. Convinced that he did not have the ability to succeed academically and professionally, he devoted himself to God, believing that to be his only alternative. Soon afterwards, he enrolled in a fundamentalist Bible college. At first, his involvement with the supernatural did not seem abnormal in the context of the religious community in which he lived. But gradually Paul began claiming to receive direct messages from heaven. His messages came from the apostle whose name he bore. One morning, Paul's roommate found him under his desk, naked, proclaiming something unintelligible about "orders from Paul and Jesus, and the frauds of the devil and communism." The college officials persuaded Paul to enter a psychiatric hospital, where he was treated with phenothiazines. After a few months in a halfway house, Paul was well enough to live on his own. He obtained a good job as a laboratory technician and has kept it for over 10 years. He continues to take phenothiazines. Occasional experiments with drug-free periods have resulted in psychotic relapses.

Antipsychotics worked effectively for Paul; without them, he would probably have spent his entire life in the hospital. But Paul is not completely well. His affect is still blunted; he still fails to respond to other people's facial expressions or words. His own expressions oscillate between stony and giggly. In a conversation, Paul responds to his own remarks, never to the words of another speaker. When he tells a story, Paul's performance is as unvarying as a tape recording; the responses of his listeners do not alter his speech. Yet Paul does not appear sedated. His soliloquies are lively; he is energetic. In many ways, Paul behaves very much as he did before his schizophrenic episode. He is still emotionally immature and self-centered. He still has no relationships with women. He still has intellectual ability and perseverance.

In some ways Paul typifies the recovered schizophrenia patient. He can provide his own food, clothing, housing, and personal hygiene. He probably will never marry or develop intimate friendships. Even a short conversation with Paul would probably persuade an observer that he is not quite healthy. He might stand too close or too far away; he might laugh inappropriately or continue to talk when no one is listening. However, Paul's occupational success is greater than that of most recovered schizophrenia patients. He holds a job requiring professional expertise, whereas most patients with a history like his cannot handle the complexity and stress of such a position.

The overall adjustment of the recovered schizophrenia patient can be fairly well predicted from his or her adjustment before becoming ill. Antipsychotic drugs cannot create a new personality or solve the problems of living that the patient had prior to his or her illness. Treatment with antipsychotic drugs will not create a social butterfly out of a wallflower. Mark Vonnegut was socially adept and perceptive before his illness, and his illness did not destroy these skills. Paul's social competence was always marginal, and it remains marginal. To exaggerate this point, one psychiatrist said that you cannot expect a patient to write the great American novel after taking antipsychotics if he could not construct a paragraph before. In short, miracles are not recorded in the annals of psychiatry.

Unfortunately, some schizophrenia patients improve very little or not at all. Sylvia Frumkin, whom we mentioned in Chapter 4, was such a patient.[10] Sylvia's struggle with schizophrenia began when she was about 14 years old. Her parents were forced to hospitalize her a year later when she asked her uncle to adopt her. She insisted that she did not belong to her parents and Sylvia, like many schizophrenia patients, could not take care of herself. She could not eat without smearing food on herself and others. When she attempted to cook at home, she plastered the kitchen with food and dirty dishes. She would not clean her room, shower, or change clothes. She dressed inappropriately. On one occasion she attended the hospital's Jewish services in a T-shirt, half-slip, and high-heeled gold sandals. During one of her brief periods out of the hospital, she danced in the streets and gave away phonograph records while wearing only a bra and half-slip.

Because she repeatedly struck the hospital attendants and other patients, she was often put in a padded seclusion room for hours. While in seclusion, she did not control her bowel movements; the hospital attendants had to hose down both Sylvia and the seclusion room before they could release her. Sylvia never recovered enough to live independently. By 1980, 16 years after her first admission to the hospital, she had been admitted 10 times to the Creedmoor Psychiatric Center, a New York State hospital.

Did antipsychotic drugs help Sylvia Frumkin? When she received medication in sufficiently large doses, she was able to avoid seclusion. Sometimes she could even participate in the hospital's sheltered typing workshop. She wore appropriate clothing and spoke civilly with the staff and other patients. On one occasion, she stayed out of the hospital long enough to complete a medical secretary course but relapsed the day before graduation. Whenever her medication was reduced, however, her symptoms returned. She believed she carried Paul McCartney's baby. She alternately became a Buddhist and a born-again Christian. She cut up her pillowcase because demons were dancing in it. Though her condition improved at times, even at her best she could not live and work on her own. Therefore, although the drugs decreased her symptoms, we think that antipsychotics failed as a treatment.

THE NIMH STUDY OF ANTIPSYCHOTIC THERAPY

When patients enter a psychiatric hospital with symptoms of schizophrenia, the major goal of treatment is to reduce the symptoms so that they can rejoin society. The success of treatment can be measured by the amount of time the patients remain in the hospital and by the reduction in symptoms. So far we have not provided scientific evidence that antipsychotic treatment aids in accomplishing these goals. We have only provided anecdotes about patients who took antipsychotics and got relief from schizophrenia symptoms. These anecdotes are not adequate evidence that the drug causes recovery because schizophrenia, like almost every other disease, sometimes improves by itself. Sometimes, the disease goes away when patients believe they are taking a useful drug, whereas in reality they are taking a placebo, a pill containing sugar or starch instead of a therapeutic agent. A few patients will recover with nearly any treatment. Their recovery, however, does not prove that the treatment is a specific remedy for the disease.

To show that antipsychotics are effective, researchers have to show that a group of patients receiving the drugs either improves more or leaves the hospital sooner than another similar group receiving a placebo. Because of the unreliability of psychiatric diagnosis, the same physicians must diagnose both drug and placebo patients. The patients must be randomly assigned to the drug group and to the placebo group. Finally, the studies must be double blind; that is, neither the patients nor the doctors and nurses evaluating them must know who is receiving active drug and who is receiving placebo.

In 1964 the National Institute of Mental Health Pharmacology Service Center engaged nine hospitals in a collaborative study to find out whether antipsychotics really helped schizophrenia patients.[11]

Since this study antedates the *DSM-III*, all the patients may not have met the *DSM-III* or *DSM-III-R* criteria for schizophrenia. We think, however, that the diagnostic problem in this study is not serious because the investigators included all patients who had a certain set of symptoms. Although some of these patients may not have met the *DSM-III-R* criteria for schizophrenia, their symptoms were similar to those in the *DSM-III-R*.

The patients in the NIMH study were randomly assigned to one of four groups. Each of the first three groups received a different antipsychotic drug; the fourth group received a placebo. Neither the patients nor the hospital staff knew which pills contained an active drug and which contained a placebo. Three hundred forty-four patients completed the study, about 90 in each of the three drug groups and 74 in the placebo group.

At the beginning of the study, the hospital staff made a global judgment of the severity of each patient's illness and then placed each patient in one of seven categories ranging from "extremely ill" to "normal." In addition, the staff described the specific symptoms of each patient and noted their severity. For example, a patient could have been described as "moderately ill" (category four) and suffering from hallucinations, lack of personal hygiene, and incoherent speech.

After six weeks of treatment with either an antipsychotic or placebo, the patients were reevaluated. This time the staff rated each patient's improvement as well as the current severity of his illness. Based on improvement or lack of it, they put each patient into one of seven categories ranging from "very much worse" to "very much improved." As the graph in Figure 6–1 illustrates, the drug patients improved much more than the placebo patients. Over three-quarters of the drug patients were "much improved" or "very much improved" (the two categories reflecting the most improvement), while only one-third of the placebo patients fell into these two categories.

In what ways did the patients show improvement? Did the drugs actually help them think more normally? To answer these questions, the NIMH group examined the effects of the drugs on specific symptoms of schizophrenia. While virtually all symptoms decreased with the use of antipsychotics, the decrease in symptoms of confusion and disorganization was the greatest. For example, incoherent speech became coherent. Personal hygiene improved; patients dressed themselves, washed, combed their hair, and used the toilet. Patients

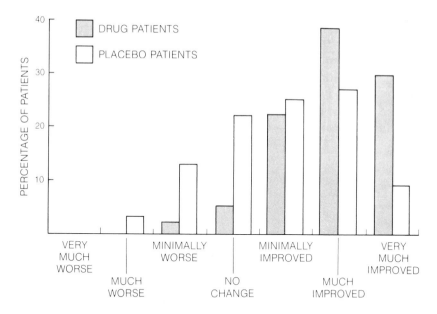

FIGURE 6–1   The effect of treatment with antipsychotic drugs or placebo on patients with schizophrenia. (Data from National Institute of Mental Health, Pharmacology Service Center. Collaborative Study Group, Phenothiazine treatment in acute schizophrenia. *Archives of General Psychiatry* 10:246–261, 1964.)

who had not spoken or responded to others became responsive to questions and requests. The drugs were less effective in combating thoughts that, though somewhat grammatical and logical, were unrelated to reality. Antipsychotics do not always eliminate delusions and hallucinations, but the drugs usually permit the patient to recognize hallucinations or delusions as such and to know that they are symptoms of disease.

How healthy were the patients at the end of the treatment? Even if they were not well enough to leave the hospital, so long as they were cleaner, calmer, and better nourished, the drugs were beneficial. Of course, the benefits are much more impressive if antipsychotics permit a patient to resume a relatively normal life outside the hospital. Because antipsychotics, like all drugs, have risks and side effects as well as benefits, people need to know just how great the benefits are. After six weeks of treatment, the hospital staff described almost 50 percent of the drug patients as "borderline ill" or "normal," the two categories indicating the greatest degree of health.

Only about 15 percent of the placebo patients fell into these two categories; the rest remained more seriously ill.

Because the NIMH study continued for only six weeks, the total length of hospitalization of the drug and placebo patients could not be compared. In other similar studies, ample evidence has been gathered indicating that the average hospital stay is greatly decreased by drug therapy. In one of the most detailed studies, the patients receiving drugs stayed in the hospital only about half as long as the patients not receiving drugs.[12]

The actual effectiveness of the drugs compared to placebo is probably underestimated by the NIMH statistics. Some of the placebo patients became so much worse during the treatment period that they had to be eliminated from the study and given some other type of treatment. Had these very ill patients been included in the statistical results, the percentage of improved placebo patients would have been smaller.

The conclusions of the NIMH study have been confirmed by hundreds of double-blind studies performed by many teams of researchers.[13] One point of controversy has been whether negative symptoms, such as flat effect and social withdrawal, improve in response to antipsychotic treatment as much as positive symptoms, such as hallucinations and delusions. Some researchers have found that they do not.[14] This finding would suggest that patients whose symptoms are primarily negative ought not to be treated with antipsychotic drugs. Other studies, however, agree with the original NIMH studies that both positive and negative symptoms are helped by antipsychotic drugs.[15] The data suggest to us that the predominance of negative symptoms is not a good reason to withhold antipsychotic drugs from a patient with schizophrenia.

WHEN THE STANDARD TREATMENTS FAIL

As Figure 6–1 shows, about 8 percent of patients fail to improve in response to antipsychotics, and another 22 percent do not improve very much. What additional help can psychiatrists provide for these patients? One possibility would be to give these patients much larger doses of antipsychotics than are usually prescribed. While a few patients have improved on megadoses of antipsychotics, most evidence indicates that if standard doses do not work, higher doses will not either.[16] Moreover, using extremely high doses increases the risk of serious side effects.

Another possibility is to give a different drug. Although a few respond well to a second antipsychotic, after failing to respond to the first one, such patients are, unfortunately, rare. Usually failure to improve on one drug predicts failure to improve on another.

The development of new treatments is the best hope for patients who do not respond to the currently available drugs. One recently developed drug, clozapine, provides some hope for patients who remain ill in spite of receiving adequate doses of conventional antipsychotics. Trying clozapine is not merely another example of trying a second drug when a first has failed because the biology of clozapine is quite different from that of most other antipsychotic drugs.

The most extensive study of clozapine compared this drug with chlorpromazine in 268 patients from 16 different hospitals.[17] All patients had been ill for the previous five years and had never enjoyed a period of normal functioning during that time in spite of antipsychotic treatment. Patients were randomly assigned to chlorpromazine or clozapine for the six weeks of the study. Their progress was rated in several different ways. In the most global rating, patients were categorized as improved if their symptoms decreased and they were only mildly ill at the end of the study. As might be expected from their histories, the chlorpromazine patients improved very little over the six weeks of the study; in fact, only 4 percent improved. But 30 percent of the clozapine patients improved. Clozapine was superior to chlorpromazine in decreasing both positive and negative symptoms. Clozapine's side effects were also quite different from the side effects of conventional antipsychotics (see Chapter 8). This may make clozapine a superior drug not only for patients who do not respond to conventional antipsychotics, but also for those who cannot tolerate their side effects.

USE OF ANTIPSYCHOTIC THERAPY TO PREVENT RELAPSE

Does a recovered patient require continued medication in order to stay out of the hospital? To answer this question, researchers compare relapse rates of patients who are maintained on antipsychotic drugs after release from the hospital with relapse rates of patients who are maintained on placebo. Gerald Hogarty and his colleagues found that recovered patients maintained on antipsychotics had about a 55 percent chance of remaining in the community for two years after leaving the hospital, whereas patients maintained on placebo had only a 15 percent chance (Figure 6–2). Thus, maintenance therapy with antipsychotics more than doubles a patient's chances of remaining out of the hospital for two years.[18] Some of the

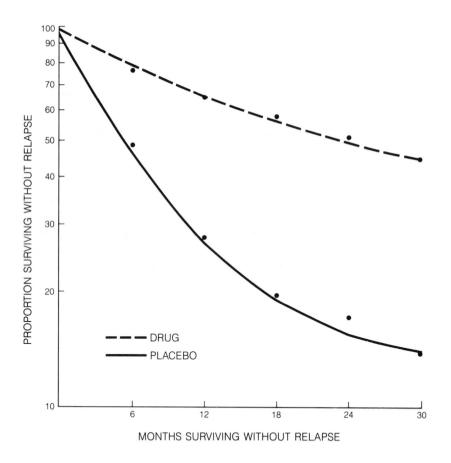

FIGURE 6–2   Proportion of patients remaining well with drug therapy and with placebo. Figure modified from Hogarty, G. E. and Ulrich, R. F. Temporal effects of drug and placebo in delaying relapse in schizophrenic outpatients. *Archives of General Psychiatry* 34:297–301, March 1977. Copyright © 1977 American Medical Association.)

drug patients who relapsed may not have taken their medicine at all or may have decided on their own to reduce their dose. To determine whether these factors contributed to relapses, the same group of researchers compared, over a two-year period, the relapse rates of patients taking oral antipsychotics with the relapse rates of patients receiving antipsychotics by injection. The researchers had accurate drug records of the patients who received injections but had no way of knowing whether the patients receiving oral medication took their drugs as directed. At any rate, there was no significant difference in the relapse rates of the two groups.[19] Failure to take medications does not seem to contribute very much to relapse.

Because antipsychotics can have serious side effects, researchers are looking for ways to minimize their use without jeopardizing recovery. The use of antipsychotics can be decreased in three ways: by decreasing the number of people taking the drugs, by decreasing the dose taken by individual patients, and by decreasing the duration of drug use by individual patients.

Of patients who have had a schizophrenic episode, 20 to 30 percent do not need maintenance antipsychotic therapy to prevent another one. If psychiatrists had a way to identify those people, the number of people taking maintenance antipsychotics could be vastly reduced. Unfortunately, physicians have not succeeded in identifying particular features of patients' history or symptoms that predict continued health in the absence of maintenance drug therapy.[20]

A new pharmacological test holds some promise of predicting who is likely to relapse soon after stopping medication. All the patients participating in studies of this pharmacological test were recovering well and taking antipsychotics. A few weeks later, they were given small doses of amphetamine, a drug that exacerbates schizophrenia. Some patients had no response to amphetamine; others had a transient exacerbation of schizophrenic symptoms. On the average, patients who responded to amphetamine with schizophrenic symptoms relapsed much sooner than did patients who had no response.[21] Patients who do not have schizophrenic symptoms in response to amphetamine may have a lower risk of rapid relapse and may be able to stop antipsychotic therapy if they have access to frequent mental health care. In such cases the psychiatrist can start medication at the first sign of an impending relapse. This test for probability of relapse is still a research tool; it is not available for clinical screening of patients.

Until very recently patients leaving the hospital received doses of antipsychotics that were very similar to the doses they received in the hospital during the acute phase of their illness. During the past few years psychiatrists have been studying the effectiveness of much smaller doses, usually about a quarter of the standard dose.[22] Although there is some disagreement, most studies found that lower doses did not substantially increase the risk of full-blown relapses requiring rehospitalization. But increases in schizophrenic symptoms did occur more often in the low-dose patients. The recurrence of symptoms rarely required hospitalization and could usually be managed by temporary increases in medication. Most important, the low-dose patients functioned better in their families and in the community. They felt better, were less withdrawn, performed better occupationally, and were less anxious. In addition, they suffered fewer side effects of medication. Low-dose maintenance therapy may substantially increase the quality of life for people recovering from schizophrenia. But it can only be used when the patient can be monitored closely so that impending relapses can be treated rapidly with increased medication. Low-dose therapy is not *no*-dose therapy: Patients receiving placebo relapse much more rapidly than do patients receiving low doses of antipsychotics.

While progress is being made in identifying patients who may not need maintenance therapy and in reducing the dosage for those that do, we have no way to determine when, if ever, a patient can safely stop maintenance therapy. The risk of relapse is probably greater in newly discharged patients than in patients who have been in remission for several years. Nevertheless, discontinuing medication always increases the risk of relapse, even for patients who have been healthy while taking antipsychotics for over three years.[23] At present we cannot suggest a limit for the duration of antipsychotic medication.

Because of the risk of side effects with long-term use of antipsychotic drugs, most patients should have the opportunity to find out whether they are among the 25 percent that will remain in remission without maintenance antipsychotics. The following strategy seems reasonable for most patients. First, the patient receives a low dose for six months to a year. If the patient remains healthy, a complete termination of medication might be considered. The patient is closely supervised during all dose adjustments so that medication can be increased if symptoms begin to reappear. Since most patients relapse with no medication complete cessation should be considered only if the patient and the patient's family are willing to take the risk.

LONG-TERM RECOVERY

Can a person who experiences a schizophrenic episode expect to lead a normal life for the next 20 to 30 years? Can drugs help an individual achieve that goal? Answers to these questions require long-term studies that follow drug and placebo patients for many years. Unfortunately, such studies are difficult to conduct. The research psychiatrist usually has no control over treatment after the patient leaves the hospital. Also, many patients disappear over a long period of time, leaving no forwarding address. However, researchers have done follow-up studies, attempting to locate all patients who were diagnosed as having schizophrenia at a given hospital within a particular period and then evaluating the mental health of the people they located. All these studies antedated the *DSM-III*, so the consistency of the original diagnoses is open to question. To judge the mental health of the patients, the researchers usually used information from psychiatric interviews and considered patients' marital status, employment status, and ability to live without institutional help. Not surprisingly, the results of such studies are not in precise agreement, so figures for long-term recovery are only rough estimates. The information we present in this section summarizes the findings of several studies.

The most optimistic estimates are that only about 10 percent of the patients fail to respond to drugs and remain chronically ill inside psychiatric hospitals for much of their lives. Approximately 30 percent experience partial recovery; these people remain outside the hospital and are employed much of the time, but they still need some help in caring for themselves. Approximately 30 percent do not recover completely but are not obviously ill. They can care for themselves, but their occupational level may have decreased, and they may be social isolates. Approximately 30 percent appear to recover completely. These people are almost continuously employed and stay out of institutions; some are married. It is not obvious that they previously suffered from schizophrenia. More pessimistic authorities estimate that as few as 2 to 4 percent enjoy a full and permanent recovery.[24]

Some authorities believe that long-term recovery is more likely for some types of patients than for others. The prospects are best for patients who have had only one episode of schizophrenia, who were relatively old (over 25) when the illness began, and who had the paranoid or catatonic type of schizophrenia. The prospects are less favorable for patients who have had many schizophrenic attacks, who were in their teens when they first became ill, and who had extremely disorganized thought and speech patterns.[25]

Certainly, long-term recovery rates for schizophrenia have improved over the past 50 years.[26] Emil Kraepelin who first described the disease in 1896, said that only 13 percent of patients improved even temporarily and that most of these eventually relapsed.[27] In 1941 rates of recovery were reported to be between 1 and 7 percent.[28] Today's long-term recovery rate of approximately 60 percent represents a dramatic advance, even if many of these recoveries are not complete.

In view of antipsychotics' demonstrable effectiveness over the short term (two years or less), it seems hard to believe that the drugs have not contributed to the increase in long-term recovery rate. However, the contribution of the drugs to long-term recovery cannot be proved rigorously. A rigorous proof requires that patients be randomly assigned to drug and placebo groups and studied for 10 to 30 years. Such studies have not been done and are almost impossible to carry out.

OVERUSE AND MISUSE OF ANTIPSYCHOTICS

Antipsychotics, like other drugs, can be incorrectly and carelessly prescribed. Usually the physician, not the patient, is responsible for overuse and misuse. Here we discuss some of the ways antipsychotics can be misused and how that misuse has led many people to believe that the drugs are nothing more than chemical straitjackets with dangerous side effects.

In *One Flew Over the Cuckoo's Nest*, Ken Kesey illustrates the popular idea that psychiatric drugs make life easier for the hospital staff but do not help the patients.[29] Kesey describes a psychiatric hospital where many of the patients stare at the walls or aimlessly pace back and forth. The more alert patients argue pointlessly over a card game. Their day is marked primarily by the line-up for medication, the perpetuator of their minimal and meaningless activity.

Unfortunately, Kesey's portrayal contains a grain of truth. Many state hospitals are grossly understaffed. Drugs are dispensed mechanically, without sufficient regard for accurate diagnosis and without thorough evaluation of their effectiveness for each individual. There is rarely time to evaluate patients individually to determine the best drug therapy for each. In addition, the ward staff may not be adequately trained to recognize overdose and side effects. Staff members are responsible for running the hospital in an orderly manner, and they are concerned about keeping the patients under control; they constantly fear that a patient will break into psychotically violent or destructive behavior. Under these conditions, it is hardly surprising that the staff may take comfort in overly sedated patients.

When patients receive the proper dosages of antipsychotics, they remain reasonably alert. Although the drugs have a pronounced sedative action during the first few days of treatment, after a week or so they produce antipsychotic effects without sedation. In fact, psychotic symptoms usually begin to disappear just as the sedative effects begin to wear off. At this point, the drugs appear to normalize activity levels: Agitated patients may appear tranquilized, and stuporous catatonic or withdrawn patients become more active and sociable. The drugs decrease abnormally high activity and increase abnormally low activity.[30]

In the United States about 20 different drugs are used to treat schizophrenia. They vary in their antipsychotic and their sedative potency. Their potency against psychotic symptoms does not always correspond to their potency as sedatives. In fact, some of the drugs most effective in relieving psychotic symptoms are the least effective as sedatives.[31] It is also worth pointing out that sedation, in itself, is not antipsychotic. Barbiturates and other sleeping pills are of little use in controlling psychotic symptoms.

It is unfortunate, we think, that the antipsychotic drugs are often referred to as major tranquilizers. This description probably originated early in the development of antipsychotics, when Laborit used chlorpromazine to calm surgical patients and to improve surgical anesthesia. Moreover, Delay and Deniker's first clinical use was to calm manic patients. Before the antipsychotic properties of the phenothiazines were well understood, the term *major tranquilizer* may have seemed appropriate, but it is inaccurate.

Patients and their relatives may complain that antipsychotic medication makes people emotionally unresponsive or reduces drive and energy. Mark Vonnegut espouses this view about Thorazine, while admitting that the drug had its uses. He feels that the drug deprived him of his ability to care or to make judgments: "While I very likely owe my life to Thorazine, I doubt if I will ever develop much affection for it or similar tranquilizers. . . . I knew that Dostoyevsky was more interesting than comic books, or, more accurately, I remembered that he had been. I cared about what happened at the farm [a communal farm that Vonnegut had founded], but it was more remembering caring than really caring." [32]

Thorazine might have produced Vonnegut's emotional wasteland. On the other hand, flat affect, a classic symptom of schizophrenia, might have been responsible for his inability to distinguish nuances of emotions. In such situations it is difficult to know whether the emotions had been dulled by Thorazine or by the underlying disease, only partially relieved by the drugs.

Patients' self-reports do not provide good evidence that a drug works. Often patients report that placebos are effective. If people with schizophrenia take snake oil and then get better, they may conclude that snake oil cured schizophrenia. Furthermore, patients may feel that a drug has cured their disease merely because it makes them feel better. Alcohol has this capacity, but it has no genuine therapeutic benefit. In fact, many of the patent medicines popular in this country in the nineteenth century owed their popularity to their high alcohol content.

To reject a treatment because of alleged side effects can be a mistake. In some patients, the alleged side effects may really be exacerbations of the illness and not caused by the drug at all. In other patients, the benefits may compensate for the side effects. For example, we think relief from incapacitating psychotic symptoms compensates for a few weeks of moderate sedation.

Antipsychotics are overused if a physician continues to prescribe them even though they are no longer useful. One situation that encourages this kind of overuse is failure of drug treatment. The physician may continue to prescribe an antipsychotic merely because that is his or her usual policy, even when the patient shows no signs of improvement. This practice is particularly likely to occur in an understaffed state hospital. Sometimes medication is continued because the patient has a history of violence or extreme excitement. Antipsychotics are usually fully effective in three to six weeks. A patient who fails to improve after six months of treatment is probably not going to improve in twelve. The only consequence of continued medication is an increased risk of side effects.

Theoretically, overuse can also occur when long-term antipsychotic treatment is prescribed for the rare patients who will recover with brief drug treatment or with none at all. In practice, this sort of overuse is inevitable because psychiatrists cannot identify these patients except by observing the consequences of withholding drugs.

Even at the risk of receiving unnecessary prescriptions, we think that almost all schizophrenia patients should receive antipsychotics early in their hospital stay. The exceptions would be those patients who show immediate signs of rapid recovery. We make this recommendation because very few patients will recover without drugs, and there are risks in allowing a person to remain in a psychotic state. After the symptoms are relieved, most patients should receive maintenance antipsychotics, and reduced dosages should be tried when adequate supervision makes this feasible.[33]

Antipsychotics are misused, as opposed to overused, when they are prescribed in the absence of an appropriate diagnosis. Schizophrenia is the most common indication for antipsychotic drugs, but there are others. For example, a short course of antipsychotic therapy is often effective for a manic patient who is severely agitated or for a depressed patient with psychotic symptoms. In the early 1960s chlorpromazine was occasionally misused as a treatment for morning sickness in pregnancy, a clearly inappropriate use, especially since there was no evidence that the drug was safe for the unborn baby. Perhaps because of their designation as tranquilizers, antipsychotics have also been prescribed for all sorts of psychiatric problems involving excessive agitation, including schizophrenia, mania, depression, anxiety, and insomnia. However, antipsychotics are not the safest or most effective treatment for anxiety, insomnia, or most types of depression. For these illnesses, other drugs or psychotherapy should be tried before resorting to antipsychotics.[34] Antipsychotics have also been used to calm violent or disruptive patients in nursing homes and in facilities for the mentally retarded. Whether this is an appropriate use is a complex question whose answer depends on many variables, including how unmanageable the behavior is and what alternatives are available.

THE EFFECTS OF PSYCHOTHERAPY

If the environment contributes to the genesis of schizophrenia, a well-chosen environmental change might reverse the disease process. Psychotherapy provides the traditional change in the environment. Vonnegut elegantly explains the preconception that therapy for schizophrenia should be verbal: "It's such a poetic affliction from inside and out, it's not hard to see how people have assumed that schizophrenia must have poetic causes and that any therapy would have to be poetic as well." [35]

Unfortunately, understanding and changing the environment may not reverse the damage it causes. When a skier falls on an icy patch of snow and breaks a leg, the damage is done. No lesson in ski safety can undo it; no change in the snow conditions will put the leg in a cast; no understanding of the forces that break bones will cause them to heal any faster. Similarly, there is no reason to assume that, just because schizophrenia is partially caused by environmental factors, psychological treatment will help the patient with schizophrenia. Neither is there any reason to assume that understanding schizophrenic thinking will lead to a curative change in the brain. Vonnegut provides another apt analogy: "People suffering from high fevers also sometimes suffer from hallucinations and delirious thinking, but I have yet to hear anyone suggest that understanding the content of such delirium could bring down the fever." [36]

Rather than jumping to the conclusion that psychotherapy can help the schizophrenia patient, we must look at the evidence. Two questions should be considered separately. First, is psychotherapy alone an effective treatment? Second, is psychotherapy plus drug therapy more effective than drug therapy alone? Attempts to answer these questions are fraught with difficulties.

One difficulty is that the psychotherapeutic techniques used to treat schizophrenia (in contrast to those used in depression, described in Chapter 13) are not precisely specified. Three hundred mg of chlorpromazine is 300 mg of chlorpromazine, no matter who hands out the pill, but psychotherapy changes with the psychotherapist. If psychotherapy fails, its ineffectiveness can be attributed to the inadequacy of the particular therapist. However, to be practical, a treatment must be useful when delivered by any qualified therapist. A patient cannot evaluate the effectiveness of every potential practitioner before selecting one to administer psychotherapeutic treatment.

Another difficulty in studying the effectiveness of psychotherapy is that some patients get better without any treatment at all. Novels, occasional case histories, and anecdotes do not provide evidence that psychotherapy (or any other treatment, for that matter) works. Though a patient might have recovered without any treatment, recovery is gratuitously credited to the treatment in progress. Like any other medical treatment, psychotherapy can be evaluated only by comparing the progress of patients receiving psychotherapy with the progress of similar patients receiving other treatments or no treatment at all. Each group of patients must have the same symptoms, diagnosis, and prognosis. This caveat may seem obvious, but it is not always heeded, even in studies that have been published in respected psychiatric journals. For example, in an article published in the *American Journal of Psychiatry* the recovery of two groups of patients is compared. One group received psychoanalytically oriented psychotherapy and milieu therapy but minimal drug therapy, while the other group, in a different hospital, received only drug therapy. The patients receiving the psychological treatment recovered somewhat faster and were somewhat better adjusted two years after leaving the hospital. So far this sounds like substantial evidence for the effectiveness of psychotherapy. But a careful reading of the article reveals that only patients who were well-adjusted prior to their illness were selected for psychological treatment. Many psychiatrists think that these are just the patients who are most likely to recover and have the best post-illness adjustment, regardless of treatment. The authors of the article admit that their work was not designed to compare drug and psychological treatment; nevertheless, they imply that they are presenting evidence for the effectiveness of psychological treatment.

While admitting the flaws in their research plan, the authors conclude that their "observations in a biologically oriented clinical research program employing psychosocial techniques argue for the feasibility of treating acute schizophrenic patients with minimal use of medication. The experience can be gratifying for patients and staff. Patients in such a program have not fared poorly compared with patients treated in more conventional settings." [37]

We disagree with their conclusions. Comparing the rapid recovery of patients with good prognoses and the slower recovery of patients with average prognoses cannot provide any information about treatment effectiveness. It is like comparing recovery from a cold without treatment and recovery from pneumonia with penicillin treatment and then arguing that the results demonstrate the feasibility of using nondrug techniques in the treatment of respiratory infections, and concluding that the experience can be gratifying for patients and physicians.

A third difficulty in evaluating the effectiveness of psychotherapy is that, in many studies, the people evaluating the recoveries are the therapists themselves — far from the ideal observers. Psychotherapy requires hard work and emotional investment, and precisely because they have worked so hard, psychotherapists cannot give an unbiased evaluation of the effectiveness of their own work.

The most thorough comparison of pharmacological and psychological treatments was performed by Philip R. A. May, a psychiatrist at the University of California, Los Angeles. He studied five treatments for schizophrenia: antipsychotics, milieu therapy, individual insight-oriented psychotherapy, a combination of antipsychotics and individual psychotherapy, and electroconvulsive therapy. (We do not discuss electroconvulsive therapy for schizophrenia because it is now rarely used for this diagnosis.) In milieu therapy, patients learned occupational skills and improved social competence through recreational activities and group meetings; patients' illnesses were not treated on individual bases. In insight-oriented psychotherapy, patients spent several hours each week with their therapists, investigating the psychological origins of the illness and the problems to be faced outside the hospital. The 228 schizophrenia patients in May's study were randomly assigned to one of the five treatments. Their progress was rated in three ways: evaluation by doctors and nurses, performance on a battery of standardized tests, and length of hospitalization. The evaluation teams did not deliver treatment and were asked not to try to find out what kind of treatment a patient received. The evaluation results were straightforward: Psychotherapy and milieu therapy were about equally ineffective when compared to drug therapy, which was quite effective (Figure 6–3).[38]

Philip R. A. May, A. Hussain Tuma, and Wilfrid J. Dixon studied these same patients two to five years later to find out whether drug therapy or psychotherapy had long-term advantages or disadvantages. (After patients left the hospital, drug treatment was no longer controlled by the researchers, but the patients' physicians could prescribe drugs and/or psychotherapy as needed.) The drug patients were rehospitalized less often than the psychotherapy or milieu patients and spent the fewest days in the hospital during the two to five years following their initial release. With these facts, the authors

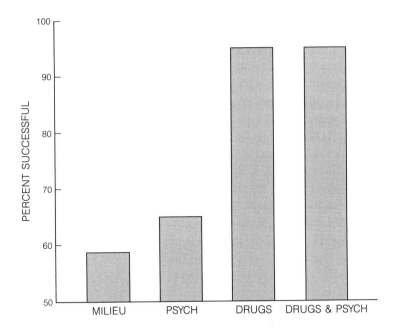

FIGURE 6–3 Percent of patients treated successfully with each of four treatment methods. Successful treatment was defined as release from the hospital within one year. Milieu: milieu therapy. Psych: psychotherapy. Drugs: antipsychotic drug therapy. Drugs and psych: both antipsychotic drug therapy and psychotherapy. Data from P.R.A. May, *Treatment of Schizophrenia* (New York: Science House, 1968).

could argue against the notion that antipsychotics create "revolving door" mental patients, patients who are released into the community only to be rehospitalized in a few weeks or months.[39]

Certainly, many patients relapse, but patients treated with antipsychotic drugs relapse less frequently than do patients treated with individual psychotherapy or milieu therapy. We do not know the reason for this difference in relapse rates. Perhaps increasing the amount of time that the brain remains in a schizophrenic state increases the likelihood that it will return to that state. If that is the case, rapid relief of symptoms may be important.

Critics of May's study argued that his therapists—psychiatric residents—were too inexperienced to provide adequate psychotherapy for schizophrenia patients. But Milton Greenblatt, a professor of psychiatry at UCLA, conducted a similar study using more experienced psychiatrists and obtained essentially the same result: Psychotherapy alone produced little change, whereas drugs produced obvious improvement.[40]

Nowhere in the massive literature on schizophrenia is there clear evidence that psychotherapy or milieu therapy alone is effective in decreasing schizophrenic symptoms.[41] Those studies reporting positive results have methodological errors: They lack control groups, or the researchers gave psychotherapy only to patients with good prognoses for spontaneous recovery. Granted, a behavioral or psychotherapeutic technique effective for schizophrenia may yet be developed; at present, however, no psychological treatment for schizophrenia has been proved effective. Vonnegut sums it up: "The poets in the business gave little hope and huge bills."[42]

When they compared the patients receiving both drugs and psychotherapy with those receiving only drugs, May's team found no difference between the two groups (Figure 6–3). As long as the patient has blatant symptoms of thought disorder, adding psychotherapy to drug therapy accomplishes nothing.[43] This result is obtained whether effectiveness is measured by doctors' and nurses' ratings of patient improvement or by length of hospital stay. In fact, psychotherapy slightly increases the amount of time the patient spends in the hospital. Perhaps, as May explained, therapists become attached to their patients and do not want them to be discharged.

It is hardly surprising that a schizophrenia patient who is catatonic, disorganized, mute, withdrawn, or paranoid does not benefit very much from psychotherapy, since psychotherapy requires the patient to have reasonably normal thought processes. Therefore, only after antipsychotics have restored some degree of rationality is it appropriate to ask whether psychotherapy helps.

That question is important because maintenance therapy with antipsychotic drugs alone decreases the frequency of relapses but cannot prevent them. During the first year, 30 to 40 percent of recovering schizophrenia patients relapse, even if they receive their medication by injection.[44] Can psychotherapy decrease this relapse rate, and if so, what kind of psychotherapy is most effective? Psychiatrists have compared several types of psychotherapy, including insight-oriented psychotherapy, social skills training, and family therapy. Insight-oriented psychotherapy was described earlier. In social skills training the patient learns skills for getting along with others. Family therapy instructs family members about schizophrenia, teaches them strategies for managing more effectively, and helps them to avoid expressing intense emotional responses to the patient.

We found only one study using insight-oriented psychotherapy. It compared insight-oriented therapy with training in social skills and management of other real-life problems. The difference between the two groups was not large, but the group receiving training in real-life problems did somewhat better. This group spent somewhat less time in the hospital, presumably because its members had fewer relapses. This group also did better occupationally.[45] The study is difficult to interpret, however, because it did not include a no-treatment control group, so we cannot tell whether both treatments were effective or neither was.

Both family therapy and social skills training are effective when compared with nonspecific supportive therapy.[46] A combination of family therapy and social skills training appears to be remarkably effective. In a study by Gerald Hogarty and colleagues at the University of Pittsburgh, not a single one of the 20 patients receiving both treatments relapsed during the first year (Figure 6–4). The combined effectiveness of the two treatments is not surprising. Social skills training teaches the patient to get along with the family. Family therapy teaches the family to get along with the patient. Both together ought to be better than either one alone. Hogarty and his colleagues caution, however, that the combined treatments have delayed relapse but not prevented relapse. As the researchers continue to follow these patients, relapses continue to occur.

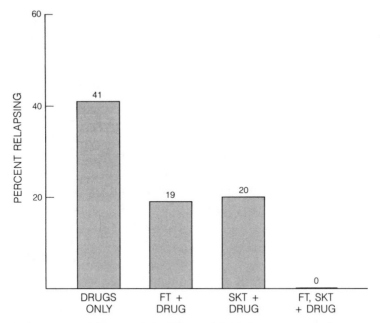

FIGURE 6-4 Comparison of the effects of four treatments on relapse rate in schizophrenia. Drug only: antipsychotic drug. FT and drug: family therapy and antipsychotic drug. SKT and drug: social skills training and antipsychotic drug. FT, SKT, and drug: family therapy, social skills training, and antipsychotic drug. (Data from G. W. Hogarty et al., "Family Psychoeducation, Social Skills Training, and Maintenance Chemotherapy in the Aftercare Treatment of Schizophrenia. I. One-Year Effects of a Controlled Study on Relapse and Expressed Emotion. *Archives of General Psychiatry* 43:633–642, 1986.)

The evidence that teaching social skills decreases relapse rates is convincing. We do not know why people recovering from schizophrenia have poor social and life management skills. Maybe people who are susceptible to schizophrenia also lack such skills. Maybe these skills decrease as a result of preoccupation with voices and delusions. Maybe these skills decrease because of the way other people respond to schizophrenic behavior. Teaching the family how to manage the patient also helps, but, again, we do not know why. Perhaps the patient is better able to keep in touch with reality if reality does not consist of frequent criticism.

Family therapy and social skill therapy are clearly effective. In view of the financial cost of psychotherapy, we believe that psychotherapy for schizophrenia or any other condition should include only those treatments known to be effective.

7

HOW ANTIPSYCHOTIC DRUGS WORK

—

A ntipsychotic drugs are not an ideal treatment for schizo-phrenia. They do not work for every patient. They have serious side effects. They control symptoms but are not a cure: Most patients relapse within a year or two of ceasing to take their medication. However, antipsychotics are the best available treatment for schizophrenia. By studying their effects on the brain, we may be able to learn why they work as well as they do, why they do not work better, and how we might make improved anti-psychotics.

After an overview of the effects of antipsychotics on dopamine receptors, we present evidence in this chapter that antipsychotic drugs block these receptors. We then describe two types of evidence that blocking dopamine receptors is required for the therapeutic effect of antipsychotics. One is the relationship between antipsychotic potency and potency in blocking dopamine receptors. The other is the effect of excessive activation of dopamine receptors. In the next sections we describe some of the effects of this blockade on brain cells. Finally, we discuss the hypothesis that schizophrenic brains have abnormal dopamine receptors.

OVERVIEW OF THE EFFECT OF ANTIPSYCHOTIC DRUGS ON NERVE CELLS

Most knowledge about the biology of schizophrenia has come from investigations of the effects of antipsychotic drugs on nerve cells. Scientists understand only the first few steps in the series of events between the time when antipsychotic drugs reach the brain and the time when the patient's symptoms begin to remit. But these first few steps are important because they suggest hypotheses about how the drugs eventually change behavior.

The first action of antipsychotic drugs on the brain is the blockade of dopamine receptors.[1] As shown in Chapter 2, receptors are protein molecules embedded in the membrane. Their function is to attach, or bind, to molecules of transmitter that are secreted by presynaptic nerve cells. The binding of a transmitter to its postsynaptic receptors triggers changes in impulse rate and metabolic activity in postsynaptic nerve cells. At most dopamine synapses dopamine is inhibitory; that is, it decreases impulse rate. Dopamine receptors are not confined to postsynaptic cells, however. Presynaptic cells, that is, the cells releasing dopamine, also have dopamine receptors that can be blocked by antipsychotics.[2] When activated by dopamine, these receptors suppress the release and synthesis of dopamine. Antipsychotic drugs bind to both presynaptic and postsynaptic receptors for dopamine.[3] While the drug molecule is bound to a receptor, the dopamine secreted by the presynaptic cell cannot bind to that receptor. The drug molecule actually gets in the way and blocks the access of dopamine. A blocked postsynaptic receptor cannot contribute to either inhibition of nerve impulses or alterations in the metabolic activity of the cell. A single synapse, of course, has many receptor molecules. If all of them are blocked, transmission will fail completely, and all biochemical effects will be prevented. If only some receptors are blocked, the effects of dopamine will be decreased, but they will not disappear completely.

EVIDENCE THAT ANTIPSYCHOTIC DRUGS BLOCK DOPAMINE RECEPTORS

Certain regions of the brain are particularly rich in dopamine synapses. These regions contain the axon terminals of cells that produce dopamine. Dopamine receptors abound on these presynaptic terminals and on the postsynaptic membranes they contact.

Scientists can measure in the rat brain the number of receptors available to the transmitter. They remove cells from a particular region of a brain, separate them from one another, and place them in a test tube. Separation ensures that all the receptors are exposed to the fluid in the test tube. A large amount of radioactive dopamine is then added to the fluid. Some of this dopamine binds to receptors on the cells' membranes, and some remains in the fluid. After gently washing out the unbound radioactive dopamine, scientists can determine the amount that is bound to the membranes by using an instrument designed to measure radioactivity. The number of molecules bound depends on the number of cells in the test tube and the part of the brain that the cells were taken from. The experiment is then repeated, but this time a radioactive antipsychotic is used rather than radioactive dopamine. The antipsychotic also binds to the cell membranes.

This experiment shows that dopamine and the antipsychotic bind to the same types of *cells*, but it does not show that they bind to the same *receptors*. Perhaps the cells in the test tube have two different types of receptors: one type that binds dopamine, and another that binds the antipsychotic. Perhaps either the dopamine or the antipsychotic attaches to all membranes regardless of whether the membranes contain specific receptors for any transmitter. To disprove these hypotheses, biochemists have shown that dopamine and antipsychotics compete for the same receptors, by comparing the amount of radioactive dopamine bound when only dopamine is added to the cells with the amount bound when nonradioactive antipsychotic is also added. When antipsychotic is present, less dopamine binds. This means that antipsychotic is occupying some receptors that would otherwise be available for dopamine. Dopamine and the drug compete for the same receptors (Figure 7–1).[4]

If antipsychotics block dopamine receptors, they should prevent the effects of dopamine on the impulse activity of nerve cells. This prediction has been tested by applying both dopamine and antipsychotic drugs to living nerve cells. Chemicals are applied through a

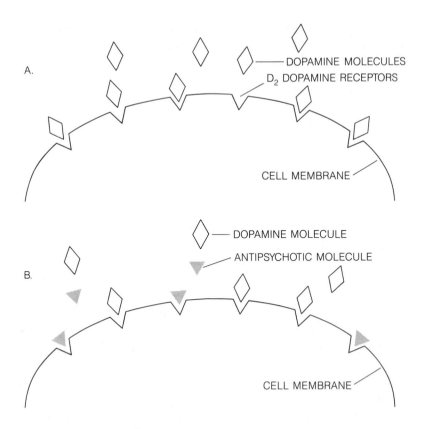

FIGURE 7–1 A. Nerve cell membrane with dopamine receptors. Only dopamine is present in the immediate vicinity of the cell. Most receptors are occupied by dopamine. B. Both dopamine and antipsychotic are present in the immediate vicinity of the cell. Some receptors are occupied by antipsychotic; fewer are occupied by dopamine.

tiny glass tube to a living nerve cell in the rat brain. At the same time, microelectrodes record the electrical response of the cell. Many cells with dopamine receptors emit nerve impulses spontaneously at a fairly steady rate in the absence of dopamine. Since dopamine is inhibitory, when it is applied to one of these cells, the rate of nerve impulses decreases. However, if an antipsychotic drug is applied along with dopamine, the drug prevents the response to dopamine; the rate of impulses does not decrease.[5] The drug alters the cell's capacity to respond to input from presynaptic cells releasing dopamine and hence alters its capacity to transmit information to other nerve cells.

THE BLOCKADE OF DOPAMINE RECEPTORS AND ANTIPSYCHOTIC POTENCY

Although we have presented evidence that antipsychotic drugs are antagonists at dopamine receptors, we still cannot assume that blocking dopamine receptors is the first step in relieving the symptoms of schizophrenia. The drugs may have other effects on nerve cells that are still unknown. One of these unknown effects may be responsible for alleviating schizophrenic symptoms.

The wide variety of antipsychotic drugs on the market provides a tool for determining the relation between receptor blockade and relief of schizophrenic symptoms. The drugs vary widely in clinical potency; that is, they vary in the size of the dose required to alleviate schizophrenic symptoms. (The larger the dose required, the less potent the drug.) However, less potent drugs are not necessarily inferior to more potent ones. Considerations governing choice of drug for a particular patient are discussed in the next chapter. The drugs also vary widely in their receptor-blocking ability. If blockade of dopamine receptors is required for therapeutic effectiveness, the drugs that are most potent in the psychiatric clinic should be the best dopamine receptor blockers. Similarly, the drugs that are least potent clinically should be the poorest dopamine receptor blockers. On the whole, these predictions are valid.[6]

Surprisingly, researchers can better predict clinical potency by a drug's ability to displace haloperidol, a potent antipsychotic drug, from dopamine receptors than by its ability to displace dopamine from these same receptors. To measure haloperidol displacement, the researcher first measures the amount of radioactive haloperidol that binds to calf nerve cells dispersed in a test tube. He then repeats the experiment but now adds the test drug as well as radioactive haloperidol to the test tube. If the test drug binds to dopamine receptors, it will displace some of the radioactive haloperidol from the receptors, decreasing the amount of haloperidol already bound. Many antipsychotic drugs have been tested in this way. The graph in Figure 7–2 shows the relationship between drugs' clinical potency and their ability to compete with haloperidol for receptors. If a drug's ability to block haloperidol binding is weak, its clinical potency is low. If a drug's ability to block haloperidol binding is powerful, its clinical potency is high.[7]

Why should displacement of haloperidol, a drug, be a better predictor of antipsychotic efficacy than the ability to displace dopa-

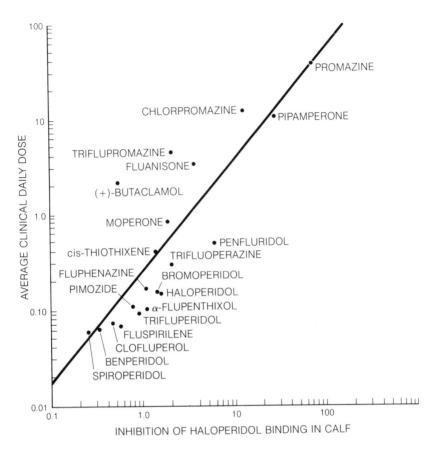

FIGURE 7-2 Correlation between the ability of antipsychotic drugs to decrease haloperidol binding and their clinical potency. (From S. H. Snyder, D. R. Burt, and I. Creese, "The Dopamine Receptor of Mammalian Brain: Direct Demonstration of Binding to Agonist and Antagonist Sites." In *Neurotransmitters, Hormones, and Receptors: Novel Approaches*, edited by A. J. Ferendelli, B. S. McEwen, and S. H. Snyder. Bethesda, Md,: Society for Neuroscience, 1976.)

mine, the natural transmitter? The puzzle was solved when scientists found that all dopamine receptors are not the same. There are two subtypes, called D1 and D2.[8] Dopamine binds to both of these subtypes. If it did not, both subtypes would not be dopamine receptors. Some antipsychotics also bind to both D1 and D2 receptors. But others, like haloperidol, bind only to D2 receptors. Since antipsychotics do not bind to D1 receptors, the blockade of D2, but not of

D1, receptors is probably related to antipsychotic potency. Therefore, the ability to displace haloperidol, which binds only to relevant
(D2) receptors, should be better related to clinical potency than the
ability to displace dopamine, which binds to both relevant (D2) and
irrelevant (D1) receptors.

THE EFFECTS OF EXCESSIVE ACTIVATION OF DOPAMINE SYNAPSES

If blocking dopamine receptors alleviates schizophrenia, then a drug
that activates dopamine receptors excessively should produce symptoms of schizophrenia. At the very least, the drug should exacerbate
schizophrenic symptoms in people who already suffer from the disease. It might even cause schizophrenia-like symptoms to appear in
healthy people. In addition, the schizophrenia-like symptoms produced by such a drug should be reversed by treatment with antipsychotics like chlorpromazine and haloperidol. These suppositions can
be tested by using amphetamine, a drug that increases the activity at
dopamine synapses in two different ways: First, it causes the release
of dopamine from the presynaptic terminal; second, it blocks dopamine reuptake into the presynaptic terminal, increasing the amount
in the synaptic cleft.[9]

Ingestion of high doses of amphetamine (50 to 500 mg over 24
hours) can induce a psychosis that can easily be mistaken for schizophrenia, even by an experienced psychiatrist. Burton Angrist and
Abraham Sudilovsky described a volunteer who had no symptoms of
schizophrenia before taking amphetamine. After taking the drug, the
volunteer proclaimed that he had become a "prophet" who was
being addressed directly by God. He stated: "In my human form he
might let me act human for the rest must still wonder at my actions
which make them doubt my having been used to enlighten. Every
thought that stops me from accepting all knowledge more than man
has ever known."[10] Another example is provided by D. S. Janowsky
and his colleagues at Vanderbilt University. They describe a patient
who entered the hospital claiming that spirits rose out of people's
heads and spoke to him. After treatment with antipsychotics, he
admitted that his talk about spirits had been "crazy talk," but within
one minute of an amphetamine injection, he again claimed that the

spirits were rising out of the interviewer's head.[11] It is hard to imagine more typical examples of schizophrenic behavior.

People who abuse amphetamine sometimes bring such a psychosis upon themselves. Jessica, a 41-year-old divorced pharmacist, took advantage of her easy access to amphetamine, using the drug to counteract lethargy and boredom. Eventually she became addicted. Jessica had always been friendly and open, but now she became hostile and suspicious. She accused her son of spying on her and hiring detectives to follow her. One day she told her son that the announcer on the evening news had sent coded messages to her brain that would enable her to outwit the detectives. At first, Jessica's son was irritated at her suspiciousness. Later, he became angry. Finally, he realized that his mother was seriously ill. Like most people suddenly confronted with serious mental illness, he had no idea what might be wrong or how to get help. He knew nothing of her amphetamine abuse.

It took much wheedling to get Jessica to a psychiatrist, and once she did meet with him, she successfully concealed her drug use. The psychiatrist thought she had schizophrenia and needed antipsychotic therapy, but Jessica refused to enter the hospital. Because initiating antipsychotic therapy on outpatients is risky, the psychiatrist could not offer her much help. Several days later, Jessica walked into a camera store and smashed a movie camera that she believed had been spying on her from the window. She was then hospitalized on a two-physician certificate. (In many states, a person can be involuntarily committed to a psychiatric hospital for a few days if two physicians certify that the person is a danger to him- or herself or others or cannot care for him- or herself.) In the hospital Jessica had no access to amphetamine and was given antipsychotics. Her symptoms cleared up unusually fast. When medication was removed, she did not relapse. As soon as Jessica stopped taking amphetamine, she stopped suffering from apparent schizophrenia. As we discussed in Chapter 4, the proper diagnosis of schizophrenia requires that the psychiatrist rule out the possibility that the symptoms are caused by drug abuse. Amphetamine and cocaine, which is very similar to amphetamine, are the possible culprits in cases of apparent schizophrenia. In Jessica's case, the psychiatrist should have immediately suspected drug abuse because Jessica had no history of schizophrenia, and the disease seldom develops for the first time in a person Jessica's age.

The effects of amphetamine are specific to schizophrenia. A small dose can exacerbate symptoms in patients who are suffering from this disorder but does not increase the symptoms of patients with other psychiatric diseases, such as affective disorders.[12] Conversely, the ability of drugs to exacerbate schizophrenia is specific to amphetamine. Other psychoactive drugs do not exacerbate schizophrenia. The hallucinations produced by LSD are clearly different from those in naturally occurring schizophrenia or in the schizophrenia-like syndrome produced by amphetamine.[13]

If amphetamine psychosis results from the overactivation of dopamine receptors, amphetamine-induced symptoms, like Jessica's, should be reversed by antipsychotic drugs, and, indeed, they are: the treatment is quite specific to antipsychotics. Sedatives, such as barbiturates, do not alleviate psychotic symptoms; they merely sedate the patient.[14] Since amphetamine and antipsychotic drugs pose some risks, researchers do not experiment on humans by inducing amphetamine psychosis and then examining the potency of various antipsychotic drugs in alleviating it. They can, however, experiment on rats. Rats and humans treated with amphetamine exhibit some similar symptoms. People who abuse amphetamine frequently engage in ritualistic, stereotyped behavior. For example, they may spend long hours on tasks that require repetitive small movements like disassembling the electronic components of radios. Not surprisingly, reassembly requires more concentration than they can muster. Rats given high doses of amphetamine develop a similar syndrome called stereotypy. They pace back and forth, sniffing the corners of their cages; they chew repetitively on the bars. Predictably, the antipsychotic drugs that are most potent in reversing the effects of amphetamine in rats are those that bind best to D2 receptors.[15] Recall that the antipsychotics most potent in treating schizophrenia in humans are also those that bind best to D2 receptors. This finding suggests that similar abnormalities might be present in the brain of a schizophrenia patient and in the brain of an amphetamine abuser. Understanding more about how amphetamine affects brain cells might yield new hypotheses about the biochemical defects in the schizophrenic brain.

L-Dopa is another drug known to cause schizophrenia-like symptoms. Like amphetamine, it increases dopamine transmission. L-Dopa is normally present in the body and is used in the synthesis of dopamine. Given large amounts of L-Dopa, the brain makes abnormally large amounts of dopamine. The amount of dopamine released from presynaptic terminals in the brain will also be abnormally high. L-Dopa is used to treat Parkinson's disease, a type of palsy caused by deficient dopamine transmission. Occasionally, patients with Parkinson's disease who are treated with this drug develop symptoms of schizophrenia as side effects. Finally, when the drug has been given experimentally to schizophrenia patients, their symptoms have gotten worse.[16] These facts about L-Dopa support the conclusion that antipsychotic drugs are effective in the treatment of schizophrenia because they can block transmission at dopamine synapses.

THE BRAIN'S RESPONSE TO RECEPTOR BLOCKADE

The conclusion that antipsychotic drugs act by blocking dopamine receptors has led researchers to form the dopamine hypothesis of schizophrenia, which simply states that schizophrenia is *caused by* abnormalities at dopamine synapses. Obviously, however, relief from the symptoms of schizophrenia involves more than changes at dopamine synapses. Cells directly affected by antipsychotic drugs transmit altered messages to other cells; the changes in dopamine synapses spread, domino fashion, throughout the brain. Unfortunately, neuroscientists are ignorant about where the dominoes fall. They do not yet understand the sequences of synaptic events that produce even the simplest normal behaviors, much less behaviors as complex as speech. Until they understand how the normal brain can organize thoughts and execute speech, they probably will not be able to understand how the schizophrenic brain produces delusional and disorganized thought and speech or how blocking dopamine receptors reorganizes thought and speech. If scientists have only the barest outline of how the brain produces normal posture or movement, how can they understand catatonia? If they do not know which synapses fire in which order when we laugh or cry, how can they understand the synaptic changes underlying flat affect? One thing neuroscientists are sure of, though, is that none of these complex, distinctly human behaviors can be produced by just one or even a few types of synapses working alone. Each behavior requires nerve circuits involving many different types of synapses.

EVENTS THAT FOLLOW THE BLOCKADE OF DOPAMINE RECEPTORS

While scientists cannot follow the chain of drug-induced events from blockade of dopamine receptors to the relief of schizophrenic thought, emotion, and speech, they do understand two changes that follow closely from the blockage of dopamine receptors. One of these changes may be important in understanding why several weeks often elapse between the initiation of antipsychotic therapy and the decrease in symptoms. The other may be important in understanding one of the most serious side effects of antipsychotic drugs.

Changes in Impulse and Metabolic Activity of Dopamine Cells

Antipsychotic drugs block dopamine receptors almost immediately, but often two to three weeks elapse before the symptoms of schizophrenia are substantially improved. Studies of the biochemical and electrical responses to antipsychotic drugs have suggested a solution to this puzzle. The basic idea is that during the first stage of treatment with antipsychotics, the drugs increase the firing of dopaminergic cells, that is, cells that release dopamine. But the cells cannot maintain this increased activity for long. A subsequent large decrease in activity is the basis for the relief of schizophrenic symptoms.

To imagine how this might happen, recall that there are dopamine receptors both on the postsynaptic cells and on the presynaptic dopamine-releasing cells. The receptors on the presynaptic cells are called autoreceptors and are of the D2 type that is responsive to antipsychotics.[17] These autoreceptors detect the availability of dopamine in the synaptic cleft. When antipsychotics block the autoreceptors, the autoreceptors signal that there is little dopamine in the cleft, and this increases the rate of firing of dopaminergic cells. After a few weeks of this accelerated activity, the majority of dopamine cells suffer "depolarization block": The initial frantic activity alters the state of the cell membrane so that it can no longer continue to fire (Figure 7–3). Depolarization block takes about three weeks to develop, just about the time it takes for antipsychotic drugs to alleviate schizophrenic symptoms in humans.[18] This suggests that it is a decrease in activity at dopaminergic synapses that alleviates the symptoms.

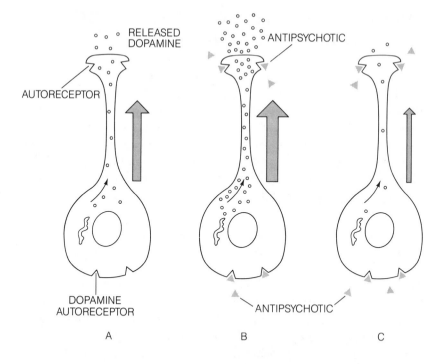

FIGURE 7–3 Diagram of a nerve cell before (A), immediately after (B), and three weeks after (C) institution of treatment with an antipsychotic. Initially the antipsychotic increases impulse traffic and synthesis and release of dopamine. Three weeks later depolarization block has decreased all three. The amount of impulse traffic is indicated by the thickness of the arrow pointing in the direction of the nerve impulses.

Antipsychotics do not modify the activity of dopamine cells sending their axons to the prefrontal cortex. At first this seems surprising because regional blood flow and PET scan studies indicate that schizophrenia patients have abnormal activity in the prefrontal cortex. But there are complex, indirect connections between the frontal lobe and the caudate nucleus, a component of the basal ganglia. Therefore, depolarization block in cells projecting to the caudate may cause changes in the prefrontal cortex (Figure 7–4).

Changes in dopamine synthesis are consistent with changes in impulse activity.[19] Dopamine synthesis is controlled both by the amount of dopamine in the cleft and by the concentration of dopamine in the nerve cells. The immediate response to antipsychotics is an increase in the rate of dopamine synthesis because the blockade of autoreceptors signals that there is little dopamine in the synaptic

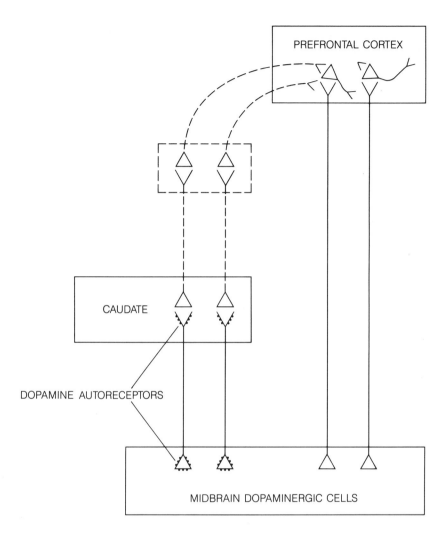

FIGURE 7–4 Simplified block diagram of connections of midbrain dopaminergic cells. Some of these cells connect to the caudate nucleus, others to the prefrontal cortex, but only the cells connecting to the caudate have autoreceptors. Caudate cells connect indirectly to the prefrontal cortex. This indirect connection, which traverses several brain regions, is indicated by dotted lines and an unnamed dotted box.

cleft and because the intracellular stores of dopamine are depleted by the high release rate.

At about the time that the initial increase in electrical activity is replaced by depolarization block, the initial increase in dopamine synthesis also disappears. Now the synthetic machinery is controlled by dopamine concentration in the cells. If dopamine is not being released, additional synthesis is not needed.[20]

Scientists do not have direct evidence in humans that depolarization block and the concomitant decrease in dopamine synthesis is part of the chain of events leading from antipsychotic treatment to relief of schizophrenic symptoms. Getting such evidence is difficult because scientists cannot record electrical activity in human brains and because they cannot use living humans for direct measurement of dopamine synthesis.

There is, however, indirect evidence. First, depolarization block, the decrease in dopamine synthesis, and improvement of symptoms all take about two to three weeks of antipsychotic treatment. Second, scientists have attempted to compare the improvement of schizophrenic symptoms with indirect measurements of dopamine synthesis. The rate of dopamine synthesis can be inferred from measurements of a dopamine metabolite (breakdown product) called homovanillic acid. Several groups of investigators measured changes in plasma homovanillic acid during antipsychotic treatment. Some, but not all, found an increase in homovanillic acid during the first few days of treatment; all found a persistent decline over the next several weeks. Homovanillic acid change in humans had the same time course as dopamine synthesis changes in rats. In addition, the human patients with the greatest decline in homovanillic acid concentration also had the greatest improvement in schizophrenic symptoms.[21] These results suggest that clinical effectiveness of antipsychotic drugs is, at least in part, due to their ability to decrease the activity of dopaminergic cells and to decrease dopamine synthesis and release.

Changes in Dopamine Receptors

Under the influence of antipsychotic drugs, the postsynaptic cells make extra dopamine receptors.[22] This overproduction is the postsynaptic cells' attempt to compensate for the weakening of synaptic transmission caused by drugs. The extra receptors tend to restore the cells' sensitivity to dopamine in the face of partial receptor blockade and the lower level of dopamine release due to depolarization block. Just as a sensitive photographic film with more silver salt is more likely than a less sensitive film with less silver salt to "see" an object in dim light, a cell with more dopamine receptors is more likely than a cell with fewer receptors to "see" a small amount of transmitter. If a switch is made from a less sensitive to a more sensitive film but the amount of light allowed through the camera's lens, is not reduced, the photographs will be overexposed. Discontinuing an antipsychotic drug after long-term treatment is similar to switching to a more sensitive film: The increase in dopamine receptors produced in reaction to the drug causes an abnormally large response to dopamine.

The compensatory increase in receptors has been measured in rat brains. The first step in the experiment was to inject rats with an antipsychotic drug over a period of several weeks. Next, the researchers let a few days elapse, giving the drug time to leave the receptors, since the number of dopamine receptors could not be measured while the drug was blocking them. Then the researchers removed a region of the brain known to contain dopamine receptors. In order to compare the number of dopamine receptors in treated and untreated rats, they also removed the identical region of the brain from rats that had not been treated with an antipsychotic. Finally, the researchers separated the cells removed from each group of rats and added radioactive haloperidol to each. By measuring the amount of haloperidol bound to cells from each rat, they calculated the number of dopamine receptors on the cells from the treated rats and on the cells from the untreated rats. The cells from the treated rats had more dopamine receptors.[23]

This increased sensitivity to dopamine might not be important if depolarization block were complete. If no dopamine cells were releasing any dopamine, it would not matter how many receptors there were. But, of course, no drug totally prevents transmitter release. The extra receptors, particularly those in the caudate nucleus, may be partially responsible for tardive dyskinesia, one of the most serious side effects of antipsychotic drugs (see Chapter 8).

THE SCHIZOPHRENIC BRAIN

We would hope that understanding what antipsychotic drugs do to synapses would provide some hints about the nature of the defect in the schizophrenic brain. What scientists have learned so far about antipsychotic drugs and amphetamine suggests that overactive dopamine synapses may be a cause of schizophrenia. Overactivity at dopamine synapses could result either from the release of too much dopamine at the presynaptic terminal or from an excess of dopamine receptors at the postsynaptic cell.

Most experiments on the role of dopamine synapses in schizophrenia have concentrated on the hypothesis that schizophrenic brains have too many dopamine receptors. Until very recently, all analyses of dopamine receptors were done on brain samples obtained at autopsy. Most studies found many more dopamine receptors in brains taken from schizophrenic patients than in brains taken from healthy people.[24] Unfortunately, these studies are difficult to interpret because the increase in dopamine receptors could be the result of antipsychotic medication rather than a manifestation of disease. Although most patients had been off medication for at least a few months prior to the study, drug-induced dopamine receptors may have remained in their brains; scientists do not know how long it takes for these extra receptors to disappear following drug termination. Only a few of the patients used in these studies had never received antipsychotic medication. Postmortem studies of large numbers of never-medicated patients will probably never be possible because withholding an effective medication from ill patients is not ethical medical practice.

Positron emission tomography (PET) may eventually enable us to find out whether nonmedicated schizophrenics have an abnormally large number of dopamine receptors. In these studies a living patient is given a small dose of a radioactive D2 antagonist. The antagonist binds to dopamine receptors. PET detects the binding in each region of the brain, and a computer calculates the density of dopamine receptors. Since this technique does not require removal of tissue, it can be used on live patients as soon as their schizophrenia is diagnosed and before they receive any mediation. The technique is, however, still experimental; scientists disagree on the antagonist that should be used and on the way the data should be analyzed. Scientists in three laboratories have attempted to compare dopamine receptor density in never-medicated schizophrenia patients with that in healthy people. One group has found that the schizophrenia patients had more dopamine receptors[25]; the other two found no difference between the patients and the healthy controls.[26] Eventually PET will provide a definitive answer. At present, some evidence suggests that victims of schizophrenia have an abnormally large number of dopamine receptors, but this evidence is not conclusive.

The hypothesis that the schizophrenic brain contains excessive dopamine receptors explains some of the effects of antipsychotics. It explains why blocking dopamine receptors and the subsequent decrease in dopamine synthesis and release alleviates the symptoms. It explains why antipsychotics control schizophrenia but cannot cure it. The analogy with diabetes used earlier is instructive here. Insulin does not cure diabetes; it cannot induce the pancreas to make insulin. Similarly, an antipsychotic does not cure schizophrenia; it cannot induce the nerve cells to make normal dopamine synapses. In both diseases the drug compensates at least partially for a biochemical abnormality, but the underlying abnormality is still present.

Some facts cannot be explained by the dopamine hypothesis. For example, the hypothesis does not explain why all patients are not helped. A recent PET study supports the view that there are dopamine-dependent and non-dopamine-dependent types of schizophrenia. This study found that antipsychotics block dopamine receptors equally effectively in patients who are helped by the drugs and in those who are not.[27] This rules out the hypothesis that the drug simply does not reach the relevant brain sites in the nonresponders. These patients must have a disorder that is not related to dopaminergic activity.

The hypothesis also fails to explain why discontinuing treatment does not make the disease worse than it was before treatment. During treatment with antipsychotics, the patient becomes extremely sensitive to dopamine because both the old and new dopamine receptors are exposed. Surprisingly, removal of the drug and recovery from depolarization block does not worsen the disease. Relapses of schizophrenia after drug holidays are not obviously worse than the initial episodes or than relapses occurring while the patient is on medication.

Clearly, neuroscientists do not completely understand what is wrong with the schizophrenic brain, but progress has been made. Studying the effects of antipsychotic drugs has taught us that dopamine synapses are an important factor. Refining the research methods and investigating other transmitter systems may tell us more precisely how the schizophrenic brain differs from the healthy one.

In Chapter 5 we discussed global changes seen in some schizophrenic brains, such as increased ventricular size and abnormalities in cerebral blood flow. Are these changes related to the excess of dopamine receptors postulated here? We do not know with certainty. Some scientists have hypothesized two different types of schizophrenia. One type is characterized by predominance of positive symptoms, normal ventricular size and overactive dopamine systems. A second type is characterized by predominance of negative symptoms, enlarged ventricles, and a normal or even underactive dopamine systems.[28] Others disagree with this classification because some research indicates that both positive and negative symptoms respond to antipsychotics.

SIDE EFFECTS OF
ANTIPSYCHOTIC DRUGS

—

I f you were to look up the side effects of the antipsychotic drugs in a standard medical pharmacology text, you would be appalled at the number listed and at the severity of some of them.[1] You would find that these drugs can affect virtually every organ of the body, from the skin to the liver. The severity of these side effects ranges from just annoying to life threatening. We discuss only the most common ones in this chapter; physicians watch for many other side effects, whose likelihood is extremely small. If you do consult a complete list, try to keep the information in perspective. A cloud of side effects hangs over every significant drug, but that cloud should not obscure the benefits. For instance, patients with bacterial infections are treated with penicillin even though on occasion a person is allergic to the drug and dies from it. Before deciding whether to use a particular treatment, the physician and the patient must weigh both its risks and its benefits. How damaging is the disease? Is the patient willing to live untreated even if treatment is available? How serious are the side effects? How likely are the most serious side effects?

Our discussion of the side effects of antipsychotic drugs emphasizes the neurological side effects because they are the most common and because one of them, tardive dyskinesia, is among the most serious. Furthermore, knowledge of how antipsychotic drugs affect the brain aids our understanding, at least partially, of why these side effects occur. Other medically important side effects will be discussed briefly.

PARKINSONIAN SIDE EFFECTS, DYSTONIA, AND AKATHISIA

Antipsychotic drugs can cause several different kinds of movement disorders.[2] One of these disorders is very similar to Parkinson's disease. Patients with Parkinson's disease typically have an expressionless face, move very slowly with a shuffling gait, and have a severe tremor. The cause of Parkinson's disease is a deficiency of transmission at dopamine synapses in the basal ganglia, forebrain structures involved in the control of posture and movement. When schizophrenia is treated with antipsychotic drugs, the dopamine receptors in the basal ganglia are partially blocked and synaptic transmission is impaired. It is not surprising, then, that parkinsonian symptoms result as a side effect of the drugs.

As we mentioned in Chapter 7, L-dopa is an effective treatment for Parkinson's disease. This drug increases the amount of dopamine in the basal ganglia and relieves the symptoms. But L-dopa cannot be used to treat parkinsonian symptoms that are a side effect of antipsychotic therapy. L-Dopa enhances transmission at dopamine synapses throughout the brain. Therefore, it counteracts the effect of the antipsychotic drug and may exacerbate schizophrenia.

The dopamine deficiency of Parkinson's disease results in an imbalance between activity at dopamine synapses and activity at acetylcholine synapses. The balance shifts in favor of acetylcholine synapses. This balance can be restored either by decreasing transmission at acetylcholine synapses or by increasing transmission at dopamine synapses. Therefore, parkinsonian symptoms caused by antipsychotics are usually treated effectively with drugs that partially block acetylcholine synapses. Two of the drugs most commonly used to alleviate these symptoms trihexyphenidyl hydrochloride and benztropin mesylate (trade names are Artane and Cogentin, respectively).

Sometimes abnormal movements that look like drug-induced parkinsonism are actually symptoms of schizophrenia that are not controlled by the antipsychotic drug. Slow and reluctant movement may be schizophrenic withdrawal. The expressionless face may be a manifestation of flat affect. Peculiar postures and grimaces are both parkinsonian side effects and schizophrenic symptoms. Even a psychiatrist may have difficulty distinguishing between parkinsonian side effects and a reemergence of schizophrenia. Merely observing the patient may not suffice. Usually, but not always, a psychiatrist can make this distinction by giving the patient antiparkinsonian medication. If this treatment helps, the patient is suffering from side effects of medication and not from an increase of schizophrenic symptoms.

Some patients suffer from dystonia, involuntary muscle contractions that cause bizarre and uncontrolled movements of the face, neck, tongue, and back. A particularly distressing form of dystonia is oculogyric crisis, in which the eyes roll uncontrollably. Like the parkinsonian side effects, dystonia can be confused with an increase in the symptoms of schizophrenia because schizophrenic patients often assume peculiar postures. Dystonia can also be mistaken for seizures. When dystonic symptoms are, in fact, a side effect of antipsychotic drugs, they respond dramatically to antiparkinsonian drugs.

Other patients suffer from akathisia, which looks, at first glance, like severe restlessness and agitation. In fact, akathisia is sometimes mistaken for schizophrenic agitation. The patients complain of severe discomfort in their arms and legs and move them about continually. They cannot describe or localize any specific pain, but no position—sitting, standing, or lying down—is comfortable for very long. They continue to move about in the vain hope of finding a comfortable position. Antiparkinsonian medication is the usual treatment, but it is not always successful. Reduction in the dose of the antipsychotic medication may be necessary.

Dystonia and akathisia, like Parkinson's disease, probably result from subnormal synaptic transmission at dopamine synapses in the basal ganglia, but it is not known why some patients experience parkinsonian side effects, others dystonia, and yet others akathisia. Most of the neurological side effects occur early in treatment, decreasing in severity after a few weeks. Again, it is not known why the side effects diminish while the drugs continue to block dopamine receptors throughout treatment.

TARDIVE DYSKINESIA

Schizophrenia is usually a chronic disease, and antipsychotic medication is the only effective treatment. Unfortunately, one devastating side effect prevents many victims of schizophrenia from taking medication indefinitely.[3] These patients are haunted by the specter of tardive dyskinesia (TD). *Tardive dyskinesia* means "late-appearing movement disorder"; unlike most neurological side effects of antipsychotics, TD usually does not appear until a patient has taken antipsychotics for many years. It begins as jerky, tic-like movements in the tongue and face.[4] As the disease progresses, the entire body may become affected, making either tic-like or writhing movements. These movements are virtually continuous during waking hours but cease during sleep. Patients with TD may flick their tongues in and out of their mouths as often as 20 times in 30 seconds. Their gait becomes unsteady as the disease progresses. If the disease becomes extremely severe, they may start rocking back and forth at the hips. Irregular breathing gives them the appearance of gasping for breath. Fortunately, they do not lose complete control of the muscles used in breathing; patients with TD do not die of respiratory failure. This fact may be small consolation, though, for TD can be so socially debilitating that it is to be feared nearly as much as schizophrenia itself. On the other hand, some cases of TD are mild and are diagnosed by the psychiatrist before they are noticed by patients or their families. Some cases do not progress beyond mild tongue movements even if antipsychotic medication is continued.

Since TD was first described in 1957, its reported prevalence among schizophrenia patients has increased. Part of this increase is real; TD has increased with the use of antipsychotics. Part of the increase results from the fact that psychiatrists have become increasingly aware of the problem and accurately diagnose a larger proportion of the cases. Until 1965 the reported prevalence of TD was about 5 percent of chronically hospitalized schizophrenia patients.[5] Current estimates of the prevalence of TD vary widely. One reason for this is that the diagnostic criteria vary. Only since 1976 has a scale been available for quantifying abnormal movements,[6] and even when this scale is used, there is no accepted criterion for deciding how much abnormal movement constitutes TD. Obviously, if even slight abnormal movement is diagnosed as TD, the reported prevalence will be much higher than if only dramatic abnormalities are diagnosed as TD.

TD probably occurs in about 20 to 25 percent of hospitalized schizophrenic patients.[7] It is caused by antipsychotics, not by schizophrenia, and occurs in patients who take antipsychotics for other psychiatric diagnoses.[8] All cases of abnormal movement are not, however, TD. Symptoms resembling TD probably occur in about 5 percent of the population that has not taken any antipsychotic drugs[9]; therefore, the true prevalence of drug-induced TD is about 15 to 20 percent.

All patients taking antipsychotic drugs do not develop TD. Female sex and advanced age are the greatest risk factors. About 63 percent of TD patients are female. Estimates of the prevalence of TD in elderly patients taking antipsychotics hover around 50 percent. In contrast, the overall prevalence of TD in patients under 40 is about 10 percent.[10] The logical inference that TD prevalence is greater in older patients because they have taken antipsychotics longer is not correct. Patients whose psychotic disorder begins late in life have the greatest risk. In this group of patients the greatest risk occurs during the first two years of treatment. In younger patients, however, the risk is fairly constant with time. The incidence of new cases is about 3 percent each year.[11]

Negative schizophrenia symptoms may also be a risk factor for TD. Patients who are mute, have flat affect, and have cognitive dysfunctions, such as inability to do the card sorting tasks described in Chapter 5, are more likely to develop TD than are patients who do not have these symptoms. Because these are also the patients who tend to have abnormal computed tomographic (CT) scans, investigators have hypothesized that brain damage may predispose a patient to develop TD. Direct evidence for this theory would require evidence that the same patients have both TD and abnormal CT scans. Some studies support this prediction, but the results are not yet conclusive.[12]

Psychiatrists would like to know how to minimize the risks of TD while still treating their patients for schizophrenia. Carefully selecting the antipsychotic probably will not help. All the commonly used antipsychotics probably produce TD at about the same rate. There is evidence, however, that clozapine (see Chapter 6) does not produce TD. It does not produce parkinsonian side effects, and clinical studies of clozapine have not reported any new cases of TD.[13] Unfortunately, as shown later in this chapter, clozapine produces other side effects, such as agranulocytosis, that preclude its frequent use.

It seems logical that patients taking higher drug doses would be more likely than patients taking lower doses to develop TD, but there is not much evidence that this is the case. One possible explanation for this is that the risk is maximal at all effective drugs doses. Another is that blood level, rather than dose, may be related to the development of TD. Yet blood level may be poorly related to dose, because individual rates of drug metabolism are quite variable. It would also seem logical that intermittent drug holidays would decrease the likelihood of TD because they decrease total drug exposure. Surprisingly, drug holidays are probably not helpful and may even make TD less reversible.[14]

Even though TD is clearly caused by antipsychotic drugs, the amount and duration of drug treatment is not a good predictor of which patients will be afflicted. Age and negative symptoms are much better predictors. This suggests that some property of the brain makes a person vulnerable to TD. The presence of antipsychotic drugs interacts with that vulnerability to produce the disorder.

CAUSES OF TD

One hypothesis is that TD results from the extra dopamine receptors that are produced in response to antipsychotic drugs. The extra receptors make the postsynaptic cell supersensitive to dopamine.[15] In a sense, TD may be the converse of Parkinson's disease. Both diseases result from abnormalities in the basal ganglia. In Parkinson's disease, dopamine transmission is inadequate and acetylcholine synapses dominate. This imbalance causes slow and shaky bodily movements. In TD, extra dopamine receptors may increase the strength of dopamine synapses to the point where they dominate acetylcholine synapses. Dopamine domination may cause the writhing and twitching of TD. According to this hypothesis, TD results when the basal ganglia overcompensate for the partial dopamine blockade caused by the antipsychotic drug.

A number of facts about TD are consistent with the dopamine supersensitivity hypothesis.[16] First, TD gets worse if antipsychotic drugs are suddenly terminated. Presumably, drug withdrawal unblocks receptors, increasing the number available to dopamine. Second, TD gets worse if the patient is given L-dopa, which causes the brain to make extra dopamine. The increased supply of dopamine increases the number of receptors activated. Third, TD can be temporarily suppressed by increasing the dose of antipsychotic drug. The increased amount of drug available to the dopamine receptors may block many of the extra receptors. This suppression is, however, short lived. The higher dose probably causes the slow development of even more dopamine receptors and a corresponding worsening of the underlying condition.[17]

In spite of these facts, dopamine supersensitivity is probably not the complete explanation for TD. Presumably, all patients receiving antipsychotics develop extra dopamine receptors, but only some develop TD. Postmortem measurements of receptor densities do not indicate that patients with TD had more dopamine receptors than patients without TD.[18] Some other property of the brain must interact with the increased number of dopamine receptors to produce TD. We do not know what this property is, but the fact that patients with negative symptoms are more likely to have TD provides a hint. Perhaps the brain damage that often accompanies negative symptoms interacts with dopamine supersensitivity to produce TD.

TREATMENT OF TD

There is no successful pharmacological treatment for TD. Although articles appear from time to time in medical journals, claiming successful pharmacological treatments, rigorous testing has unfortunately failed to show that any of these provide reliable help.

The appearance of TD presents a dilemma. If the patient's psychiatric condition can tolerate cessation of antipsychotic treatment, this is probably the best course. Younger patients have a good chance of remission once the drug is stopped, but even in elderly patients TD sometimes improves.[19] The symptoms will not improve immediately upon withdrawal of antipsychotics and may even worsen for a few weeks. Restoring antipsychotic medication will relieve the symptoms, and increased doses may suppress them entirely for a few weeks or months.[20] But antipsychotics should not be considered a treatment for TD. For the first few months after drug withdrawal, there is little to do but wait. Some authorities believe that if the patient does not improve within three months of antipsychotic withdrawal, the TD is probably irreversible. Other scientists have reported substantial improvement several years after drug withdrawal.[21]

Sometimes the patient's psychiatric condition does not permit withdrawal of antipsychotic medication. In this case, the outcome is more variable. Continuing medication does not always cause TD to become debilitating. The TD may remain stable, it may get worse, or it may improve. Again, young patients are more likely to improve than are older ones.[22]

A compromise solution has been suggested by a group of psychiatrists studying TD in Japan. They found that the involuntary movements often improved if the physicians attempted to find the smallest dose of antipsychotics that would be effective for each patient and then reduced the dose to this amount.[23]

ADDITIONAL NEUROLOGICAL SIDE EFFECTS

Another neurological side effect of antipsychotic drugs is the secretion of milk from the breasts, occasionally even in men. The blockade of dopamine receptors in a portion of the brain called the hypothalamus can increase production of prolactin, the hormone controlling milk secretion. Sometimes the increase in prolactin is so great that milk is produced. Although this side effect of antipsychotic medication is annoying and embarrassing, it is not dangerous. It can even be useful to the physician, because the level of prolactin in the blood is an indicator of how effectively an antipsychotic drug has blocked dopamine receptors. Interestingly, blood prolactin increases almost immediately after antipsychotic therapy begins, demonstrating again that antipsychotic drugs block dopamine receptors immediately, even though their therapeutic effects are not fully expressed for two to three weeks.[24]

When a physician prescribes a drug, he usually would like to confine its action to a specific target. Unfortunately, this is rarely possible, and antipsychotics are no exception to this rule. In addition to blocking dopamine receptors, they can also block certain norepinephrine receptors and some, but not all, acetylcholine receptors.[25] Fortunately, antipsychotic drugs do not block the acetylcholine receptors on skeletal muscles and hence do not cause muscle weakness or paralysis. They do, however, block acetylcholine receptors at the junctions between nerve fibers and internal organs. Blockade of these synapses causes many side effects, known collectively as anticholinergic side effects. For example, blockade of synapses at the salivary glands causes dry mouth, and blockade of synapses at the iris of the eye causes blurred vision. Anticholinergic side effects are usually more annoying than serious (but see Chapter 13 for some exceptions). They complicate the treatment of movement disorders because the antiparkinsonian drugs also decrease transmission at acetylcholine synapses and therefore exacerbate anticholinergic side effects.

Some side effects are caused by the blockade of norepinephrine receptors.[26] One such side effect is orthostatic hypotension, a sudden decrease in blood pressure when the patient stands up suddenly after having been sitting or lying down for a while. The drop in blood pressure prevents the brain from receiving enough blood and hence enough oxygen. The patient feels dizzy or faint and may experience a partial blackout of vision. These effects usually disappear in a few seconds. Healthy people experience orthostatic hypotension from time to time, but the antipsychotic drugs make it occur more often. Furthermore, the decrease in blood pressure can be dangerous to people with cardiovascular disease and to people whose blood pressure is already low. Older patients are at greatest risk. Obviously, people taking antipsychotic drugs should avoid situations where loss of balance is particularly dangerous, and they should not stand up suddenly in a situation where a fall would be disastrous. For example, they should not paint the gutters while squatting on a steeply pitched roof because they might be unable to stand up slowly enough to avoid dizziness and a dangerous fall.

The sedative effect that patients and their relatives so often complain about is probably caused by the blockade of receptors for transmitters other than dopamine. Several different transmitters and receptors may be involved. Most antipsychotic drugs cause some sleepiness at first, but in most patients, this sedation gradually disappears after the first few weeks of therapy. Nevertheless, patients and their relatives may continue to insist that medications turn patients into "zombies." In Chapter 6 we heard Mark Vonnegut's complaint, for example, that drugs had impaired his ability to make judgments and feel emotion. Sometimes these complaints are justified: If the drug dose is large enough, the sedative effects will be incapacitating and may not disappear completely with time. Often, however, symptoms that appear to arise from drug overdose are, in fact, a reassertion of the active disease. Patients suffering from schizophrenia often do not have normal emotional expressions. They may look more like "zombies" when not taking the drug than when taking it. Before concluding that a patient has been overmedicated, one needs to know how the patient behaved in the absence of medication and whether the patient's psychosis could be controlled with a lower dose.

TWO NONNEUROLOGICAL SIDE EFFECTS

Neuroleptic Malignant Syndrome

Neuroleptic (another name for antipsychotic) malignant syndrome affects about 0.5 to 1.0 percent of patients receiving antipsychotics.[27] It usually occurs in the beginning of treatment and lasts five to ten days. It begins with motor abnormalities, such as rigidity or dyskinesia. A high fever and inability to regulate the cardiovascular system follow.

The cause of neuroleptic malignant syndrome is not understood, but it clearly involves the brain's mechanism of temperature regulation. Because dopamine is involved in temperature regulation, neuroleptic malignant syndrome may be a direct result of dopamine receptor blockade in temperature-regulating regions of the brain. We do not know why a few patients are afflicted with this syndrome while most are not. The first treatment is to discontinue the antipsychotic. Because antipsychotics are metabolized slowly, they may remain in the brain for a long time, and several days may pass before the patient shows substantial improvement. Additional treatments may be necessary to counteract specific symptoms, for example, cooling for fever and assistance with respiration. While most patients recover completely, some have died. Early studies reported that about 20% of those patients who suffer from this syndrome, or about 1 in 1000 of all patients given antipsychotic drugs, died. Fortunately, a more recent study has reported much better results from vigorous treatment. In this recent study, there were no deaths in 24 cases that were vigorously treated.[28]

Agranulocytosis

Agranulocytosis is another rare but serious side effect of antipsychotics.[29] This condition is a loss of white blood cells, which are important in fighting infection. Patients with agranulocytosis must be kept away from possible sources of infection until their white cell count returns to normal. Occasionally, patients with agranulocytosis die from infection. In patients treated with chlorpromazine the risk of agranulocytosis is about 1 in 2,000 patients, and it is somewhat lower in patients treated with haloperidol. With clozapine, agranulocytosis is a much greater risk, occurring in from about 1 in 50 to 1 in 200 patients. This is unfortunate because clozapine is effective for some patients who do not respond to other antipsychotics and because the risk of TD is probably less with clozapine than with other antipsychotics.[30]

ADDICTION AND TOLERANCE

Because many patients take antipsychotic drugs for months or years, it is appropriate to ask whether patients may become addicted as people become addicted to alcohol, tobacco, and opiates. We present a detailed discussion of addiction in Chapter 18, but a brief definition is in order here. One suffers from addiction to a drug if one (1) uses the drug in greater amounts than can be medically justified, (2) brings harm to oneself or others as a result of excessive use, and (3) cannot voluntarily stop one's excessive use. Most addictive drugs produce physiological dependence; that is, withdrawal from the drug causes the long-time user to become ill. In addition, most addictive drugs produce tolerance; that is, the addict must increase his or her dose over time, or the drug loses its effectiveness.

The behavior of cigarette smoking fits this definition of addiction. Smokers use more tobacco than is medically justified. They harm their health and the health of others as a result of their excessive use. They usually find it difficult or impossible to quit smoking. Over several months or years, they increase their consumption from a few cigarettes a week to a pack or even two packs a day. The definition also encompasses the addictive behaviors associated with heroin, alcohol, sleeping pills, and many other substances. It does not apply, however, to the pattern of use associated with antipsychotic drugs. First, patients with schizophrenia do not tend to increase their drug use beyond what is medically required. In fact, the side effects of the antipsychotic drugs are sufficiently unpleasant that many patients are inclined to defy doctor's orders and refuse to take the drugs. Second, although it could be said that the side effects of the drug harm the patients, the therapeutic effect prevents even greater harm, both to the patients and to others. Third, patients taking antipsychotic drugs have no difficulty discontinuing their drug use when the psychiatrist instructs them to do so; they feel no craving for the drug, and they do not suffer a distressing withdrawal illness when they stop using it. Although some patients experience mild discomfort if medication is stopped abruptly, gradually tapering the dose to zero creates no problems. Finally, tolerance does not occur for the antipsychotic effects of the drugs. Clearly, the long-term use of antipsychotic medication can cause problems. Drug addiction, however, is not one of them.[31]

MINIMIZING SIDE EFFECTS

Drug Selection

There is no evidence that one antipsychotic drug is more effective than any other. Although antipsychotic drugs vary in potency, less potent drugs can be just as effective as more potent ones, even for the sickest patients. That one drug is more potent than another means only that the more potent drug is effective in smaller doses.

For example, trifluoperazine (Stelazine) is a more potent drug than chlorpromazine (Thorazine). About 5 mg of trifluoperazine is equivalent in antipsychotic efficacy to about 100 mg of chlorpromazine. When the doses are properly adjusted, both are equally effective.

Since there are many antipsychotics with similar therapeutic effectiveness on the market, a physician usually selects an antipsychotic for a patient because of its particular side effects rather than its particular therapeutic effects. All antipsychotics cause movement side effects, sedation, and orthostatic hypotension, but the intensity of each varies from drug to drug. A psychiatrist who wants to minimize the movement disorders — for example, parkinsonism, dystonia, or akathisia — is likely to select chlorpromazine. Unfortunately, the movement side effects can be minimized only at the expense of increasing sedation. On the other hand, a psychiatrist who wants to minimize sedation will probably select haloperidol or trifluoperazine. However, decreasing sedation increases the risk of movement abnormalities. For each case, the physician and patient must choose the drug that will cause the least annoyance and discomfort. If the side effects are too onerous, the patient will refuse to take the drug.

At one time, psychiatrists supposed that sedating phenothiazines would be the best treatment for patients who were excited or hyperactive, whereas the so-called activating phenothiazines would be best for those who withdrew socially, failed to talk, or moved very little or very slowly. However, there are no controlled observations to substantiate this conjecture. Current medical opinion is that both hyperactive and withdrawn patients are helped by both activating and sedating drugs.

Someone who fears that a relative or friend is suffering unnecessarily from side effects of antipsychotic drugs should consult with the patient's psychiatrist to answer several fundamental questions:

- Are the symptoms indisputably side effects? Could they be symptoms of the underlying disease?
- Has the patient been taking the drug long enough for some of the initial side effects to wear off? Most patients will be disagreeably sedated during the first ten days or so on medication; this side effect is a necessary evil.
- Could the situation be improved by lowering the dose? This remedy may be feasible after the acute symptoms have abated.

- Would it help to change drugs? Each patient tolerates some drugs better than others, but there is no antipsychotic without bad side effects. The psychiatrist cannot try the entire pharmacopeia. Two or three drugs, each with a different spectrum of side effects, can reasonably be tried. Moreover, the effects of a change in drugs may not be immediately apparent because it takes months for all traces of an antipsychotic to leave the body, so the friend or relative must not be impatient. Changing drugs rapidly would only lead to confusion: If the side effects were to improve, the psychiatrist would have no idea which drug caused the improvement.

The patient's friend or relative must bear in mind how sick the patient was without treatment. The patient may have to tolerate some unpleasant side effects to get the therapeutic benefit: the return to rationality.

If a patient has been taking antipsychotic medication, but his or her symptoms have not improved, is the patient likely to respond to a different drug? Perhaps — but then again, perhaps not. One authority recommends that a second drug should be tried, if a patient does not respond to the first in a few weeks, but there is no point in changing drugs every few days.[32] Another authority recommends that, if a patient fails to respond to a second antipsychotic, drug therapy should be discontinued and the diagnosis reevaluated.[33] Unfortunately, about 10 percent of schizophrenia patients fail to respond to conventional antipsychotic medication[34]; some of these will respond to clozapine. Patients who still fail to respond should not continue taking drugs that have only risks for them and no benefits.

Dosage

The minimum effective dose is often called the threshold dose. A patient who receives less than the threshold dose does not benefit from the drug. Doses much greater than the threshold usually do not bring increased benefits; furthermore, they may bring increased side effects at first and perhaps an increased risk of TD later. The optimal dose is therefore only slightly more than the threshold dose.[35]

Determining the correct drug dose for each patient is important but difficult. Drug dosages are given by weight, usually specified in milligrams. (A milligram is one one-thousandth of a gram.) The dosage will be higher for patients receiving a low-potency drug than for patients receiving a high-potency drug. Nevertheless, a higher dose of a low-potency drug may produce the most acceptable combination of therapeutic effects and side effects for some patients. When a patient receives a new antipsychotic drug, we cannot determine that the effective amount of medication has been increased or decreased simply by knowing that the number of milligrams has been increased or decreased. We must also know the relative potencies of the new and old drugs. This seemingly obvious point can be overlooked even by psychiatrists. Some of Sylvia Frumkin's unexplained improvements and relapses (see Chapter 6) may have resulted from irrational changes in medication. She failed to improve on 1,800 mg of chlorpromazine per day but improved rapidly when switched to 90 mg of haloperidol. Haloperidol is not a better drug than chlorpromazine, but 90 mg of haloperidol is the effective equivalent of 4,500 mg of chlorpromazine. Although a psychiatrist would not intentionally triple a patient's medication in one step, Sylvia Frumkin's physician did just that when he switched her from chlorpromazine to haloperidol.[36]

A proper dose depends on the particular patient as well as on the drug because different people metabolize drugs at different rates. Even when two patients of the same sex and weight receive equal doses of chlorpromazine, the levels of the drug in their blood may be very different. Psychiatrists could compensate for these individual differences by adjusting each patient's dose after measuring the amount of chlorpromazine in the blood. But because this procedure is expensive and not available everywhere, blood concentrations of antipsychotic drugs are not routinely measured.

The slow onset of action of antipsychotic drugs impedes the determination of correct dose. Typically, the relief from schizophrenic symptoms does not occur for several weeks after beginning drug therapy. This delay does not mean, however, that the dose is too small. Because of the slow elimination of antipsychotics, patients who stop taking these drugs may go several weeks without a relapse. This does not mean, however, that they do not need drug therapy. Active metabolic products of the drug may remain in their bodies for several months. Furthermore, the slow action makes it difficult to determine if any increase in dose has caused improvement or if any decrease has caused a relapse.

We end by repeating the message at the beginning of this chapter: All drugs have risks. Some risks are more severe than others; some are more common than others. The existence of risks does not mean that antipsychotics should not be used, however; it means that the risk and benefits should be assessed as precisely as possible, that antipsychotics should be used only for appropriate diagnoses, that use should not continue if the patient is not benefiting, and that frequent medical management is essential.

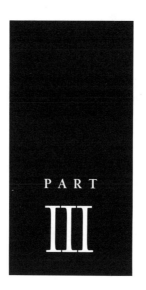

MOOD DISORDERS

9

DIAGNOSING MOOD
DISORDERS

—

But I have that within which passeth show;
These, but the trappings and the suits of woe.
HAMLET, ACT I, SCENE 2

I n this chapter we describe the essential features of bipolar
disorder and major depressive disorder, the two most debilitating types of mood disorder. Cases are presented to
convey a general picture of the disorders and to illustrate how the
criteria given in the *DSM-III-R* help to distinguish them from other
categories of mental illness.

A mood is a long-lasting emotion that pervades and colors all
aspects of mental life. Enduring joy, tranquility, and anxiety are
moods. In mood disorders, also called affective disorders, the patient
suffers from inappropriate and/or excessively intense moods. Psychiatrists and psychologists recognize two types of mood disorders,
depression and mania. Adjectives that describe depression include
pessimistic, sad, withdrawn, fatigued, guilty, discouraged, worthless and
hopeless. Adjectives that describe mania include *optimistic, expansive,
energetic, sociable, generous, overconfident,* and *reckless.*[1]

Other moods can, of course, be troublesome, but the difficulties they cause are not usually discussed under the category of mood disorders. Excessive and long-lasting anxiety is usually considered under the separate category of anxiety disorders (Chapter 16). Other abnormal moods are characteristic of mental disorders other than mood disorders. For example, suspiciousness is characteristic of schizophrenia; pervasive anger that precipitates vandalism or violence is characteristic of personality disorder.

B.B., a woman of 39 who had studied operatic singing, suffered from manic episodes. During one of her episodes B.B. started keeping her family up all night with prayer and loud singing. When interviewed by personnel at the psychiatric hospital to which her family took her for treatment, she was wearing a flamboyant long red skirt with a peasant blouse and was regally adorned with heavy earrings, multiple necklaces, bracelets, and medals pinned to her bosom. She talked very fast, frequently breaking into song. She could not be interrupted to answer questions. Her talking and singing concerned her intimate relationship with God; she said that her beautiful singing voice was God's gift, allowing her to share her joy with less fortunate others. B.B. has been hospitalized 10 times during the past 20 years, sometimes for suicide attempts, sometimes for mania, and sometimes, in her words, "just because I was crazy." Although B.B. does have a beautiful voice, she has been unable to organize a career in singing due to the intrusion of mental illness.[2]

Bob, an accountant in a hospital, suffered bouts of excessive and inappropriate depression. On three occasions during the past five years Bob had been overcome with feelings of worthlessness and guilt accompanied by the idea that he was incompetent at his work. In fact, because of his poor mood, he did become inefficient as an accountant; he became inaccurate and forgetful. During these times he would run his hands through his hair in anguish, berate himself for being foolish, and issue sighs of desperation. It became impossible for him to enjoy pleasures that he was normally enthusiastic about, such as good food and skiing. His interest in sex was diminished. In fact, he lost his energy for almost all activities. He had difficulty falling asleep in the evenings and had an especially hard time getting started in the mornings. Fortunately, his wife Jane could tolerate these periods and could help Bob survive, but the strain on the marriage was significant.

Mood disorders can be distinguished from schizophrenia by appealing to the intuitive distinction between thoughts and emotions.

In mood disorders inappropriate emotions are conceived to be the primary problem; in schizophrenia invalid thinking and perception are thought to be the primary problems. Of course, people with depression or mania may also have disturbed thinking, but psychiatrists believe that the abnormal mood evokes these disturbances, rather than vice versa. B.B.'s excessive feelings of high spirit evoke her belief that she is God's messenger; the belief disappears when she calms down. Bob's conviction that he is worthless and incompetent disappears when his depression lifts. In the thought disorder of schizophrenia, patients usually also have maladaptive emotions, but these inappropriate emotions do not seem to explain the associated delusions and hallucinations. Indeed, the delusions and auditory hallucinations of schizophrenia can occur at times when the patient is emotionally calm or even during periods of flat affect.

Mood disorders tend to be less debilitating than schizophrenia. One reason for this is that the bad moods come in episodes of a few weeks or months. Between episodes the person may be normal both socially and occupationally. During periods of mild mania (called *hypomania*), the person may even be more than normally productive due to his or her high energy level, optimism, and self-confidence. But a person with hypomania stands on a shaky pedestal. At any time this person's mood may escalate into full mania, in which case the person might recklessly quit his or her job to write the great American novel, overconfidently squander the family savings on high-stakes gambling, or arrogantly destroy his or her good marriage to pursue a new love affair.

Mood disorders are common. They occur in many different societies and are even described in the writings of the ancient Greeks.[3] Numerical estimates of the prevalence of mood disorders give only approximate figures. The epidemiological catchment area studies administered by the NIMH suggest that about 3 percent of the U.S. population suffers from a mood disorder during any six-month period. About twice that number report having suffered a mood disorder at some time during their lives.[4] Forty-five to 85 percent of people who have one episode have another.[5] Perhaps lack of treatment contributes to relapse and chronic depression. Only about one in five victims receives treatment from a mental health professional.[6]

These prevalence figures are based on diagnostic structured interviews conducted with a random sample of about 10,000 people living in households in St. Louis, New Haven, and Baltimore. The diagnosis was based on criteria of the *DSM-III* (see Chapter 3), which are very similar to the criteria of the *DSM-III-R* (see below). Interviews were conducted only with people living in households; people living in hospitals, mental hospitals, dormitories, jails, or other institutional settings were excluded. Since there are many people with mood disorders in mental hospitals, the numerical estimate is probably on the low side. Other surveys, at other times, relying on other criteria, in this and other countries, have come up with figures as much as threefold higher.[7]

Few people will escape contact with mood disorders. Therefore, one should learn to recognize the symptoms so that one will know when treatment is appropriate for oneself, a friend, or a family member. Too often, mood disorders invade a person's life insidiously; the victim or the victim's family is not fully aware that a mental health problem has been gradually developing.

DIAGNOSTIC CRITERIA

In the *DSM-III-R* mood disorders are divided into two categories: bipolar disorders and depressive disorders. *Bipolar disorders* are illnesses that include at least one manic episode or an episode of hypomania. They usually include one or more episodes of depression as well, but this is not strictly required. *Depressive disorders* contain one or more depressive episodes or one or more episodes of a less severe depressive condition called *dysthymia*; there are no manic or hypomanic episodes in depressive disorders.

Diagnostic Criteria for a Manic Episode

A manic episode is defined in the *DSM-III-R* by six criteria, A through F. All six criteria must be satisfied.

Criterion A

A distinct period of abnormally and persistently elevated, expansive, or irritable mood.

This criterion places three requirements on mood elevations that can be called manic episodes. First, the elevated mood occurs as a change in the person's behavior, a distinct period or spell that is different from the person's typical personality. Second, the mood is of abnormal intensity, outside the bounds of behavior that is sensible and customary in this person's life and culture. Third, the episode persists for considerable time. The criterion does not say how long it must persist, but manic episodes are expected to last from a few days to a few months. An episode lasting only an hour would not do.

Between the manic episodes there may be long periods either of normality or of depression. In some cases mania or hypomania switches directly to depression without intervening normality. In these cases the patient's personality is dominated by wide swings of mood from mania to depression. Usually, each phase lasts for weeks or months, but sometimes the switching occurs much more rapidly. Cases have been reported in which the person's mood swings daily from one extreme to the other.[8] In most cases the switching occurs at erratic times and not in regular cycles. Still other patients may experience depressive symptoms mixed with mania.

The experience of two abnormal moods that superficially seem to be polar opposites is the origin of the *DSM-III-R* term *bipolar disorder*. It is also the origin of the older term, *manic depression*, that Emil Kraepelin applied to the illness when he first described it nearly a hundred years ago. The *DSM-III-R* definition of bipolar disorder differs from earlier definitions of manic depression in that a manic episode alone is sufficient to make the diagnosis. The earlier definitions required episodes of both depression and mania. In the *DSM-III* and *DSM-III-R* there is no reference to depression in definition of bipolar disorder because the committee believed that all or almost all patients who suffer a manic episode will also suffer from depression at some other time. Also, the optimal treatment for manic episodes is the same as the treatment for manic episodes accompanied by depressive episodes, so there is no impact of co-occurring depressive episodes on treatment of mania (see Chapter 15).

In some patients mania is an irritable mood; the person is chronically angry, arrogant, belligerent, or impatient. For example, a woman may stamp her foot and angrily announce, "I'm just furious," when she sees that her visiting mother, who is trying to be helpful, has used a piece of steel wool to scour a pan. The angry daughter declares, "It's perfectly obvious that steel wool sheds filthy rust particles all over the kitchen." With that, she marches to her bed-room and slams the door. In another example, a woman may come home from work expecting to begin making dinner immediately, but upon finding that the kids have left a pot in the sink with burned refried beans stuck to the bottom, she flies into an angry tirade, demanding that the negligent children be punished. She then an-nounces her categorical refusal to have anything more to do with cooking—ever.

When expansiveness predominates, the person with mania can be grandiose, overconfident, gregarious, loquacious, and probably too loud. For instance, a man may announce to you that he has just talked the bank loan officer into lending him $200,000 to start a new company to manufacture his invention, a circuit board for home computers. He also offers you a golden opportunity to become one of the original stockholders. He claims, "There's no way you can make less than a million!" He may even succeed in persuading you to invest in the business.

Criterion B

During the period of mood disturbance, at least three of the following symptoms have persisted (four if the mood is only irritable) and have been present to a significant degree.

1. inflated self-esteem or grandiosity
2. decreased need for sleep, e.g., feels rested after only three hours of sleep
3. more talkative than usual or pressure to keep talking
4. flight of ideas or subjective experience that thoughts are racing
5. distractibility, i.e., attention too easily drawn to unimportant or irrelevant external stimuli
6. increase in goal-directed activity (either socially, at work or school, or sexually) or psychomotor agitation
7. excess involvement in pleasurable activities which have a high potential for painful consequences, e.g., the person engages in unrestrained buying sprees, sexual indiscretions, or foolish business investments

This criterion distinguishes the manic mood from other excited states. Almost invariably, people in a manic episode are overconfident and have an exaggerated opinion of their importance and power (symptom 1). B.B. thought that she had a particularly intimate relationship with God. A woman may think she is ravishingly beautiful and sexually irresistible. She may try to use her sexual powers to influence important people like her boss, minister, or psychiatrist. A man may believe he can succeed in any undertaking whether it be in business, politics, gambling, or lechery. The grandiosity can be delusional; that is, it can be absurd. A woman may believe that she has been anointed by God to accomplish His mission on earth by giving her body sexually to famous people. A man may believe he has discovered a new form of energy that can be harnessed to accelerate spaceships to previously unachievable velocities. The idea for the invention, he thinks, was received by radar from superintelligent beings. He thinks that his discovery has not been accepted by engineers at NASA because the agency administrators are not as smart as he is and have a vested interest in the entrenched military-industrial complex.

During a manic episode the person may have a decreased need for sleep (symptom 2). He or she may toss and turn in bed, becoming furious with frustration because of the inability to sleep. The person may work or play indefatigably for days, scarcely sleeping at all. B.B. sang and prayed all night and was not tired. In *Moodswing* Ronald Fieve has described the work habits of a number of artists who, he believes, experienced manic or hypomanic episodes. Among these are Honoré de Balzac, Vincent Van Gogh, and Ernest Hemingway. These men all had spells during which they worked furiously for weeks without seeming to get tired. During one excited period lasting 42 days, Hemingway slept only two-and-a-half hours a night.[9]

It is easy to spot overactivity in speech (symptom 3). In the manic mood, the patient talks too much, too loudly, and too fast. B.B. had this symptom. Verbal output can be so rapid that it cannot be understood; it can be so insistent that others never get a chance to speak. Nonstop, noninterruptable talking is such a striking and frequent symptom of mania that it has been given a name, *pressure of speech*.

Thinking, like speaking, is accelerated. Ideas seem to come in swarms. The patient does not complete one line of thought before starting another. This symptom is called *flight of ideas* (symptom 4).

When the ideas fly too fast, they become disorganized and worthless, but when the symptom is only mild, the rapid thinking can be productive. Balzac, Van Gogh, and Hemingway experienced periods of frenetic productivity when their ideas came with unusual rapidity and ease. A mild, but qualifying, form of this symptom is merely the subjective experience that thoughts are racing. The racing thoughts need not be expressed overtly for all to see.

Distractibility (symptom 5) is another sign of mania. The rushing stream of thought easily changes direction. During a full manic episode patients often have difficulty keeping their attention on a single subject for an effective length of time. Minor stimuli in the environment may distract them. Words may be chosen for sound rather than meaning. A patient might start ranting about what should be done to punish the school board for hiring a fourth assistant superintendent, but when he hears the sound of a barking dog, he changes the subject to the scandal in the county over the animal control program. Before this indictment is complete, however, the sound of his own voice saying "dog" may make him begin lecturing about the problem of *log* exports to Japan that is causing the loss of sawmill jobs in his home state of Oregon. While the patient believes that he is brilliant and in complete control, his undisciplined thinking significantly impairs his ability to manage his business and social affairs.

Increased activity (symptom 6) may show up in numerous ways. The patient may make grandiose plans and begin multiple projects that he or she cannot possibly complete. He may be restless and constantly in motion — wiggling, walking, moving in quick-step. The increase in activity is often expressed sexually. For example, a man may exhibit a change in his typical sexual behavior, demanding that his wife have intercourse with him several times a day; a woman may have an affair when it is not her usual style to be promiscuous.

During a manic episode, the patient may become astoundingly reckless in the pursuit of pleasure or other goals (symptom 7). Overconfidence may lead to total obliviousness to the possibility that pleasure seeking may turn out badly. Careless gambling sprees, irresponsible sex, and squandering of money are common. Fieve tells of a patient named William Smythe, a wealthy businessperson. One of Mr. Smythe's manic episodes included the following escapade. Feeling absolutely on top of the world, he hired a young man to parade him down Fifth Avenue, dressed in a white uniform, in a white carriage drawn by a white horse. Along the way, Mr. Smythe picked up a young couple just engaged to be married and offered to take them to dinner. When they politely refused, he went to his bank and obtained $50,000—in silver dollars, twenty-, fifty-, and hundred-dollar bills. As the three rode down the avenue, they threw money to people on the street. This caused a tremendous commotion. Everyone from beggars to well-dressed matrons scurried to grab as much as they could. This taste of Mr. Smythe's generosity apparently softened the young couple's reluctance about dinner, for the party of three then went to an elegant restaurant. There, Mr. Smythe gave the young man $500 to buy a tie and jacket to satisfy the restaurant's dress code. He gave another young man $1,000 to buy a new guitar. The meal ended with a circle of newspaper reporters around Mr. Smythe's table. All the money was gone. Mr. Smythe had to pay the restaurant with a check.[10]

Criterion C

Mood disturbance sufficiently severe to cause marked impairment in occupational functioning or in usual social activities or relationships with others, or to necessitate hospitalization to prevent harm to self or others.

A major objective of this criterion is to distinguish between full mania and hypomania. Full mania is unquestionably harmful. It is serious enough to cause "marked impairment in occupational functioning or in usual social activities. . . ." B.B. and Mr. Smythe clearly satisfied this criterion. Hypomania is similar to mania except that it fails to cause unquestionable harm. Sometimes hypomania may contribute to success. When self-confidence and grandiosity are not too severe, they can be infectious and inspiring to others. In their productive periods, Hemingway, Balzac, and Van Gogh presumably did not satisfy criterion C.

Criterion D

At no time during the disturbance have there been delusions or hallucinations for as long as two weeks in the absence of prominent mood symptoms (i.e., before the mood symptoms developed or after they have remitted).

n rules out the diagnosis of manic episode in com-
ich schizophrenia-like symptoms occur at one time
toms at another. Such cases exist and should be
_ate diagnostic category called schizoaffective dis-
___. Diagnostic criteria for schizoaffective disorder are given in a
separate section of the *DSM-III-R*. Schizoaffective disorder may be
biologically and medically distinct from uncomplicated mood disorders, being, instead, more similar to schizophrenia.

It is hypothesized that in genuine mood disorders delusions and
hallucinations occur only during acute episodes of mania or depression. As mentioned earlier, the disordered mood is supposed to
trigger or evoke the disordered thoughts and perceptions. After the
mood episode has passed or before it starts, the patient is not
supposed to be troubled with hallucinated voices and bizarre delusions. Bizarre behaviors, such as failure to talk or move, are also
thought to occur only during the acute episode of altered mood.[11]

Criterion E

Not superimposed on Schizophrenia, Schizophreniform Disorder,
Delusional Disorder, or Psychotic Disorder NOS.

This criterion prohibits diagnosing manic episode and a schizophrenia simultaneously in complex cases in which schizophrenia-
like delusions and hallucinations occur at the same time as manic
symptoms. Schizophreniform disorder, delusional disorder, or psychotic disorder not otherwise specified (NOS) are all disorders of the
schizophrenia family that are described elsewhere in the *DSM-III-R*.
When symptoms of mania and schizophrenia occur at the same time,
the diagnostician must choose between manic episode or schizophrenia. When delusions and hallucinations are present, the first
inclination is to diagnose schizophrenia. But, as we have seen, mood
disorders can also involve delusions and hallucinations. Distractibility is a useful symptom for distinguishing between the manic and
the schizophrenic state. In schizophrenia, many patients are preoccupied with their delusional belief system and cannot be distracted;
in mania, patients remain sensitive to inputs from other people, and

they can usually be distracted from their inner thoughts. In some cases, the decision between schizophrenia and mania cannot be made with certainty, however. In such cases, the diagnosis has to be based on a judgment about which symptoms are more prominent or whether biological relatives of the patient have had schizophrenia or bipolar disorder.

Criterion F

It cannot be established that an organic factor initiated and maintained the disturbance. . . .

As we have already mentioned in Chapter 4, with respect to the diagnosis of schizophrenia, it would be a tragic mistake to misdiagnose a behavior pattern as a manic episode when it is actually a symptom of drug intoxication, vitamin deficiency, or hormone imbalance. Proper treatment could be delayed for months or years.

DIAGNOSTIC CRITERIA FOR A MAJOR DEPRESSIVE EPISODE

Sorrow, disappointment, and discouragement are natural and healthy responses to important losses, such as a death in the family, divorce, or career failure. People usually recover without psychiatric treatment.

Depression resembles normal sadness, but its duration and intensity are not justified by any corresponding loss or failure. In its milder forms depression can be difficult to spot. When people are sad, they usually think they are sad about something. The something may be the death of a friend, failure to be promoted at work, difficulty getting along with in-laws, or absence of a child who has gone away to college. There are always ready reasons for sadness. But are they justifications or rationalizations? When depression is mild, it can be difficult to tell whether it is a healthy response to problems of living or an unfortunate condition of the brain that is imposing suffering and disability upon the person's life. When depression is severe, however, the magnitude of the incapacity and suffering clearly indicate the presence of illness. In some cases, though far from all, patients report that feelings of depression are distinctly different from the feelings they experience following a serious loss or disappointment.

After review and discussion of the scientific literature, the *DSM-III-R* committee agreed on four criteria for diagnosing a *major depressive episode*. The illness is called major depressive episode rather than just depressive episode to distinguish it from normal depressive emotions and from milder depressive conditions (dysthymia) that are also defined in the *DSM-III-R*.

Criterion A

At least five of the following symptoms have been present during the same two-week period and represent a change from previous functioning; at least one of the symptoms is either (1) depressed mood, or (2) loss of interest or pleasure. (Do not include symptoms that are clearly due to a physical condition, mood-incongruent delusions or hallucinations, incoherence, or marked loosening of associations.)

1. depressed mood (or can be irritable mood in children and adolescents) most of the day, nearly every day, as indicated either by subjective account or observation of others
2. markedly diminished interest or pleasure in all, or almost all, activities most of the day, nearly every day (as indicated either by subjective account or observation by others of apathy most of the time)
3. significant weight loss or weight gain when not dieting (e.g., more than 5% of body weight in a month), or decreased appetite nearly every day (in children, consider failure to make expected weight gains)
4. insomnia or hypersomnia nearly every day
5. psychomotor agitation or retardation nearly every day (observable by others, not merely subjective feelings of restlessness or being slowed down)
6. fatigue or loss of energy nearly every day
7. feelings of worthlessness or excessive or inappropriate guilt

(which may be delusional) nearly every day (not merely self-reproach or guilt about being sick)
8. diminished ability to think or concentrate, or indecisiveness, nearly every day (either by subjective account or as observed by others)
9. recurrent thoughts of death (not just fear of dying), recurrent suicidal ideation without a specific plan, or a suicide attempt or a specific plan for committing suicide

Criterion A defines a depressive syndrome with a list of nine possible symptoms. The patient must have a total of five symptoms to obtain the diagnosis. One of the first two symptoms is mandatory; the remaining seven are optional. In order to count, a symptom must be a change from the person's customary behavior. The symptoms must all be present during the same two-week period. A symptom does not count if the psychiatrist believes that the symptom is a response to some other illness. It would not count, for example, if the symptoms of depression occurred mainly while the patient was suffering from the flu and had a fever. Nor would it count if the symptoms developed in response to delusions or hallucinations experienced in connection with schizophrenia. (Diagnosing a mental disorder with the *DSM-III-R* is like figuring out whether you have satisfied the requirements for a bachelor's degree.)

The first two symptoms, which define the core features of depression, state that the person must show (1) depressed or irritable mood or (2) diminished pleasure. Although bad mood or loss of pleasure always occur to some extent, these symptoms need not be the most troublesome. Inability to concentrate, make decisions, or sleep could be of greater concern to the patient. Patients can report their own depression and loss of pleasure, or a psychologist or family members may observe them. People with depressed mood are likely to describe themselves with words like *sad, blue, depressed, discouraged, down in the dumps*, etc.

Psychiatrists use the Greek work *anhedonia* ("inability to experience pleasure") as the name for symptom 2. For example, a man who usually loves to take a woman to an elegant restaurant and the theater may find himself "too tired for it now." Bob, the hospital accountant, who usually loves to ski and usually spends more on ski trips than his recreation budget allows, may decide that skiing is "too expensive.'' A woman who is normally sociable and enjoys parties may become withdrawn and uncommunicative.

A reduction in the desire for and enjoyment of sex is especially common in depression. Bob experienced this symptom. He and his wife Jane were normally quite exuberant sexually. But when Bob got depressed, he became sexually passive. Sometimes he even felt resentful at the prospect of having intercourse. He would become a bit hostile toward Jane near bedtime when he sensed that she was feeling sexy. During one of his sexually apathetic periods, he actually found himself wishing that sex did not exist. He imagined he would then be free of the conflict caused by his lack of enthusiasm.

Changes in appetite and sleep pattern (symptoms 3 and 4) are often called the biological or vegetative symptoms of depression. Of course, all the symptoms are biological because they are expressions of neural activity in the brain. But symptoms 3 and 4 seem to lack conscious psychological content. It is important to note that symptoms 3 and 4 specify changes from the normal pattern. People who have always been thin and eaten little do not have a depressive symptom just because they customarily do not eat much; although depression is usually associated with reduced appetite and weight loss, sometimes it is associated with overeating and weight gain. Either too much or too little sleep qualifies as a symptom. A depressed person who sleeps too little usually wakes up too early in the morning, but failure to fall asleep at night or wakening in the middle of the night also qualify. Sometimes the patient may sleep more than usual and may even stay in bed almost around the clock. Another common feature is that mood and other symptoms may be worse in the morning than later in the day. This is often referred to as the diurnal variation of depressive symptoms and is regarded as an indicator of the biological source of depression. Bob experienced a worsened mood in the morning.

Psychomotor agitation or retardation (symptom 5) refers to changes in the speed and reactivity of movements that express emotion. With psychomotor agitation, the movements are more obvious and faster than normal. With retardation the movements are slower or absent.

When agitated, the depressed person has nervous mannerisms and is overactive in speech, behavior, and emotional expression. There may be too much wailing, worrying, crying, pacing, and hand wringing. We know a woman with agitated depression who scratched her head so much while worrying about spending too much money that she actually wore all the hair off her scalp in two spots, each about an inch in diameter.

The movements and speech of patients with psychomotor retardation are abnormally slow rather than abnormally fast. Normal people may become impatient trying to converse with the patient because he speaks with the speed of molasses in January. In severe cases, there may be no speech at all. Perhaps the retarded speech in depression is the antithesis of pressure of speech in mania.

Bob suffered from retardation. His wife Jane, who was a nurse at the same hospital where Bob was an accountant, could always tell when Bob was entering another active phase of his illness because he became uncommunicative. When she tried to discuss plans about how they each would get to work the next day (they had only one car and worked different shifts), Bob seemed unable to talk. He tried to speak up and would say, "Well . . .," but then no ideas came to him. He seemed confused. His mind was stuck while Jane waited. Sometimes Jane had to give up on joint planning and make the arrangements herself.

Activities other than speech are affected, too. The patient performs less work and participates in fewer activities; in fact, the patient's whole body moves more slowly. Bob often rode his bicycle to work. Ordinarily, he was a strong rider and worked up a sweat on the way home. But when Bob got depressed, he rode slowly. When he came to a hill, he would get off his bike and walk. Once he stopped moving entirely and just sat down and stared at the street for several minutes.

Symptom 6, loss of energy and fatigue, fits into the concept of depression as a deactivation or slowing down of mental and behavioral processes. Loss of energy does not mean quite the same thing as retardation, although the two may have a common cause in the brain. A person with agitated depression and without retardation is capable of feeling "just exhausted" and may proclaim, in an agitated way, an imperative need for sleep. Such a patient may show an angry rush to get ready for bed and jump under the covers furiously. Loss of energy can be combined with retardation, of course. Bob sometimes spent the better part of entire weekends in bed. He did not have the energy to wash the car and mow the lawn. Jane would eventually do these chores for him. It took all the discipline Bob could muster just to get to work on weekdays.

Bob also experienced feelings of worthlessness, self-reproach, and guilt (symptom 7). His colleagues regarded him as competent, but when he was depressed, he became obsessed with the idea that he was not doing a good job anymore and that his colleagues had no respect for him. Sometimes, when he thought no one would hear, he exclaimed aloud, with hateful self-reproach, "You're stupid!" Inevitably, Jane overheard him berating himself and tried to stop him. She wondered if he was angry at her or if there was something she could do to help him relax. But her concern was of no avail, for it only caused Bob to be overcome with guilt about damaging their marriage by being an albatross around her neck.

In about 10 percent of depressed patients, the feelings of worthlessness and guilt can become so intense that they activate delusions or even hallucinations. A hallucinating depressed person may hear a voice that berates him and calls him names because of his past errors and shortcomings. In depression, however, the voice is not as talkative as in schizophrenia.

Diminished ability to think or concentrate (symptom 8) is one of the most common complaints of people with depression, especially if their occupation calls for much listening, reading, writing, or thinking. A depressed college professor, despite heroic efforts, may find it impossible to pay attention to the doctoral thesis he is supposed to be evaluating. A competent lawyer, when depressed, may be unable to listen attentively to the client and unable to assimilate the details of the case. A depressed author may stare at the typewriter for weeks without producing a paragraph worth keeping. Bob, the hospital accountant, worked more slowly and made more computational mistakes when he was depressed.

Thoughts of death, suicide plans and suicide attempts (symptom 9) emphasize the clinical significance of depression. Approximately 15 percent of the people who suffer from depressive episodes die by suicide, and suicide is the second most frequent cause of death between the ages of 15 and 24. Suicide, however, does not always indicate depression. Suicidal thinking and behavior frequently accompany schizophrenia and anxiety disorders.[12] Suicide may occur in the absence of mental illness, of course: Sometimes a soldier, for example, consciously gives up his or her own life as an act of heroism.

An overt suicide attempt is a severe symptom. Having morbid thoughts of one's own death also qualifies but is less intense. Bob frequently had suicidal thoughts. While driving home from the hospital, he would imagine that he was going to get killed by steering his little car into a bridge abutment or under a log truck. When sitting at

home or at work, he would brood gloomily on the f
had to live through another 30 years, a prospect that
grinding ordeal.

Criterion B

1. It cannot be established that an organic factor initiated and maintained the disturbance.
2. The disturbance is not a normal reaction to the death of a loved one. . . .

When the depressive syndrome described in criterion A is caused by drugs, other illnesses, or the death of a loved one, the syndrome is not considered a major depressive episode. A depressive response to bereavement may be diagnosed as a depressive episode if it is unusually prolonged, say, longer than two months.

Criterion C

At no time during the disturbance have there been delusions or hallucinations for as long as two weeks in the absence of prominent mood symptoms (i.e., before the mood symptoms developed or after they have remitted).

This criterion is a word-for-word copy of criterion D for manic episode. Its purpose is the same: to distinguish between major depressive episode, a mood disorder, and schizoaffective disorder, which may be more similar to schizophrenia than to mood disorders. The vast majority of depressed patients do not experience schizophrenia-like hallucinations or delusions, and so they easily satisfy criterion C.

Criterion D

Not superimposed on Schizophrenia, Schizophreniform Disorder, Delusional Disorder, or Psychotic Disorder NOS.

This criterion duplicates criterion E for manic episode. It prevents the diagnosis of major depression and schizophrenia-like conditions as simultaneous disorders in the same person. As in the case of criterion E for manic episode, the diagnostician must choose whether to use the name major depression or schizophrenia to describe a case that shows both depressive and schizophrenic symptoms simultaneously. This is done by judging which set of symptoms came first, which are more prominent, and which are more enduring.

Criterion D emphasizes that occasionally a patient who has bizarre delusions and prominent hallucinations may not have schizophrenia and may appropriately carry the diagnosis of depression. Such a case is described by Spitzer and colleagues. A young man with depression heard three voices, one of a child, one of a woman, and one of a man impersonating a woman. The voices spoke extensively among themselves about the patient. Sometimes they referred to him in the third person, and sometimes they spoke directly to him. The voices spoke about many different subjects, not just about depressive themes like guilt and death. The voices disappeared when effective treatment relieved the depressed mood, reappeared when the bad mood returned after treatment was discontinued, and disappeared again when treatment resumed. This case was diagnosed as a major depressive episode *with psychotic features* because the hallucinations appeared only in conjunction with the depressive symptoms.[13]

Unlike the three voices, most depressive delusions and hallucinations are recognizably different from the psychotic symptoms of schizophrenia. The delusions and hallucinations of depression typically concern poverty, illness, guilt, sin, and punishment. They only rarely have the bizarre, magical quality that is the trademark of schizophrenia.

CRITERIA FOR DEPRESSION
WITH MELANCHOLIA

There is a long tradition of belief that depression in response to stressful circumstances is distinct from depression that springs up without obvious environmental provocation. The validity of this distinction is an unsettled issue. The *DSM-III-R*, however, does honor the traditional belief by defining a variety of depression called the melancholic type. Various authors have considered the melancholic type of depression to occur mainly in cases that are not provoked by stress, respond better to drug treatment, and produce more occupational and social impairment than the nonmelancholic type.

To conserve space, we do not present a detailed discussion of the criteria for the melancholic type. Since it is mentioned several times in later chapters, however, we list the criteria here for your reference. To obtain the diagnosis of major depressive episode, melancholic type, the patient must satisfy criteria A through E for major depressive episode and, in addition, express five symptoms from the following list of nine:

1. loss of interest or pleasure in all, or almost all, activities
2. lack of reactivity to usually pleasurable stimuli (does not feel much better even temporarily, when something good happens)
3. depression regularly worse in the morning
4. early morning awakening (at least two hours before usual time of awakening)
5. psychomotor retardation or agitation (not merely subjective complaints)
6. significant anorexia or weight loss (e.g., more than 5% of body weight in a month)
7. no significant personality disturbance before first Major Depressive Episode
8. one or more previous Major Depressive Episodes followed by complete or nearly complete recovery
   previous good response to specific and adequate somatic antidepressant therapy (e.g., tricyclics, ECT, MAOI, lithium)

MEASURING THE SEVERITY OF DEPRESSION

The above discussion of diagnostic criteria for mania and major depression largely ignores the problem of assessing the severity of the disorder. The *DSM-III-R* concentrates on naming the disorder, not on telling how severe it is. Within the diagnostic scheme of the *DSM-III-R* it is possible to rate severity according to the number of symptoms and the degree of occupational impairment. For example, a case of depression that showed only five of the nine symptoms and little occupational impairment would be rated mild. If the case showed several symptoms in addition to those minimally required to make the diagnosis and included substantial interference with occupational functioning, it would be called severe.

More sensitive methods of rating the severity of depression have been devised. These methods usually take the form of a semistructured interview administered by a trained diagnostician or a self-rating symptom checklist that is filled out by the patient.

One of the most well-known severity scales is the Hamilton Depression Scale, abbreviated HAM-D. This scale was developed and validated by Max Hamilton of the University of Leeds in England.[14] Using the HAM-D, the diagnostician records a number of points for each of a list of 17 symptoms. Nine of the symptoms are rated on a scale of 0 to 4; eight are rated 0 to 2. On the 0–4 scale, 0 is recorded if a symptom is absent. The doubtful or trivial presence earns a 1, a mild presence a 2, an obvious presence a 3, and a severe presence a 4. One of the symptoms, for example, is suicide, which is rated 0 to 4. Suicide is scored as 0 if suicidal thinking is absent, as 1 if the patient thinks life is not worth living, as 2 if the patient expresses a desire to be dead, as 3 if the patient has made suicide plans or half-hearted and ineffective attempts, and as 4 if the patient has made serious attempts. Bob would have scored 2 on suicide. The overall severity score is the sum of the points assigned to all 17 symptoms. The maximum possible score is 52. A score of 18 is considered to indicate significant depression in need of treatment. A score of 25 or more indicates severe depression. Normal people obtain scores well below 10.

The HAM-D is frequently used as a research tool for assessing the effectiveness of treatments for depression. A sample of depressed patients who score an average, say, of 25 prior to treatment, may drop to an average of 12 after six weeks of treatment with a new drug. By contrast, a similar group of depressed patients may drop their average HAM-D score from 25 to only 18 following six weeks of treatment with placebo sugar pills.

We have described the two most debilitating mood disorders, bipolar disorder and major depression. Depressive episodes are a component of both disorders, but only bipolar disorder has both manic episodes and depressive episodes. It is an interesting question to what extent the depressive episodes of bipolar disorder are biologically the same as those of depressive disorders. The *DSM-III-R* recognizes no distinction between them. As we will see in future chapters, however, there must be some distinction since treatments that are highly effective for controlling depression in bipolar patients are not as effective in major depression patients.

In Chapters 10 through 13 we discuss research on the possible causes and current treatments for major depression. Four chapters are required because this has been an active research area in recent decades. In Chapter 14 we discuss bipolar disorder and its treatment with lithium. As you will see, the use of lithium for bipolar disorder can fairly be called the greatest success thus far achieved in biological psychiatry.

PSYCHOSOCIAL AND
BIOLOGICAL CORRELATES
OF DEPRESSION

—

We begin this chapter with an epidemiological analysis of depression, discussing whether depression can be accounted for by the social circumstances of a vulnerable population. Then we discuss the relationship between life stresses and depression. This is followed by a discussion of cross-cultural studies.

In the second half of this chapter we discuss biological correlates of depression. We begin with a discussion of data obtained by brain imaging and genetic techniques. These data suggest that the brain of a depressed person is metabolically and genetically different from the brain of a normal person. These methods do not at present provide information on cellular mechanisms of depression. We defer discussion of cellular correlates of depression until we have discussed the effects of antidepressant drugs; studies of the action of these drugs contribute to our understanding of the cellular basis of depression.

In this chapter we primarily discuss unipolar depression (without manic episodes), but we include some material on bipolar disorder when it parallels the material on unipolar depression.

DEPRESSION: A PERSONAL AND A PUBLIC HEALTH PROBLEM

Many symptoms of schizophrenia, like the devils that danced in Sylvia Frumkin's pillowcase,[1] are so bizarre that the patient's illness is beyond dispute. When a person has depression, however, the existence of an illness is less obvious. Usually, a depressed person's thoughts are neither bizarre nor patently incorrect. The reasons given for feeling depressed make sense in comparison to the explanations given by a schizophrenia patient for his or her strange behaviors. When a person suffers from depression, both the afflicted person and his or her family are often unsure whether problems of living are causing the depression or whether the depression is causing the problems of living. Probably neither is the sole cause of the other. Problems of living interact with a vulnerable brain to cause depression. Not surprisingly, both pharmacotherapy and psychotherapy are effective treatments for depression. Unlike most acutely ill schizophrenic patients, most depressed patients can benefit from psychotherapy. Depressed patients use language normally and can communicate with a therapist. However, psychotherapy is not always effective. Depressed patients may have abnormal brain biochemistry that makes them vulnerable to depression. Drugs that alter this biochemistry may help.

When we first encounter a friend or relative who has become depressed, it is natural to try to help. It seems so obvious that he is not as worthless as he thinks, that his life is not an unrelenting shower of failures. A logical examination of his situation should persuade him that his life is actually quite successful and enjoyable. We may try to improve his mood by providing some pleasurable experiences. Then we expect him to "snap out of it." When our efforts to help do not work, we feel dismayed. As our friend continues spending his days in tears, berating himself for nonexistent sins, and refusing pleasure because he believes that he does not deserve it, we begin to realize that he is afflicted with something more than the sadness that all people experience from time to time. Suicide attempts may convince us that he is seriously ill. Our friend's depressed mood is not as easy to cure as we expected. Common-sense treatments do not help.

Depression is a serious mental health problem both because it is very prevalent and because it can have serious consequences. The most obvious consequences of depression are deterioration of work performance, marital unhappiness, and personal misery. Fortunately, both pharmacological and psychotherapeutic treatment of depression have improved greatly over the last 30 to 40 years. In 1940 only about 40 percent of hospitalized patients recovered within one year. This statistic shows that available treatments were virtually ineffective since about 40 percent of all depressed patients recover without treatment. Now, however, the rate of recovery within one year approaches 85 percent. This does not mean that 85 percent of depressed people are permanently cured. About half of them will suffer at least one relapse. Nevertheless, modern treatment has made it possible for people who have recovered to spend months or years without episodes of depression.[2]

Occasionally, depression is a fatal illness. The overall mortality rate for depressed patients is substantially higher than that for the general population. Accidents and suicides account for most of these additional deaths.[3] Depression dramatically increases the risk of suicide. Accurate figures are difficult to find, but the best estimates we have indicate that 7 to 15 percent of people suffering from depression commit suicide.[4] In the total population, only 1.0 to 1.4 percent dies by suicide.[5] Since about half the suicides in the entire population occur in people suffering from depression,[6] only 0.5 to 0.7 percent of the nondepressed population commits suicide. Thus, depression increases the risk of suicide about twentyfold. Depression is not the only psychiatric disorder that increases the risk of suicide. A large number of suicide victims suffer from schizophrenia or panic disorder.

WHO GETS DEPRESSED?

Depression is so prevalent that it has been called the common cold of mental illness. As mentioned in Chapter 9, recent epidemiological studies using *DSM-III* criteria estimated that about 5 percent of the U.S. population has suffered a major depressive episode.[7]

METHODS FOR STUDYING DEPRESSED POPULATIONS

In an attempt to understand environmental causes of depression, social scientists have studied the relation between the disorder and a variety of social and demographic factors. Most of these studies are retrospective; that is, they compare the past lives of depressed people and those of normal people. The problem with these studies is that in most cases we do not know the direction of causality. For example, depressed people report more stress than nondepressed people, but this does not mean that stress causes depression. Depression may be the cause rather than the result of stress. Depression certainly creates marriage problems. It can cause job performance to deteriorate, perhaps resulting in loss of the job. It can alienate friends and spouses. It can influence perception of past stress. The problem of determining the direction of causality in retrospective studies is illustrated by an experiment done by Peter Lewinsohn and Michael Rosenbaum at the University of Oregon. They asked depressed people, people who had recovered from depression, and normal people questions about their parents' behavior. Both the normal people and the recovered depressives reported their parents as more warm and loving than did the depressed people.[8] Clearly perception of stress changes with mental state.

A prospective study is the best way to get information about demographic variables or life events that might cause depression. In prospective studies on the development of depression, investigators diagnose a large population of people. They ask both normal and depressed people a wide variety of questions about stress and other aspects of their lives. During this first interview the subjects' responses are not colored by depressed mood and their life situation has not yet been altered by depressed behavior. Six months to a year later, they reinterview the population and find out who has become depressed during the time between the two interviews. In this way they can ask what symptoms present at the first interview predict future depression. Prospective studies are hard to carry out because subjects must be followed for a long time. Therefore, although the studies usually begin with a large sample of subjects, they often have many fewer subjects at the end.

Both prospective and retrospective studies can be useful. Prospective studies are logically more suited to separating cause and effect. Retrospective studies can often produce more reliable correlations between depression and the environment because they can use much larger numbers of subjects.

Demographics

Using both prospective and retrospective studies, scientists have examined demographic variables such as age, sex, and social class, as well as social variables such as stress, perception of one's control over life, thought patterns, and social support. Prevalence of depression clearly varies with age and sex. Depression is uncommon in children but strikes with approximately equal probability throughout young and middle adulthood. Surprisingly, adults over 65 report very little depression. We are suspicious, however, that the data from older adults is inaccurate, because not only do very few older adults report current depression, but very few report past episodes.[9] Perhaps older adults do not remember past episodes or are reluctant to report depression.

Sex is the most reliable demographic predictor of depression. Depressed females outnumber depressed males by about two to one.[10] This sex difference cannot be explained by the fact that women visit doctors more often and so are more likely to receive a diagnosis of depression. Studies by the National Institutes of Health using random samples of the entire population, not of the physician-visiting population, have confirmed this sex ratio.[11]

In our opinion, feminists do not need to search for societal excuses for this sex difference. Such a search might be prompted by the notion that unless a societal cause can be found for the sex difference, its very existence implies that women are inferior. However, we do not think that sex differences in the prevalence of a disorder imply a value judgment. No one treats the greater incidence of heart disease in men, for example, as evidence of inferiority. Some investigators think that the traditional role of women in society contributes to the greater prevalence of depression among women. They point out that having three or more children at home increases the risk of depression.[12] Others do not agree with this theory; they find no evidence that women experience more stress than men. Lewinsohn and his colleagues find that some of the often cited disadvantages of being female, such as low family income or the role of housewife do not predict depression.[13]

The relation between depression and social class is less clear. Some scientists find a strong relationship; others do not.[14] If people in lower socioeconomic classes suffered more depression, one might argue that the stresses and privations of lower-class status cause depression. An alternative explanation might reverse cause and effect, arguing that depressed people have lower socioeconomic status because they behave in a depressed fashion. Prospective studies could suggest which explanation is correct.

One of the largest surveys relating depression to social class found that while a greater percentage of people in the lower social classes were currently depressed, a greater percentage in the upper classes had at least one episode of depression. This suggests that poor people have longer episodes and more relapses because they cannot afford treatment.[15]

Lifelong prevalence of depression is not related to race. The rates are similar in blacks and whites.[16]

Stress, Social Support, and Depression

The hypothesis that stress and misfortune cause depression is intuitively reasonable, but getting scientific evidence for it is difficult. Stress is clearly correlated with depression. Depressed people report more recent stress and less marital social support than normal people.[17] About 25 percent of depressed people say that they recently experienced one or more severe stresses, such as death in the family, divorce, birth of child, or change of job. Only about 5 percent of nondepressed people report similar stress.[18] None of these facts provides evidence, however, that stress causes depression. Many of these stresses might be results of depression.

Death is one stress we rarely control by our behavior. So the relation between bereavement and depression provides some indication of whether this particular type of stress can cause depression. People who experienced the death of a loved one in childhood are about two to three times more likely to suffer from depression than are those who did not experience childhood bereavement. However, only about 30 percent of depressed adults suffered bereavement as children.[19] So while childhood bereavement may contribute to depression, it is not the only cause, and it may not be a major cause. Bereavement, like other factors, probably interacts with biological vulnerability.

Because depression causes so much stress, prospective studies are probably the only way to find out whether stress might cause depression. Both Lewinsohn and his colleagues at the University of Oregon and Scott Monroe and his colleagues at the University of Pittsburgh have found that stressful life events predict depression.[20] Each team of investigators gave psychiatric interviews to a large population of women (500 to 800 people) at two different times 8 to 12 months apart. They also questioned women about social support and a variety of major and minor life stresses. They were most interested in the people who were not depressed at the time of the first interview but were depressed at the time of the second interview. Both groups of investigators found that stressful life events and a difficult marriage during the interval between the two interviews increased the probability of depression at the time of the second interview. This is the first good evidence that stress is a likely cause of depression.

One might hypothesize that many social and psychological features besides stress and marital support would influence the development of depression. Lewinsohn's group looked at some, including the effect of social support outside marriage, income, engagement in pleasant activities, expectation of positive and negative events, and feeling in control of one's own life. None of these was clearly related to the development of depression.[21]

Cross-Cultural Studies

Like schizophrenia, depression probably occurs in all cultures. Until very recently, diagnostic procedures were not sufficiently uniform to permit a comparison of prevalence in different societies. Recently, WHO has provided data that enable scientists to make one-month prevalence estimates for a number of cultures. The prevalence of major depression is similar in most Western countries, but is considerably higher (19 percent) in Uganda, the one non-Western country for which data are available.[22] WHO also found that the same symptoms are present in all cultures studied, but the frequency of particular symptoms varies with culture.[23] In the West, the depressed patient is likely to talk about guilt and self-reproach ("If only I hadn't yelled at him, he wouldn't have left"; "If only I had studied harder in school, I would be able to properly provide for my family"). In non-Western countries, patients are more likely to describe physical symptoms such as weight loss, sleep disturbance, loss of appetite, dry mouth, and headaches; they rarely express feelings of guilt.

Depression probably occurs in all cultures, and the similarities across cultures are more striking than the differences.[24] This suggests that stresses that are peculiar to our culture are not responsible for depression in our culture. If stress causes depression, the responsible stresses are probably endemic to the human condition. We probably could not decrease depression by becoming less industrial, less capitalist, less sexist, or less racist.

BIOLOGICAL BASES FOR DEPRESSION

Data from brain-imaging studies suggest that the brains of depressed people are different from the brains of normal people. Genetic studies suggest that the genes of depressed people make them susceptible.

Brain Imaging

Brain-imaging techniques, especially PET scans, have provided some evidence for abnormalities in the prefrontal cortex of depressed patients. Perhaps the most interesting results have been obtained by a team of investigators at UCLA who did PET scans on six groups of patients. Three groups were depressed and three were not depressed. The depressed patients were unipolar depressives, bipolar depressives, and depressives who also had obsessive compulsive disorder (see Chapter 19). The nondepressed patients were normal people, manic patients, and patients with obsessive compulsive disorder who were not depressed. All three groups of depressed patients had a lower metabolic rate in the left prefrontal cortex (Fig. 2-1) than did any of the three nondepressed groups.[25] This is good evidence for a metabolic abnormality that is associated with depression and is not associated with a variety of other psychiatric disorders.

As noted, the anterior prefrontal cortex is the region of the brain that has abnormally low metabolism in people with schizophrenia. In fact, studies comparing prefrontal cortex metabolism in depressed and schizophrenic patients have not been able to find clear differences between the two groups.[26] The UCLA investigators point out that the prefrontal cortex is a large and complex region of the brain. The fact that people with depression and those with schizophrenia have reduced metabolism in this region does not mean that the same neural circuits are abnormal in both disorders. The imaging techniques cannot distinguish small enough areas of the brain to permit such a conclusion. Furthermore, there are not yet many of these studies, and they disagree on many details. Part of the problem is that PET scans are very expensive, so most PET-scan studies involve rather few patients. Another problem is that because a PET scan measures brain activity, the results depend on exactly what the patient does during the test. Quiet rest, performing a card-sorting task, and performing a counting task will all produce slightly different patterns of activity. Different investigators have made their measurements under quite different conditions.

Genetics of Depression

The fact that depression tends to run in families suggests that it is heritable. As discussed in Chapter 5, heredity and environment are hopelessly entangled in family studies; therefore, these studies are only suggestive. They cannot prove the role of either heredity or the environment. Evidence has to come from adoption studies, twin studies, or experiments locating the responsible gene.

Seymour Kety and his colleagues have done an adoption study on affective disorders that is similar to their adoption study on schizophrenia. They examined the adoptive and biological relatives of both adopted and control people with affective disorders and found that 2.1 percent of the biological relatives of the affectively ill adoptees had unipolar depression. The rate of unipolar depression among all the other groups of relatives was 0.6 percent or less. While most of the adoptees were depressed, some had other affective diagnoses. Therefore, this result does not show that unipolar depression per se is heritable; it only shows that affective disorders in general have a genetic component.[27] The prevalence of depression in this study is surprisingly low because diagnoses were made from hospital records;

relatives without hospital admissions for psychiatric illness were not diagnosed and assumed to be normal. In the schizophrenia study, in contrast, diagnosis was made from interviews of all the relatives the researchers could locate.

Twin studies have provided the best evidence for genetic susceptibility to depression. Different investigators have reported a concordance for identical twins of 40 to 54 percent and of 11 to 19 percent for fraternal twins.[28] This difference can be interpreted in two ways. On the one hand, if you see the genetics glass as half full, you might conclude that the difference in the concordance rates between identical and fraternal twins suggests a genetic component in depression. On the other hand, if you view the glass as half empty, you will focus on the fact that the concordance rate for identical twins is not 100 percent, and you will conclude that the environment makes a significant contribution to major depression. As we have emphasized throughout our discussion, both heredity and environment can influence the development of a mental illness; therefore, both conclusions are probably valid.

Genetics of Bipolar Disorder

The evidence for a genetic component in bipolar illness is much stronger than the evidence for a genetic component in unipolar depression. The most convincing evidence comes from adoption studies. In a study modeled after Kety's adoption studies, Julien Mendlewicz and John D. Ranier looked for affective illness (bipolar disorder or major depression) in the biological and adoptive parents of Belgian adopted children with bipolar illness. They also examined the biological and adoptive parents of healthy Belgian adopted children. Eighteen percent of the biological parents of the bipolar adoptees had an affective illness, while only 1 to 4 percent of the parents in the other groups were afflicted. Bipolar illness clearly has a genetic component.[29]

The concordance rate for identical twins is high (72 percent) for bipolar illness. In addition, the concordance rates are virtually the same for identical twins reared apart and for those reared together.[30] Again, the fact that the concordance is not 100 percent means that the defective gene *confers susceptibility* to the disorder but is not the sole *cause* of the disorder. Genetic susceptibility may explain why one person develops depression in response to minor stress or lack of optimal social support, while another remains healthy in spite of very great stress or failure of support.

In 1987 a multidisciplinary team of scientists thought they had located the gene for bipolar disorder. They made an extensive study of bipolar disorder in the Old Order Amish, a closed and highly inbred community. Using the methods described in Chapter 5 for locating disease-causing genes, they reported that a gene for bipolar disorder was very close to two abnormal DNA sequences.[31] Like the studies of DNA in schizophrenia patients, however, all studies of DNA in bipolar patients are not consistent. Two other groups of scientists studying families in Iceland and three locations in North America did not find a bipolar gene near these abnormal DNA sequences.[32] The failure of other groups to find abnormalities does not necessarily mean that one set of investigators is wrong and the other right. It might mean that more than one genetic abnormality can confer susceptibility to bipolar disorder. But in this case one of the groups turned out to be wrong. In November 1989 a group of scientists at the NIMH repeated the original molecular biology study with the addition of 39 new family members. When these new subjects were added, the entire study no longer provided evidence that the gene for bipolar disorder was in the originally proposed location.[33] New information can overturn or require the reinterpretation of older information; that is why the replication of scientific experiments is so important: One can never be certain that a result is correct until it has been repeated in several laboratories.

11

TREATING DEPRESSION WITH TRICYCLIC ANTIDEPRESSANTS

P atients suffering from depression often respond to drugs. But in contrast to schizophrenia, which requires drug treatment, depression often can be effectively treated without drugs. In recent years, several psychotherapeutic techniques have been developed specifically to treat depressed patients. However, in some severe cases neither drugs nor psychotherapy work, and electroconvulsive shock may be required. In this chapter we discuss tricyclic antidepressants, the most commonly used antidepressant drugs. This category of drugs gets its name from the chemical structure of the drugs comprising it. In the next chapter we discuss additional treatments for depression: other drugs, electroconvulsive therapy, and psychotherapy.

Antidepressants are not stimulants. Unlike caffeine and amphetamine, they do not keep the patient awake. They do not produce euphoria in either depressed or healthy people. In fact, if healthy people take these drugs, they feel sleepy, have difficulty in processing sensory information, and have decreased motor coordination and cognitive skills. They may also experience an increase in anxiety. If they take the drugs for several days, these symptoms increase.[1]

The response of depressed people to antidepressants is quite different. For the first week after beginning treatment with a tricyclic antidepressant, patients probably do not notice much change in symptoms. But sometime during the second or third week, the depression starts to lift. Sleep disturbance and appetite improve; guilt and suicidal thinking disappear.[2] As the depressed mood lightens, patients may say that they feel "normal" for the first time in many months. They begin to enjoy life again.

Of course, not all patients receive such dramatic relief. All symptoms do not improve at the same time. Sleep disturbance may improve within a few days while the depressed mood continues for three to four weeks. Sometimes one or more symptoms persist. A patient may continue to have occasional suicidal thoughts or occasional bouts of guilt. Still another may appear symptom free to family and friends yet remain aware of some remnants of his or her depression. Some people, unfortunately, are not helped at all.

Even when treatment is successful, patients may occasionally relapse. They may have episodes of sadness, irritability, or early morning awakening. These relapses should not be surprising. The effects of antidepressants, like the effects of antipsychotics, do not outlive the presence of the drug in the brain. The drug does not cause a permanent change in the state of the depressed brain; hence, the drug is not a permanent cure for depression.

CASE STUDIES

Beatrice and Derek both suffered from depression, but their symptoms were quite different. We tell their stories to illustrate the effectiveness of drug treatment on two people who had quite different patterns of symptoms.

Beatrice: Depression with Agitation

For several years, Beatrice had been irritable, but for the last six months before she saw a psychiatrist, her irritability bordered on the irrational. She screamed in anger or sobbed in despair at every dirty dish left on the coffee table or on the bedroom floor. Each day the need to plan the dinner menu provoked agonizing indecision. How could all the virtues or, more likely, the vices of hamburgers be accurately compared to those of spaghetti? A glass of spilled milk was an occasion for panic. Beatrice would bolt from her chair and run from the dining room. Ten minutes later, she would realize that the spilled milk was insignificant. She had her whole family walking on eggs. She thought they would be better off if she were dead.

Beatrice could not cope with her job. As a branch manager of a large chain store, she had many decisions to make. Unable to make them herself, she would ask employees, who were much less competent, for advice, but then she could not decide whose advice to take. Each morning before going to work, she complained of nausea. In public she was usually able to control her feelings of desperation and felt a little better when she actually arrived at work and was away from the wary eyes of her family.

Beatrice's husband loved her, but he did not understand what was wrong. He thought that she would improve if he made her life easier by taking over most of the housework, cooking, and child care. His attempt to help only made Beatrice feel more guilty and worthless. She wanted to make a contribution to her family. She wanted to do the chores "like normal people" did but broke down crying at the smallest impediment to a perfect job. Because Beatrice's volatility put a stress on her marriage, the couple went to a psychiatrist for marriage counseling. The psychiatrist failed to diagnose Beatrice's depression. He provided marriage counseling that was designed for healthy people; consequently, the counseling failed. Months passed, and Beatrice's problem became more serious. Some days she was too upset to go to work. She stopped seeing her friends. She spent most of her time at home either yelling or crying. Finally, Beatrice's husband called the psychiatrist and insisted that something was seriously wrong.

After a diagnostic interview, the psychiatrist suggested that she enter the hospital. According to her hospital records, her diagnosis was pseudoneurotic schizophrenia, a category that had always been poorly defined and is no longer used. The psychiatrist prescribed an antipsychotic drug and group therapy. During the three weeks in the hospital, Beatrice relaxed, and her husband had a needed rest. After she left the hospital, Beatrice continued to take the antipsychotic as an outpatient. The drug decreased her agitation but did not stop the crying or lift the depressed mood. Continued psychotherapy also failed to help. Two years and several thousand dollars later, Beatrice decided to look elsewhere. She asked her psychiatrist to recommend a colleague. (That was not easy for a woman who could not decide between hamburgers and spaghetti!)

The second psychiatrist did not change Beatrice's medication immediately, but she did continue psychotherapy, trying to teach Beatrice to respond more rationally to other people's behavior. Beatrice agreed with this approach in principle, but it did not keep her from yelling at her husband and children and feeling worthless and guilty afterward. Finally, after a few tearful months, the psychiatrist began to question her colleague's diagnosis and prescribed antidepressant medication for Beatrice. Ten days later Beatrice told her psychiatrist that a 100-pound weight had suddenly been lifted from her shoulders. For Beatrice, it was not "a beautiful day, but . . ." anymore; it was simply "a beautiful day." No qualifications were necessary. Either hamburgers or spaghetti was fine for dinner. The psychiatrist was almost as delighted as Beatrice.

Beatrice has been taking antidepressants for three years. She tried drug holidays twice, but each time she became depressed and agitated within about ten days after stopping the medication. She may need drug treatment indefinitely.

Beatrice's response to antidepressants sounds almost too good to be true, but Beatrice's story is not fictional. We know Beatrice and are familiar with her psychiatric history. However, her story does not end here, because antidepressants did not solve all of Beatrice's problems. She remained somewhat irritable and unable to respond rationally to the inevitable small disasters of family life — the dent in the car and the leak in the washing machine. These remaining symptoms suggested that antidepressants alone were not adequate medication. Therefore, a few months after prescribing antidepressants, the psychiatrist added lithium (Chapter 15), and Beatrice became less irritable and less agitated. Now Beatrice rarely explodes. When she does, she recovers quickly. When the house is more cluttered than she can tolerate, she gets annoyed, but she no longer screams at the children. Beatrice's husband has a mate again. Her children see their mother laugh.

Beatrice, like Jill in Chapter 3, had difficulty getting the correct diagnosis. Because effective treatment depends on correct diagnosis, both women suffered needlessly for several years. Because Beatrice did not have schizophrenia, antipsychotics did not help her very much, in spite of the fact that phenothiazines do have weak antidepressant effects. Beatrice suffered from a major depression; antidepressants changed her life. Although Beatrice did not satisfy all the *DSM-III-R* criteria for bipolar disorder, she had almost enough symptoms to satisfy them. And lithium helped. Accurate diagnosis is not just an academic nicety; the patient's health and sometimes her life depend on it.

Beatrice's story illustrates the progress that psychiatry has made during the past twenty years. No one should be too critical of Beatrice's first psychiatrist. When Beatrice first became ill in 1969, diagnosis was much more difficult than it is now. The *DSM-III* had not yet been published. The criteria for the diagnosis of affective disorder had not been as well established. Different psychiatrists used different criteria, and many had no explicit criteria at all. They relied purely on clinical judgment. If Beatrice had walked into the office of her first psychiatrist in 1982 instead of 1969, he might well have provided the correct diagnosis.

Derek: Depression with Retardation

Derek's condition was less serious than Beatrice's. His depression was not incapacitating; yet treatment greatly improved his life. Derek had probably suffered from depression all of his adult life but was unaware of it for many years. Derek called himself a night person, claiming that he could not think clearly until after noon even though he was often awake by 4:00 A.M. He tried to schedule his work as an editorial writer for a small town newspaper so that it was compatible with his depressed mood at the beginning of the day. Therefore, he scheduled meetings for the mornings; talking with people got him moving. He saved writing and decision making for later in the day.

Derek had always been a thoughtful person and was often preoccupied. His family and colleagues grew used to his apparent inattention and absentmindedness. He often failed to answer people when they spoke to him. Sometimes they were surprised to hear his slow, soft-spoken reply 20 or 30 seconds later. His wife tried to be patient when it took him 20 seconds to respond to, "Do you want coffee or tea tonight?" Derek's private thoughts were rarely cheerful and self-confident. He felt that his marriage was a mere business partnership. He provided the money, and she provided a home and children.

Derek and his wife rarely expressed affection for each other. Occasionally, he had images of his own violent death in a bicycle crash, in a plane crash, or in a murder by an unidentified assailant.

Derek felt that he was constantly on the edge of job failure. He was disappointed that his editorials had not attracted the attention of larger papers. He was certain that several of the younger people on the paper had better ideas and wrote more skillfully than he did. He scolded himself for a bad editorial that he had written ten years earlier. Although that particular piece had not been up to his usual standards, everyone else on the paper had forgotten it a week after it had appeared. But ten years later, Derek was still ruminating over that one editorial.

Although Derek was distressed much of the time, the possibility that he had a psychiatric illness never occurred to him. First of all, he did not know anything about mental illness. Second, he certainly was not incapacitated. He did his job. He and his wife did not fight; they merely failed to love each other. He took care of his family. He participated in sports, playing basketball and softball for his newspaper's team in the city league. Occasionally, he took his family on overnight bicycle trips that required much initiative, organization, and energy. He was supportive of his children and interested in their schoolwork and friends.

Derek could be cheerful when the social situation required him to be. His colleagues found him pleasant and easy to get along with. But when by himself or alone with his wife, Derek could not keep up the illusion. His thoughts and talk reflected hopelessness and self-deprecation. Life was not much fun. Even Derek's recreational activities originated in a sense of duty to family or community. He would never be offered a job on a big city paper. Most important, he could not make his wife love him.

Derek attributed his inability to enjoy himself and his methodical, passionless marriage to his severe Anglo-Saxon Protestant upbringing. He had been taught that open expressions of affection were ill mannered. He had never seen his own parents embrace in their 50 years of marriage. In his family, humility was valued more than self-confidence. He had been brought up to do the "right thing," not to enjoy himself. Raucous merrymaking was only for the irresponsible. Even a game of Go Fish had to be played in secret when he was a child.

Derek brushed off his morning confusion as a lack of quick intelligence. He had no way to know that it was a symptom of depression. He never realized that his death images might be suicidal thinking. People do not talk about such things. For all Derek knew, everyone had similar thoughts.

Derek might have continued living his battleship-gray life, had it not been for the local college. One winter Derek signed up for an evening course called "The Use and Abuse of Psychoactive Drugs" because he wanted to be able to provide accurate background information in future newspaper articles on drug use among high school and college students. The course covered psychiatric as well as recreational drugs. When the professor listed the symptoms of affective disorders on the blackboard, Derek had a flash of recognition. Perhaps he suffered from depression.

Derek consulted a psychiatrist, who confirmed his suspicion and prescribed imipramine. A week later, Derek was sleeping until his alarm went off. Two weeks later, at 9:00 A.M. he was writing his column and making difficult decisions about editorials on sensitive topics. He started writing some feature stories on drugs just because he was interested in the subject. Writing was more fun than it had been in years. His images of his own violent death disappeared. His wife found him more responsive. He conversed with her enthusiastically and answered her questions without the long delays that had so tried her patience.

Antidepressants, however, did not solve all Derek's marital problems. Derek and his wife had gotten so good at doing their duty that they could not devote a day or even an evening to enjoying themselves without feeling guilty. Even the bicycle trips had been justified as being good for the children, nonpolluting, and good exercise. Derek and his wife had to learn to enjoy each other.

Derek's marital problems had been the result of his depression, not symptoms of it. His improvement gave both Derek and his wife hope that happiness was possible, that they were not forever controlled by the asceticism of their Puritan ancestors. They also obtained marriage counseling, hoping to solve the problems created by Derek's long-standing depression. The mood of Derek's marriage suggested that his wife might also be depressed. Therefore, the therapist's first task was to examine Derek's wife for symptoms of mental illness.

If someone is incapacitated by a psychiatric illness, the need for help will probably be fairly obvious. But that person may not be able to find treatment without help from a relative. If, like Derek, the person is not incapacitated, he will not get help without deciding that he has a problem. We are not recommending self-diagnosis or nonprofessional treatment of psychiatric disorders. Diagnosis and treatment decisions are the responsibility of the psychiatrist. But the psychiatrist will not have a chance to help a patient unless that person knows enough about psychiatric illness to guess that he or she may be afflicted and then seek diagnosis and treatment. Making that guess may prevent unnecessary misery. Derek suffered for many years because he knew nothing about mental illness and concluded he was just not an optimistic person.

EFFECTIVENESS OF TRICYCLIC ANTIDEPRESSANTS

Several types of drugs provide effective treatment for depression. This chapter discusses a group of drugs called tricyclic antidepressants. These are the most commonly used and the most thoroughly studied. They get their name from the three rings in their chemical structure.

Beatrice's and Derek's stories illustrate the changes that antidepressant drugs can produce in depressed patients, but anecdotes are not evidence. If you were skeptical that antidepressants really work, you might suspect that Derek's improvement was merely a placebo effect. After all, Derek was never really sick. You might further suspect that all people have periods when they are less moody and when they can concentrate better. Of course, the possibility of a placebo effect can never be ruled out when considering a single case history, but the improvement in Derek's sleep is a phenomenon that is not under voluntary control and can be verified by someone other than the patient. This improvement suggests that the drug effect is real. In this section we present more scientific evidence that tricyclic antidepressants really work.

An adequate evaluation of antidepressants is similar to an adequate evaluation of antipsychotics. First, to distinguish between spontaneous recovery and true drug response, researchers must include a placebo group in their study. The placebo control group is even more important in studies of antidepressants than in studies of antipsychotics because about 30–35 percent of depressed patients get well spontaneously during the four to six weeks required to test an antidepressant.[3]

Determining the appropriate dose is a second problem. Effective doses are not as well established for antidepressants as for antipsychotics. In many research studies, as well as in many doctors' offices, patients receive doses that are smaller than optimal.

A third problem is patient compliance with the physician's orders. Antidepressants are frequently given to outpatients. These patients often do not understand that the drug will have no effect for a week or more. When they do not feel better in a few days, they become convinced that the drug is not working, and they quit taking it. Other patients continue medication and feel much better after a week or ten days. But because they do not realize that they are likely to relapse without the antidepressant, they, too, stop taking the drug. Thus, many are depressed again when they return to the clinic for evaluation. Antidepressants taken according to directions and in adequate amounts may be much more effective than is indicated by the early studies.

Most studies of antidepressant effectiveness proceed somewhat as follows. Patients entering a hospital or outpatient clinic are diagnosed as depressed by the specific procedure used in that particular facility. (Because most of the classic research on antidepressant effectiveness predates the *DSM-III*, the patients studied in one facility may have had somewhat different symptoms from the patients studied in another.) After diagnosis, the researchers rate the severity of each patient's depression, using a standardized procedure, for example, the HAM-D.[4]

After their depression has been evaluated, patients are randomly assigned to either the drug group or the placebo group. The patients in the drug group most commonly receive either imipramine or amitriptyline, both tricyclic antidepressants. The experiment must be double blind; that is, neither the patient nor the mental health workers who rate his or her improvement know which group the patient is in. After the drug has been taken for one to four months, the severity of the patient's depression is rated again. Finally, the researchers break the code and find out whether the patients taking tricyclic antidepressants have improved more than the patients taking placebo.

About 90 studies measuring the effectiveness of tricyclic antidepressants were published between 1958 and 1972, and their findings are not all in agreement. About two-thirds of these studies found that antidepressants were more effective than placebo; the rest found that antidepressants and placebo were about equally effective. None found that placebo was more effective than antidepressants.[5] More recent studies have usually been designed to compare standard with new antidepressants, but because they usually include a placebo group, they provide additional confirmation of the effectiveness of standard drugs.

Tricyclic antidepressants are clearly an effective treatment for depression, but this does not mean that they are a desirable treatment. If they are only slightly effective, the risk of side effects may not be worth the benefits. Alternatively, other treatments may be safer and/or more effective. During a drug trial lasting a few months, a depressed patient has about a 70 percent chance of improving on antidepressants and about a 30–35 percent chance of improving on placebo.[6] Antidepressant drugs approximately double the chance for improvement. (In comparisons to antipsychotics, antidepressants do not seem very impressive. Very few schizophrenia patients improve on placebo, but about 90 percent improve on antipsychotics.) If the patient has been depressed for only a few weeks and is not in severe distress, patient and physician may decide to wait and hope for spontaneous remission. But if the patient, like Beatrice or Derek, has been troubled by depression for years, he or she should probably begin antidepressant therapy.

WHAT SYMPTOMS ARE RELIEVED?

Do tricyclics and other antidepressants decrease all the symptoms of depression? Or do they just improve some while leaving others intact? You might intuitively predict that medication would be effective for the symptoms that people usually think of as biological, such as sleep disturbance and appetite suppression, but would not work as well on guilt and depressed mood. In fact, antidepressants improve virtually every symptom of major depression as described in the

DSM-III-R, but the changes in biological, or vegetative, symptoms are most pronounced.[7] Antidepressants decrease sleep disturbance, especially early morning awakening. Like Derek, most patients stop waking up several hours before the alarm goes off. They begin to eat more and to gain weight. Antidepressants improve mood and change hopelessness to hope. For example, Beatrice felt that the weight of the world had been lifted from her shoulders. Antidepressants also relieve guilt. Suddenly, Beatrice could accept the love her family had been giving her for so long. Derek stopped scolding himself for the bad editorial he had written ten years earlier. In addition, antidepressants can change apathy to activity. Beatrice began to share responsibilities for making dinner, helping the children with their homework, and cleaning the house, and she felt proud of herself. Antidepressants also relieve anxiety. Before treatment, Beatrice constantly anticipated failure. She was certain that a glass of milk would spill at dinner and that she would scream at the offender, spoiling the meal for the entire family. Now she has confidence that she can accept minor accidents.

With the help of antidepressants, patients not only move faster, they also think faster. Because "mood disorder" is a catchword for depression and because the depressed mood is the most pervasive symptom to an observer, the patients' complaints of cognitive confusion and an inability to make decisions tend to be neglected. Recall that Derek claimed that he was too confused to make decisions in the morning, but he felt that antidepressants decreased his morning confusion and enabled him to work effectively and make decisions throughout the day.

Derek's subjective evaluation of his improvement was probably valid. In several experiments on depressed patients, researchers measured cognitive difficulties before treatment and cognitive improvement during antidepressant therapy. In one experiment, people were asked to press one button in response to one stimulus and to press a different button in response to a second stimulus. Depressed people performed this task much more slowly than healthy people, but the patients increased their speed within a week of beginning treatment with antidepressants; in fact, their speed increased before other symptoms of depression were relieved. In another experiment depressed patients performed more poorly than healthy people in a short-term memory task, but the patient's memory became more accurate during antidepressant therapy. Memory

KVCC KALAMAZOO VALLEY COMMUNITY COLLEGE LIBRARY

often improved before the depressed mood lifted.[9] Unfortunately, cognition does not always improve. The sedative effects of some antidepressants can cause cognitive problems of their own (Chapter 13).

Derek's work and family life improved when his depression was treated. This effect, too, is supported by more rigorous studies. Measures of social and vocational performance improve when depressed patients receive a tricyclic antidepressant. Patients receiving placebo do not improve on these measures.[10]

LIMITATIONS OF ANTIDEPRESSANTS

Antidepressants are not, however, a sure cure for depression. Some patients simply do not respond. Others find the side effects, which include dry mouth, urinary retention, sexual dysfunction, constipation, and orthostatic hypotension (Chapter 8), unacceptable (Chapter 13). Some patients suffer far-reaching consequences of depression that antidepressants cannot undo. If depression has impaired work performance or damaged personal relationships, relieving the depression does not solve these problems. The patient does, however, become capable of working on them, perhaps with the help of psychotherapy.

Tricyclics and Bipolar Disorder

Antidepressants do more harm than good for some patients with bipolar illness. Even if they are given when the patient is depressed, the drugs can evoke episodes of mania. But for other bipolar patients, the combination of a tricyclic for depression and lithium for mania (Chapter 15) is very successful.[11] Therefore, a psychiatrist may prescribe a tricyclic antidepressant for a patient with symptoms of bipolar illness, such as agitation or hostility, but must watch carefully for manic or hypomanic behavior.

Tricyclics and Depression with Psychotic Features

Antidepressants help less than half the patients who suffer from depression with psychotic features (called delusional depression in the older literature).[12] Patients with depression with psychotic features believe things that are contrary to fact; for example, they may imagine that they have committed crimes or that someone is trying to murder them because they do not deserve to live. Simply believing that one's life has been worthless does not, however, qualify as a delusion. Perhaps antidepressants do not help most delusional patients because such patients have a thought disorder in addition to their mood disorder. Fortunately, almost 80 percent of patients with depression with psychotic features respond well to a combination of tricyclics and antipsychotics or to electroconvulsive therapy.[13]

Other Refractory Patients

Some depressed patients who are not delusional fail to respond to tricyclics. About one-third of the early studies found that antidepressants were ineffective, and recent studies find that 15 to 30 percent of the patients are not helped.[14] Three previously mentioned problems — inaccurate diagnosis, inadequate dosage, and poor patient compliance — may contribute to this lack of effectiveness.

The first step in evaluating a refractory patient is to determine that depression is the correct diagnosis. Improved diagnosis and selection of patients should increase the percentage of people helped. Patients who do not have an affective disorder and delusional patients treated with an antidepressant alone swell the ranks of drug treatment failures.

Second, the psychiatrist should be sure that the patient is receiving an adequate dose for an adequate period of time. A substantial percentage of patients treated with antidepressants receive an inadequate dose or have taken antidepressants for fewer than six weeks when the patient or mental health worker decides the treatment is not working.[15] Although incorrect doses are usually too small, occasionally a dose that is too large can prevent improvement.

Doses are often too small because a fixed dose of antidepressant produces widely different blood plasma concentrations in different people; some patients metabolize antidepressants faster than others. But plasma concentration is better correlated with effectiveness than is oral dose.[16] To study the effect of plasma level, plasma levels of the antidepressant imipramine and its active metabolite, desipramine, were measured in a group of patients who had all received the same dose of imipramine. The patients were then divided into three groups based on their plasma levels. The percent responding to the drug increased dramatically with plasma level (Figure 11–1).[17]

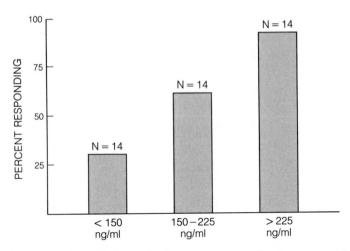

FIGURE 11–1 Effect of plasma level on percentage of patients responding to imipramine. ng/ml: nanograms per milliliter of blood plasma. (From A. H. Glassman, J. M. Perel, M. Shostak, et al., "Clinical Implications of Imipramine Plasma Levels for Depressive Illness," *Archives of General Psychiatry* 34: 197–204.) Feb. 1977. Data © 1977, American Medical Association.

A study of the effect of plasma level on response to desipramine confirmed that most patients who were nonresponders at usual doses had low plasma levels at these doses. But the investigators went on to show that these patients were not really nonresponders. In 10 nonresponding patients selected to receive larger doses, the plasma levels also increased, and 8 out of 10 patients converted from nonresponders to responders.[18]

The antidepressant nortriptyline has different requirements. The therapeutic response does not increase linearly with blood level; rather, it has a "therapeutic window": Plasma levels that are either too high or too low are ineffective.[19] When patients are taking either imipramine or nortriptyline, plasma levels can be very helpful in determining whether the dose is adequate. The usefulness of plasma levels for other tricyclics has not been established.[20]

Other studies have confirmed that 30 to 80 percent of patients who do not respond to tricyclics have received an inadequate dose and that about half of these do respond when their doses are increased.[21] If half the nonresponders receiving inadequate doses became responders when their dosages and plasma levels were raised, the effectiveness of antidepressants would increase from 65–70 percent to 85–90 percent, a substantial improvement.

Who Will Be a Refractory Patient?

Even though careful attention to providing an adequate dose decreases the percentage of tricyclic nonresponders to about 15 percent, this 15 percent represents 2 million U.S. citizens who remain depressed in spite of adequate doses of tricyclics.[22] If physicians could predict who would fail to respond to tricyclics, much grief might be avoided. A person who is unlikely to respond to tricyclics could begin an alternative treatment without spending six weeks on an ineffective one. Scientists have explored many techniques to identify both responders and nonresponders to tricyclics and other treatments, trying to base their classification on symptoms and on biological criteria, but the results have been inconclusive.

Most depressed patients who respond abnormally to dexamethasone do respond normally when their depression improves; some, however, fail to normalize. Those who fail to normalize are more likely to have an early relapse and to have a poorer long term outcome than those who do normalize.[23] There are no specific alternative recommendations for this group.

If a patient fails to respond to tricyclics, alternative treatments should be tried even if the patient does not belong to a specifically characterized group of nonresponders. Monoamine oxidase inhibitors (Chapter 12) sometimes work where tricyclics fail.[24] Patients with "atypical depression," for example, may do better on monoamine oxidase inhibitors. These patients eat and sleep too much rather than too little, they are worse in the evening rather than the morning, and they may be anxious and phobic (Chapters 17 and 19).

Adding lithium to the tricyclic sometimes helps. Although lithium is usually used for treatment of bipolar disorder (Chapter 15), it helps about half the patients with depression who do not respond to tricyclics alone.[25] Other patients who fail to improve on tricyclics respond to ECT.[26] The development of new antidepressants presents yet another possibility. Several new drugs, for example, fluoxetine (Prozac) have been introduced in the United States since 1980, but we do not have good data on the response of tricyclic nonresponders to these new drugs. Some patients may do better with psychotherapy

(Chapter 13) than with drug treatment. Unfortunately there will always be a few patients who are not helped by any of the available treatments.

PREVENTING RELAPSES

After a depressed patient has obtained relief from antidepressant medication, can he expect to remain symptom free or will he suffer a relapse? Unfortunately, without continued treatment, about 30 to 50 percent of the patients relapse within 6 to 12 months, and 75 percent relapse within two years.[27] However, this relapse rate can be decreased by continuing the treatment after the symptoms remit.[28] G. L. Klerman's group at the NIMH treated a group of depressed patients with a tricyclic antidepressant for six weeks and selected only those who responded favorably to participate in the maintenance phase of the project.[29] During the maintenance phase, one group of patients received a tricyclic for the next eight months, while two control groups received either a placebo or no treatment. Only 12 percent of the tricyclic group but about 33 percent of the control groups relapsed during the maintenance period. Other studies have produced similar results.[30]

A more recent study followed patients for a much longer time — two years. About 45 percent of the patients who continued medication but 75 percent of the patients switched to placebo relapsed over the two-year period (Figure 11–2).[31] Clearly antidepressants help prevent relapse, but many patients relapse in spite of continuing medication. We do not know how to interpret the relapses that occur in patients who continue to take antidepressants. Relapses might be due to failure to take medication or to lowering of the dose, but more likely the drug simply does not continue to work in some patients.

The high incidence of relapses suggests that patients should not stop taking antidepressants as soon as their depression is in remission. How long drug therapy should continue is not well established. The results of Klerman and his colleagues suggest that six to eight months of maintenance therapy can prevent a first-episode patient from becoming a chronic patient.[32] A recent study from the NIMH suggests that eight months may not be necessary, but a symptom-free patient should stay on medication for four to five months.[33] Perhaps

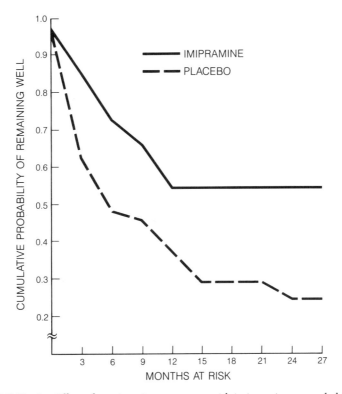

FIGURE 11–2   Effect of continuation treatment with imipramine on probability of not suffering a depressive relapse. (Modified from R. F. Prien et al., "Drug Therapy in the Prevention of Recurrences in Unipolar and Bipolar Affective Disorders," *Archives of General Psychiatry* 41: 1096–104.) Nov. 1984. Data © 1984, American Medical Association.

maintaining treatment permits a more complete recovery and forestalls the development of a lifelong problem.

In spite of psychiatrists' best efforts, depression is sometimes a chronic disease. It is for Beatrice. Antidepressants work for her, but she relapsed when she and her psychiatrist experimented with a drug-free period. About 15 to 20 percent of depressed patients have multiple relapses and thus appear to have a chronic illness.[34] Even after several years of successful treatment with psychotherapy and antidepressants, some patients relapse within a few months when the antidepressant is replaced with placebo.[35] These patients need indefinite medication. The only way to determine whether a particular patient needs continuing medication is to withdraw it and observe the consequences.

MISUSE OF ANTIDEPRESSANTS

Like any drug, antidepressants can be misused by physicians. Physicians may prescribe them without paying adequate attention to diagnosis. An incorrect diagnosis can have consequences far more serious than a few unnecessary side effects and the wasting of money. On rare occasions, antidepressants have provoked a psychotic episode in patients with schizophrenia. Careful discrimination between depression and bipolar illness is important because antidepressants used alone can provoke an episode of mania in a bipolar patient.[36] Depressed bipolar patients should receive lithium along with the antidepressant.

An inadequate assessment of the patient creates a danger of suicide by overdose. Unlike an overdose of phenothiazines, an overdose of antidepressants can be lethal. The fatal dose is usually 10 to 15 times the prescribed daily dose.[37] Acute poisoning causes excitement and seizures followed by coma. In one to three days, the coma passes into a second phase of excitement and delirium. The patient must be monitored closely during an episode of antidepressant poisoning because there is a danger of heart failure.

Antidepressants are misused when they are prescribed without careful consideration of the side effects (see Chapter 14). For some patients, these side effects are potentially dangerous.

Antidepressants are misused if the physician does not carefully explain the treatment to the patient. Because hopelessness is a symptom of depression, the patient who expects rapid relief and does not find it may despair quietly, conclude, "Nothing works for me," and then stop taking the medication. D. A. W. Johnson in Manchester, England, examined the compliance of patients receiving antidepressants prescribed by primary care physicians. Five weeks after their first visit to the doctor, 57 percent of the patients who still felt depressed had stopped taking their medication. Most of these patients stopped because they did not feel better in a few days and concluded that the drug was not working. Others stopped because of side effects, because they did not believe that medication was the correct approach to their problems, or because of fear of dependence or addiction. The physicians had little chance to correct misconceptions because the patients ignored the doctors' requests to return for follow-up care.[38] Unless pharmacotherapy is combined with frequent patient contact, even if it is not an organized program of psychotherapy, it is unlikely to be effective.

UNDERUSE OF ANTIDEPRESSANTS

Antidepressants are frequently underused; that is, they are not prescribed for patients who might benefit from them. In 1975–76 Myrna Weissman and her colleagues were interested in whether most patients suffering from depression received adequate treatment. They gave psychiatric interviews with questions about drug treatment to over 500 adults from a random sample of the population of New Haven, Connecticut. Fifty-five percent of the people suffering from depression had taken psychoactive drugs within the past year, but only 17 percent had taken antidepressants; 35 percent had taken antianxiety drugs, and 17 percent had taken barbiturates. (Some had taken more than one kind of drug.)[39]

Unfortunately, the situation has not improved very much in the past 15 years. More recent studies show that about three-quarters of depressed patients get their medical care only from primary care physicians, and only one-fourth to one-half of these patients have their depression recognized and treated.[40] Even if patients are treated for depression, the treatment is very likely to be inadequate. Over half receive antianxiety drugs rather than antidepressants. And only about one-third of those receiving antidepressants receive an adequate dose.[41] Treatment is only slightly better for patients admitted to large medical centers for treatment of depression.[42] A decision to use psychotherapy rather than drug therapy does not account for the lack of adequate drug therapy: Only half the inpatients and one-fifth of the outpatients received more than one hour of psychotherapy per week. Not surprisingly, the recovery rate for these patients is substantially lower than the recovery rate for patients in research trials where drug levels are monitored and great care is taken that drug levels are adequate.

The failure of nonpsychiatric physicians to diagnose and prescribe adequately for patients with affective disorder is illustrated in a study conducted by J. H. Barbar in Glasgow, Scotland. Researchers examined 101 patients diagnosed as depressed by physicians in general practice. The physicians spent an average of six minutes with each patient before diagnosing and prescribing. They referred only 2 percent of the patients to psychiatrists and prescribed drugs for about 90 percent of them. Although the physicians had diagnosed all of these patients as suffering from depression, they prescribed antidepressants for only about 75 percent of them. They prescribed sedatives, antianxiety drugs, and antipsychotics for the remainder. Not only was the diagnosis perfunctory, but the medication prescribed was frequently inconsistent with the diagnosis. Furthermore, when antidepressants were prescribed, the dose was often too small to be effective.[43]

Similar results were obtained in the study conducted in Manchester, England. In this study, as in the Glasgow one, researchers found that many depressed patients received an antianxiety drug rather than an antidepressant. Thirty-five percent of those receiving an antidepressant drug received a dose so small that it probably had little or no effect.[44]

As the NIMH studies show, similar prescribing practices prevail in the United States. Most physicians practicing in general hospitals prescribe antidepressants, but the average daily doses are far too small to be effective. Not surprisingly, the doctors who complained that the drugs were ineffective were those who prescribed very small doses.[45]

An interesting sidelight to the Manchester study is that the researchers asked the physicians where they got their information about the drugs they prescribed. Their answer was always "From the drug companies." Apparently, even this information never reached the patients. Patients claimed to receive their information from the mass media, not from their physicians.

It should not be surprising that nonpsychiatric physicians frequently fail to correctly diagnose patients with affective disorders. The physician will not suspect depression unless the patient gives a hint, any more than the physician will suspect appendicitis unless the patient complains of a pain on the right side. Primary care physicians may fail to diagnose depression in patients who come to the office with vague complaints that do not fit a nonpsychiatric diagnosis. Not being skilled at psychiatric diagnosis, the doctor does not recognize depression. Under pressure from the patient to "do something," the doctor may prescribe benzodiazepines, which are antianxiety drugs, not antidepressants (Chapter 17). These drugs are not very effective in the treatment of major depressive disorder.

If depression is diagnosed, failure to treat is less excusable, but the physician may not always be at fault. Some patients refuse treatment, sometimes out of fear that treatment for a mental health problem will adversely affect their insurance or employment status. In a recent survey only 12 percent of Americans said that they would take medication for depression.[46]

Failure to diagnose and treat depression not only deprives patients of adequate treatment. It may actually create a drug abuse problem if the patients self-medicate with alcohol or obtain multiple prescriptions of barbiturates or antianxiety drugs (see Chapter 17).

The NIMH is concerned about the underdiagnosis and undertreatment of depression. Physicians there are developing an educational program directed at both the public and health care professionals. Their goals include making the public more aware that depression is an illness rather than a weakness, making the public more aware of the availability of treatment, and making health care professionals more knowledgeable about diagnosis and treatment.[47]

ADDICTION AND TOLERANCE

Like antipsychotics, antidepressants do not produce addiction in the usual sense of the term. (See Chapter 17 for a full description of addiction.) They do not produce euphoria and hence do not tempt patients to take more than is medically justified. Furthermore, these drugs have no recreational value for nonpatients.[48] Usually, the drugs do not bring harm to the user or to others; the benefits of the drugs far exceed their harmful side effects. In addition, antidepressants do not cause tolerance; that is, the patient does not need to progressively increase the dose to maintain the antidepressant effect.

In a sense, antidepressants do produce physiological dependence. A patient who suddenly stops taking antidepressants may experience a withdrawal syndrome that includes muscle aches, gastrointestinal distress, and anxiety.[49] These symptoms sound alarmingly similar to the symptoms of opiate withdrawal, but the two syndromes are not the same. A patient who tapers the withdrawal of antidepressant over a two-week period usually has no discomfort, whereas even gradual opiate withdrawal over 10 to 15 weeks causes withdrawal symptoms. Further, the antidepressant patient will not crave antidepressants once withdrawal is complete. Of course, a patient who becomes depressed again may want to resume the medication, but this is rational, not addictive, behavior. In contrast, detoxification usually does not terminate the craving of the opiate addict, who continues to crave the drug for months or years or, some addicts say, forever.

12

OTHER TREATMENTS
FOR DEPRESSION

—

T ricyclic antidepressants are not the only somatic treatments
for depression. Among the other types of drugs used, monoamine oxidase inhibitors (MAOIs) are the oldest and best
studied. In this chapter we also discuss fluoxetine (trade name,
Prozac), one of the new drugs introduced in the past 10 years. This is
followed by a discussion of a nondrug somatic treatment for depression, electroconvulsive therapy (ECT). ECT is an important weapon
against severe depression that fails to respond to drugs. The last
portion of this chapter deals with psychotherapy as a treatment for
depression.

MONOAMINE OXIDASE INHIBITORS

MAOIs, the second most common chemical treatment for depression, are named for their biochemical function: They inhibit monoamine oxidases, the enzymes that break down monoamines (the transmitters norepinephrine, dopamine, and serotonin are monoamines). Although these drugs are clearly more effective than placebos in the treatment of depression,[1] psychiatrists disagree about whether MAOIs are as effective as tricyclics. Some of the early studies found that MAOIs did not work as well as tricyclics, while others showed that the two treatments were equally effective.[2] More recent studies have confirmed that MAOIs and tricyclics are equally effective.[3] One possible explanation for the conflict between earlier and more recent studies is that the earlier studies used inadequate doses of MAOI. To be certain that a dose of an MAOI is adequate, the actual inhibition of monoamine oxidase should be measured in the blood. A second possibility is that the diagnosis was incorrect in the earlier studies. These studies predate modern diagnostic procedures, and many have included patients who did not meet the *DSM-III* or *DSM-III-R* criteria for major depression or the modern criteria for atypical depression.

Studies from Columbia University and the New York State Psychiatric Institute found that patients with atypical depression respond particularly well to MAOIs. Although atypical depression is not a *DSM-III-R* category, it is used by many research psychiatrists. A diagnosis of definite atypical depression requires mood reactivity, which means that the patient feels better temporarily when something good happens. It also requires at least two symptoms from the following list: overeating, oversleeping, extreme fatigue, and chronic oversensitivity to rejection. A diagnosis of probable atypical depression requires mood reactivity and one other symptom. About 70 percent of patients with either definite or probable atypical depression responded to MAOIs, while only about 40 percent of these patients responded to imipramine.[4] In these studies the doses of both drugs were adequate.

Researchers have not performed a definitive study to test the hypothesis that MAOIs are the treatment of choice for atypical depressives while tricyclics are better for melancholic patients. Such a study would require diagnosing a group of depressives as atypical or melancholic and randomly assigning them to a tricyclic or an MAOI.

After 6 to 12 weeks of treatment, each patient would be rated by a psychiatrist who had not made the original determination that a patient was atypical or melancholic. Such a study would enable us to find out whether patients with a particular group of symptoms respond better to tricyclics or better to MAOIs.

Although most psychiatrists in the United States use MAOIs less frequently than tricyclics,[5] there are a number of good reasons to try MAOIs. First, some patients who are refractory to tricyclics respond well to MAOIs. Second, the two types of drugs have different side effects, and some patients who cannot tolerate tricyclic side effects do well on MAOIs. For example, a physician who prescribed tricyclics for an elderly male suffering from depression might find that these drugs cause urinary retention as a side effect; this physician might then prescribe an MAOI before deciding that pharmacologic treatment was not possible. Finally, people with atypical depression are more likely to respond to MAOIs. However, the greater safety of tricyclics (see Chapter 13) can be a good reason for trying a tricyclic first.

NEW ANTIDEPRESSANT DRUGS

Since the advent of tricyclics and MAOIs, a large number of "second-generation" antidepressants have been introduced. Describing all of them would be impractical. (Some not described in the text are listed in the Appendix.) When these drugs were first marketed, scientists hoped that they would be more effective than the tricyclics and would take effect more rapidly. The 7 to 21 day wait between beginning treatment and relief of symptoms is one of the tricyclics' big drawbacks. In fact, the new drugs turned out to be about as effective as imipramine and amitryptiline and to have a similar time course. But the side effects of each new drug are quite different from those of the old drugs and from those of the other new drugs (Chapter 14). The existence of the new drugs makes it more likely that each patient can find an antidepressant with an acceptable spectrum of side effects.

One of the most interesting of the new antidepressants is fluoxetine. Fluoxetine has much more specific biochemical effects than do most antidepressants (Chapter 13), and so it might be expected to have more specific psychological and behavioral effects. Surprisingly, the efficacy of fluoxetine is very similar to that of imipramine and amitriptyline. Fluoxetine, like the tricyclics, relieves most symptoms of depression in most people.[6] Even though fluoxetine is no more effective than the tricyclics, it might be a better drug for many patients because its side effects are quite different and much milder (Chapter 14).

A recent well-designed study shows that fluoxetine is also effective in preventing relapses of depression.[7] Patients who responded to the drug by decreasing their Hamilton scores to very low values continued to take it for six months; then half the patients were switched to placebo for one year while the remainder continued to take fluoxetine. Over half the placebo patients relapsed during the year, but only a little over a quarter of the fluoxetine patients relapsed. Clearly, the drug helped, but just as clearly, it was far from perfectly successful. Because fluoxetine was the only drug used in this study, we cannot tell whether fluoxetine was more or less successful in preventing relapse than the standard tricyclic.

ELECTROCONVULSIVE THERAPY

Passing large amounts of electric current through the brain seems more like a punishment than a treatment. *One Flew Over the Cuckoo's Nest* has fed public disapproval of electroconvulsive therapy (ECT), just as it has fed public disapproval of antipsychotic drugs.[8] The shock treatment described in Kesey's book inspires sheer terror. When shock hits Kesey's hero McMurphy, his convulsing muscles "bridges him up off the table till nothing is down but his wrists and ankles. . . ."[9] Chief, one of McMurphy's fellow patients, describes the aftermath of shock treatment as "that gray zone between light and dark, or between sleeping and waking, or between living and dying, where you know you're not unconscious anymore, but don't know yet what day it is or who you are or what's the use of coming back at all — for two weeks."[10] Every reader and movie patron feels the terror with McMurphy and Chief. ECT as depicted by Kesey is all risk and no benefit. And, indeed, ECT was not an appropriate treatment for McMurphy, because he had no diagnosable condition that justified it. However, modern ECT is a very effective treatment for depression and is not the harrowing experience described by Kesey.[11]

Uses and Effectiveness of ECT

A physician may elect to use ECT for a number of reasons. Depression with psychotic features is the most common indication for ECT. Only 40 percent of patients with this diagnosis improve on tricyclics, but 80 to 90 percent of the drug failures improve with ECT. Because these patients fare so poorly with antidepressants, some psychiatrists believe that it is a waste of time to try drugs and that ECT should be the first treatment.[12] Others, however, have found that almost 80 percent of delusional depressed patients improve on a combination of antidepressant and antipsychotics, suggesting that this treatment is as effective as ECT.[13] If both treatments are equally effective, it is not clear which is preferable. The drug treatments are less invasive but have more side effects than ECT.

ECT is an appropriate treatment for several other groups of patients:

1. Patients who do not improve with drugs: These patients have an 80 to 90 percent chance of improving with ECT.[14]
2. Severely depressed patients who cannot tolerate the side effects of antidepressant drugs.
3. Pregnant depressed patients: ECT is much safer than antidepressant drugs for the fetus.
4. Patients with severe medical illnesses: The cardiovascular side effects of tricyclics may be dangerous for these people.

Like the other treatments we have discussed, ECT is not a permanent cure for depression. Without maintenance treatment, about half the patients relapse within a year. If, however, ECT is followed up by prophylactic treatment with tricyclics or lithium, the rate of relapse decreases to about 20 percent.[15] In one study, patients receiving no maintenance therapy were ill for about eight weeks during the first year following ECT; those receiving lithium treatment were ill for less than two weeks.[16] Clearly, patients whose depression is severe enough to warrant ECT should receive careful follow-up care.

Risks of ECT

Just how dangerous is ECT? Certainly, this therapy is less dangerous and less frightening today than in its depiction in Ken Kesey's novel. The convulsions and resulting bone fractures have been eliminated by the use of anesthesia and muscle relaxants. The administration of oxygen and artificial respiration ensures that the patient's brain and other organs will not be deprived of oxygen if breathing stops temporarily. Patients are required not to eat or drink for four to eight hours before each treatment so that vomiting is eliminated.[17]

In spite of these precautions, ECT is not entirely safe. Occasional deaths are reported, usually due to cardiac arrest. It is difficult to compare the number of deaths caused by ECT to the number of lives it prolongs because data on mortality from depression are scanty and vary from study to study. However, David Avery and George Winokur at the University of Iowa compiled mortality data from many different studies of depressed patients. Their summary suggests that about 10 percent of untreated depressed patients die during the three years after they become ill, whereas about 3 percent of the patients receiving ECT die during the same period.[18] According to these data, ECT saves the lives of about 7 percent of the people receiving it. On the other hand, ECT kills between 0.01 and 0.8 percent of the patients who receive it.[19] These statistics indicate that ECT prolongs between 10 and 100 times as many lives as it takes. An examination of death rates also supports the notion that ECT saves lives. During the three to five years following treatment, the death rate of patients treated with ECT is less than one-third that for untreated patients.[20] These calculations probably underestimate the number of lives saved by ECT because patients receiving ECT are usually seriously ill and therefore are probably more prone to suicide and accidental death than are other depressed patients.

One might suppose that passing large amounts of current through the brain must cause permanent damage. Indeed, ECT has caused visible brain damage in animal experiments, but more shocks, more prolonged shocks, or more intense shocks were used than are used in ECT treatment of depressed patients.[21] Some autopsy reports describe brain damage in patients who had received ECT, but there is no way to know whether ECT caused the damage. Many of these patients were severely disturbed. Their psychiatric symptoms might have been the result of brain damage that occurred long before they received ECT.

If a patient with brain damage dies shortly after receiving ECT, doctors can make a reasonable guess about whether ECT is the culprit. If the pathologist believes that the brain damage is recent, ECT might well be to blame. If the damage is several years old, ECT is not the cause. But because patients rarely die soon after receiving ECT, there is not enough information to draw any firm conclusions. The few autopsy reports describing recent brain damage in ECT patients predated the use of anesthesia and oxygen. Thus, inadequate oxygenation during ECT delivery might have caused the brain damage.[22] In the modern literature, we found only one case describing brain damage in a patient who died two months after ECT. In this patient the damage had clearly been present for more than two months.[23]

Most studies on the effects of ECT on brain structure have compared patients who had ECT to another group of patients that did not have ECT. This procedure provides little information about the effects of ECT on brain structures because many psychiatric patients have abnormal brain structure before they receive ECT. To find out whether ECT causes brain damage, the same person's brain must be compared both before and after ECT. In the only study we could find with before-and-after measurements on several patients, C. Edward Coffey and his colleagues used magnetic resonance imaging to examine nine patients suffering from depression with psychotic features. Many of the patients had brain abnormalities before ECT, but brain structure did not change as a result of ECT.[24] Of course, none of this rules out the possibility of microscopic changes in the brain cells and synapses, changes that could be just as devastating to brain function as gross damage visible at autopsy or with brain imaging techniques.

The only convincing way to find out whether ECT causes significant damage to brain function is to give patients sensitive neuropsychological tests of their ability to think and remember. Although most patients are confused and disoriented immediately after ECT, they recover from this confusion in about an hour.[25] According to the patients, memory loss is the only problem that outlasts this immediate confusion. Scientists have devised elaborate tests to learn whether this complaint is justified and have found that, to some extent, it is. Patients clearly have memory deficits for the first few weeks after ECT. They have difficulty in reading and recalling a short story or in drawing a geometric design from memory. They cannot remember current events, television shows, or past events in their own lives. For the most part, memory recovers completely by six months after treatment. One remaining deficit is amnesia for the period of a few weeks before and after the ECT treatments.[26] A second deficit occurs in patients who have received bilateral ECT, that is, ECT on both sides of the brain. These patients have a persistent deficit in remembering details of their lives before ECT.[27] Many researchers believe, however, that bilateral ECT is more effective than unilateral ECT and may be the appropriate treatment for the most severely depressed or suicidal patients. Current research is now directed toward finding out how to maintain the effectiveness of ECT while causing as little memory loss and cognitive impairment as possible. Investigators have varied electrode placement, amount of current used, and stimulus waveform. Unfortunately, it is difficult to draw simple conclusions from these experiments because all the variables interact. For example, there is great disagreement about whether bilateral ECT is more effective than unilateral ECT.[28] The issue is important because memory loss is clearly much greater with bilateral ECT.[29] It is also hard to resolve because electrode placement and the amount of current used interact: If the current used is the minimum needed to induce seizures, bilateral ECT is clearly superior, but with higher currents the two methods might be closer to equivalent.[30] Recently, some psychiatrists have experimented with brief current pulses rather than sine wave ECT. If the amount of current is properly adjusted, brief pulses are just as effective as sine wave stimulation. Again, this is important because brief pulse stimulation produces less memory impairment than does sine wave stimulation.[31]

ECT is a sensitive issue. Most people are offended by the idea of sending large jolts of electric current through the brain. Frankly, so are we. However, ECT is an effective and occasionally life-saving treatment for depression. In most cases ECT should be a treatment of last resort: When tricyclics, MAOIs, and psychotherapy have been given adequate trials and have failed, when the patient is still severely depressed and requires constant surveillance to prevent self-injury, ECT should probably be tried. But there are also patients for whom ECT might properly be the first treatment; these include the severely suicidal and those with psychotic features who probably will not respond to other treatments.

PSYCHOTHERAPY FOR DEPRESSION

We did not give psychotherapy very high marks as a treatment for schizophrenia. As we pointed out, the effectiveness of traditional psychotherapy may depend on the skill and personality of the therapist. Further, because neither the treatment procedures nor the treatment goals are well specified, the technique is almost immune to evaluation. The evaluations that have been done showed that psychotherapy could not cure schizophrenia or even relieve its symptoms, although it can help prevent relapse. However, the situation is quite different for depression. Several psychotherapeutic treatments for depression have been developed in such detail that essentially the same treatment can be given by anyone who is properly trained. In addition, the development of rating scales for the severity of depression has made it possible to specify what success means and to measure that success. As Myrna Weissman, a scientist at the NIMH, remarked, comparisons of psychotherapy and drug therapy can now progress "from ideology to evidence."[32]

Several psychotherapeutic treatments have come through such evaluations with very high marks. Not only do these new treatments work, but they are an affordable choice for a large number of patients. In some treatments a therapist meets with a group of patients, decreasing costs and increasing the number of patients who can be treated. Someone entering this sort of psychotherapy program as an outpatient will probably spend a few months and a few hundred dollars. In contrast, someone entering psychoanalysis will spend years and thousands of dollars.

Three well-defined psychotherapies—interpersonal, cognitive, and behavior—have been tested on depressed patients, and all three appear to be effective. Because this book focuses primarily on drug treatments, we discuss these psychotherapeutic treatments only briefly.

Weissman, Klerman, and their colleagues used interpersonal psychotherapy, which focuses on the patient's day-to-day interactions. The therapists describe their psychotherapeutic techniques as follows:

> "The therapy was primarily supportive in nature with emphasis on the "here and now," and oriented around the patients' current problems and interpersonal relations. Patients were assisted in identifying maladaptive patterns and attaining better levels of adaptive response, particularly in family or social interactions. Therefore, no attempt was made to uncover unconscious material, modify infantile drives or induce a strongly regressive transferance.[33]

Cognitive therapists base their approach on the belief that the patient's pessimistic interpretation of life experiences leads to depression.[34] The depressed person's thoughts develop from certain attitudes and assumptions; for example, a person may think, "Unless I do everything perfectly, I am a failure." Therefore, the therapists assign tasks designed to counteract this assumption. Success at each task gives patients confidence to approach the next one and shows them that their self-reproaches are incorrect.

Behavior therapy stems from the concept that people become depressed when they do not receive sufficient positive reinforcement for their efforts.[35] A positive reinforcement is any pleasant event that is contingent upon the person's behavior. A smile in return for a compliment or a Friday night movie after a week's hard work are both positive reinforcements. Behavior therapists try to teach depressed people skills that will increase the number of positive reinforcements they receive. Learning social skills increases the reinforcements received from other people, participating in pleasant events increases the reinforcements from the environment, and learning self-control increases feelings of self-worth.

Effectiveness of Psychotherapy

While each psychotherapy was developed independently, they have common elements and very similar outcomes.[36] For example, improving a patient's skills at making new social contacts could occur in the context of any of the three types of psychotherapy. Most,

although not all, research studies comparing drugs and psychotherapy compare at least three treatments. One group of patients receives psychotherapy with or without a placebo pill. Another receives antidepressant drug, usually along with some supportive
nonspecific psychotherapy. Finally, a third receives only a placebo,
along with supportive nonspecific psychotherapy. Depending on the
design of the study, other groups may be included. These studies
have found that drug therapy and psychotherapy are both effective
treatments for depression, but they have not found a simple answer
to the obvious question, "Which is more effective?" The answer may
depend on the patient population and on the criteria for success, as
well as on the treatment itself. In some studies, psychotherapy has
been found to be as effective as drug therapy.[37] Some studies show
that it is less effective than drug therapy.[38] Still other research shows
that it is more effective than drug therapy.[39] Probably the most
reasonable summary of the evidence is that all three psychotherapies
and pharmacotherapy are approximately equally effective for most
nonpsychotic depressed populations.[40] What we would like to know
is whether specific therapies might have advantages for specific
patients.

A new study organized at the NIMH by Irene Elkin and colleagues is worth discussing in some detail because it is much larger
than most other studies and is the only one that has compared
cognitive therapy, interpersonal therapy, and pharmacotherapy.[41]
The three treatments were compared with each other and with
placebo plus clinical management (nonspecific supportive therapy).
This study is particularly noteworthy because the psychotherapies
were not given by the people who invented them and because
independent clinicians, not the therapists, evaluated the patients.
Although the methods were exemplary, the results were not startling.
The treatments had a tendency to increase in effectiveness in the
following order: placebo plus clinical management, cognitive therapy, interpersonal therapy, imipramine plus clinical management.
But the only statistically significant difference was that imipramine
was better than placebo.

Although the ordering of treatment effectiveness did not change,
there were some surprises when the results from the most severely ill
patients were analyzed separately. These severely ill patients did very
poorly on placebo. Therefore, a comparison of the active treatments
with placebo produced more dramatic results. Imipramine's superi-

ority to placebo was much greater. Interpersonal psychotherapy was now statistically superior to placebo, but probably not as effective as imipramine. Cognitive therapy was slightly less effective than interpersonal therapy and was not statistically different from placebo (Figure 12–1).

Although the data from the Elkin study do not permit firm conclusions, they confirm our earlier suggestion that any treatment is likely to work for patients who are not severely ill. When a patient is severely ill, imipramine is likely to work best. Perhaps a combination of imipramine and interpersonal or cognitive therapy would work even better (see pg 214).

The percentage of patients actually completing a treatment is an important determinant of its effectiveness, and patients are more likely to complete a psychotherapy program than a drug program. Between 40 and 65 percent of patients receiving only drug therapy complete the treatment program, compared to 70 to 95 percent of the patients receiving psychotherapy.[42] On the other hand, more patients accept drug therapy to begin with. When patients are randomly assigned to drug therapy or psychotherapy, 32 percent of the psychotherapy patients reject their original assignment, while only 17 percent of the pharmacotherapy do so.[43] When all patients are considered, including those who reject their original assignment, 48 percent of the patients assigned to psychotherapy and 33 percent of the patients assigned to pharmacotherapy complete treatment. Thus psychotherapy does have greater patient acceptability, but the difference is not as great as the attrition rates indicate.

The reasons for the high dropout rate in the drug group are not completely clear. Treatment failure indicated by worsening depression was not responsible, because about the same number of psychotherapy and drug therapy patients dropped out for this reason. Furthermore, the drug patients did not drop out because they recovered and felt no further need for treatment. Most were still depressed when they left.[44]

The patients receiving drug therapy always receive some supportive contact with a psychiatrist, but the amount varies from study to study and is never as great as that received by the psychotherapy patients. Furthermore, the research design usually specifies that drug patients not receive any specific psychotherapy. The lower dropout rate in the psychotherapy group suggests that the additional therapist contact received by these patients is important in keeping patients in the program.

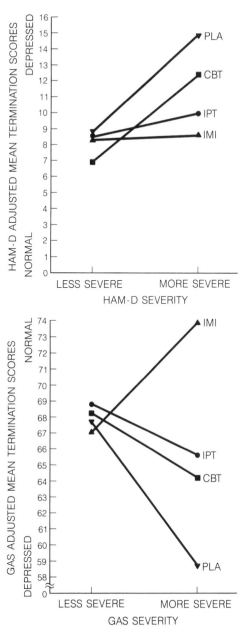

FIGURE 12-1 Effect of four different treatments for depression on less severely depressed patients and on more severely depressed patients. The top graph uses the Hamilton Depression Scale (HAM-D) as an index of effectiveness. Greater depression is indicated by high scores. The bottom graph uses the Global Adjustment Scale (GAS). Greater depression is indicated by low scores. IMI: impramine plus clinical management. IPT: interpersonal psychotherapy. CBT: a combination of cognitive and behavioral psychotherapy. PLA: placebo plus clinical management. From I. Elkin et al., "National Institute of Mental Health Treatment of Depression Collaborative Research Program," *Archives of General Psychiatry* 46: 971–82. Nov. 1989. Data © 1989, American Medical Association.

COMBINING DRUGS AND PSYCHOTHERAPY

If both psychotherapy and drug therapy are effective, is the combination better than using either one alone? Some studies suggest that the answer is yes, but others disagree.[45] Hope Conte and her colleagues at the Albert Einstein College of Medicine have tried to rate all the studies comparing drug therapy, psychotherapy, and the combination of the two based on the quality of experimental design. Using these ratings to measure the quality of the evidence that the combination treatment was better than either treatment alone, they conclude that the combination is indeed better, but only slightly so.[46]

The combination might be better than either therapy alone for either of two reasons. The two therapies might affect different symptoms, such that each treatment was effective precisely where the other was not. Alternatively, one treatment might work for some patients, while another worked for a different group of patients. Thus, more patients would be helped by the combination even though most individual patients actually responded to only one of the two treatments.

DO DIFFERENT THERAPIES AMELIORATE DIFFERENT SYMPTOMS?

We might expect drugs to have their greatest effect on symptoms that obviously reflect a biochemical problem, such as sleep disturbance and lack of appetite. Similarly, we might expect psychotherapy to be most effective in creating positive thoughts and in improving social skills.

Weissman and her colleagues at the NIMH compared interpersonal psychotherapy with antidepressants and found that these predictions were correct. Drugs had a greater and more immediate effect on sleep disturbance and appetite. They also improved depressed mood and anxiety, but the effect did not appear for several months. On the other hand, psychotherapy improved mood and anxiety within one month but had little effect on sleep disturbance. Although poor social adjustment does not contribute to a diagnosis of depression, it is worth noting that psychotherapy, but not pharmacotherapy, had the additional benefit of improving social adjustment over 6 to 12 months. Social adjustment was measured by work perform-ance, communication with others, and friction in relationships.[47]

Investigators disagree about whether cognitive therapy has specific effects on depressed thoughts compared to other depressive symptoms. Rush and colleagues found that cognitive therapy caused a greater reduction in hopelessness and a greater increase in self-esteem than did imipramine.[48] In contrast, Simons and her colleagues found that antidepressants and cognitive therapy had very similar effects on cognitive symptoms. They conclude that a change in cognition is essential to improvement and that any treatment that causes improvement of depression will cause improvements in cognition.[49]

WHICH TREATMENT WILL WORK FOR WHICH PATIENT?

How can a psychiatrist predict which patients will do best with psychotherapy, which with pharmacotherapy, and which with a combination treatment? This question is obviously important if each patient is to receive the most effective treatment without receiving unnecessary treatments. Several research teams have tried to characterize the patients that do best with each treatment. Unfortunately, their results are somewhat in conflict.

Weissman and colleagues at the NIMH found that melancholic patients did not respond to psychotherapy alone and required anti-depressants.[50] Optimal treatment for these patients was a combination of antidepressants and psychotherapy. The conclusion that melancholic patients require antidepressants is supported by a study done at the Western Psychiatric Institute analyzing dropouts from different types of treatments. People who dropped out of pharmaco-therapy tended to be only mildly depressed and nonmelancholic. The psychotherapy dropouts tended to be more severely depressed and to have melancholic symptoms.[51]

Blackburn and her colleagues came to a slightly different conclusion. They found that the most severely ill patients did best with combination therapy, but cognitive therapy alone was the treatment of choice for the other patients.[52] As mentioned, the recent NIMH study headed by Elkin also concluded that the most severely ill patients did best with drug treatment.

Blackburn and her colleagues and Rush and Beck and their colleagues all believe that severity is not necessarily the same thing as melancholia.[53] These investigators do not believe that the presence or absence of melancholia can predict which treatment will be more effective.

The disagreements among investigators make conclusions difficult to draw, but we will hazard a guess about what future research will show. Patients with severe depression accompanied by melancholia will probably respond best to a combination of antidepressants and psychotherapy. An antidepressant drug without psychotherapy will help, but is not the optimal treatment. Less severe depressions should first be treated by psychotherapy alone. Drugs should be added if the patient fails to respond to psychotherapy.

LONG-TERM BENEFITS

If a patient responds well to drugs and/or psychotherapy, are the long-term benefits greater for one type of treatment than for the others? To ask the question another way, does one treatment have only temporary effects, while another has long-term benefits? As usual, different research teams have different opinions. One year after the end of treatment, Weissman and her colleagues interviewed patients who were successfully treated with drugs and/or psychotherapy. They found that about 80 percent of them had no symptoms or only mild symptoms. If patients responded to the original treatment, their likelihood of staying well was not affected by the type of treatment they received.[54] Rush and Beck's group obtained similar, but not identical, results. One year after treatment, drug and cognitive therapy patients had similar depression ratings, but the cognitive therapy patients had less pessimistic and hopeless thinking.[55]

A more recent study came to a different conclusion. Although the initial effects of antidepressants and cognitive therapy were similar, relapses during the first year after treatment were more frequent in the groups that had received antidepressants.[56] Although the available evidence is far from conclusive, it suggests that the effects of cognitive therapy may last longer than the effects of antidepressants.

Is maintenance treatment with psychotherapy more effective than maintenance treatment with drugs? Weissman and her colleagues found that maintenance drug treatment decreased relapse rates but maintenance psychotherapy did not.[57] The difference between the two treatments was small, however, and did not demonstrate that drug treatment is consistently superior to psychotherapy in preventing relapse.

Scientists at the Western Psychiatric Institute in Pittsburgh recently reported conflicting results. They treated patients with a combination of antidepressants and interpersonal psychotherapy and then switched one group to continuation therapy with drugs and another group to continuation therapy with interpersonal psychotherapy. The relapse rate during the first year-and-a-half of maintenance treatment was much lower in the patients whose continuation therapy was interpersonal psychotherapy.[58]

CHOOSING BETWEEN DRUGS AND PSYCHOTHERAPY

The treatment chosen by a patient with chronic depression is often influenced by philosophical and emotional as well as medical considerations. Some depressed patients have a preference for one type of therapy before they enter treatment. Most of these patients are probably convinced that one is more effective, rather than that one is objectionable, because very few refuse combination therapy.[59] Patients may initially reject psychotherapy because they do not think it can possibly work for somatic symptoms, because it takes too much time, or because they do not like to take advice. Some patients refuse pharmacotherapy because they fear it will lead to a drug-dependent life or because they believe that if a drug does not effect a permanent cure, it is merely a "cover-up" and a "cop-out" and, as such, is morally reprehensible.

We do not agree with the objections to either treatment. Several types of psychotherapy have proven records as treatments for depression, and they are devoid of drug side effects. Unfortunately, the specific psychotherapies with a proven record in treating depression may not be available in every community. At any rate, for mildly to moderately depressed patients, psychotherapy, if available, should probably be the first choice.

If a patient is severely depressed, drug therapy may work better, although the evidence on this point is not yet entirely convincing. If psychotherapy does not produce substantial improvement in four weeks, drug therapy certainly should be tried. Antidepressants are not a cop-out even though they are not a cure. As we have noted, the only medical diseases that can be cured by drugs are those caused by bacteria. Most other illnesses, such as heart disease, arthritis, and ulcers, are chronic conditions. Like depression and schizophrenia, they can be controlled but not cured by drugs.

Although a chronically depressed person may need long-term antidepressant therapy, antidepressants do not create drug addicts. Most people would probably not object to a drug-dependent life if they were diabetic and dependent on insulin. Many women who refuse antidepressants probably do not mind being "dependent" on birth control pills; they may feel that chronic consumption of a drug that controls the ovaries is acceptable, but chronic consumption of a drug that controls the brain is not. (People are often unaware that birth control pills work because they affect the brain, which controls the ovaries.)

Chronic treatment with antidepressants is probably preferable to living with chronic depression. It is probably safe for medically healthy young and middle-aged adults. Some antidepressants may pose a danger to people with certain medical conditions, particularly cardiovascular disease, but some of the newer antidepressants are much safer and can be used even when these conditions exist.[60] When people with medical problems are treated with antidepressants, their medical condition must be closely monitored.

No one can know with certainty what treatment will work best for a particular patient. Beatrice (in Chapter 11) might have tried interpersonal or cognitive therapy if it had been available, but because she was severely ill, psychotherapy might not have worked. The psychotherapy that was actually available to Beatrice was not ideal, nor did it help her overcome her morning attacks of nausea, her inability to make decisions, or her irritability. When psychotherapy failed, antidepressant treatment should have been started promptly. Even if antidepressants posed some medical risk, Beatrice probably should have taken them. A person with milder symptoms might have elected not to take that risk, but depression for Beatrice was serious, and it was ruining her life: Her husband was running out of patience, her children were losing respect for her, and she was in danger of losing her job. Beatrice improved so dramatically with drugs that she did not continue psychotherapy, but continued psychotherapy probably would have helped even if it could not affect her symptoms of depression. Once Beatrice was well enough to make decisions, she could have learned through psychotherapy how to enforce them without provoking hostility. Once she managed to remain at the table when the milk spilled, she could have learned through psychotherapy how to ask for help with the cleanup.

Like Beatrice, Derek had melancholic symptoms and improved, as predicted, with antidepressants. However, his condition was not as serious. His job performance remained adequate. Because his schedule was flexible, he could work around his morning confusion. He could still enjoy his children. He could tolerate occasional bouts of inefficiency and guilt. If antidepressants had posed a serious medical risk, Derek could have rejected drug therapy. With or without drugs, Derek probably could have benefited from cognitive or interpersonal psychotherapy. Antidepressants alone could not alleviate his marital difficulties, whereas psychotherapy might help him improve his marriage, especially if his wife joined him in treatment.

It is hard to guess how long Beatrice or Derek or any other patient will need drug therapy or psychotherapy. Certainly treatment should continue for at least four months after symptoms have disappeared. And chronically depressed patients will need continual treatment throughout their lives.

THE BIOLOGY OF DEPRESSION AND SIDE EFFECTS OF ANTIDEPRESSANTS

—

T he brain of a depressed person is different from the brain of a normal person. When we discussed the causes of depression in Chapter 10, we found genetic and metabolic evidence for this assertion. But neither of these types of studies tells us about possible abnormal communication among nerve cells in depressed people. This chapter discusses three hypotheses about how the transmitters and receptors of depressed people might be abnormal. (These hypotheses are diagrammed in Figure 13–1.) The last portion of the chapter describes the side effects of antidepressant drugs.

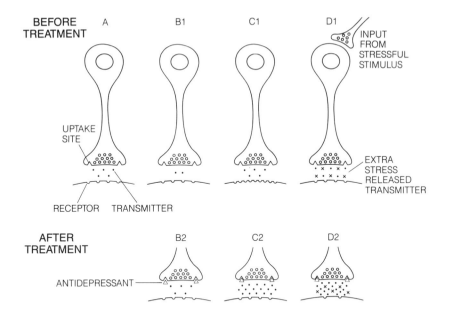

FIGURE 13-1 How antidepressants might affect synaptic transmission. A. A normal norepinephrine or serotonin synapse. B1 through D1 shows the state of the synapse before treatment; B2 through D2 shows the state of the synapse after treatment with a tricyclic antidepressant. B1. The norepinephrine/serotonin theory of depression states that depression results from inadequate norepinephrine or serotonin in the synaptic cleft. B2. Treatment with antidepressant blocks reuptake and increases transmitter in the cleft. C1. The supersensitivity theory postulates that depression results from an excess of receptors. C2. It is relieved when some receptors disappear from the membrane as a result of bombardment by extra transmitter. D1. The dysregulation theory postulates that in a depressed person stress causes too much transmitter release. D2. Antidepressants decrease the effect of this excess transmitter for two reasons. First, antidepressants increase baseline transmitter levels such that stress-released transmitter results in a smaller percentage increase. Second, antidepressants decrease receptor sensitivity such that the excess transmitter has less effect on the postsynaptic membrane.

EFFECTS OF DRUGS ON MOOD AND SYNAPSES

The major hypotheses about transmitter and receptor abnormalities originated in experiments investigating the biological effects of drug treatment. These hypotheses made predictions about how the untreated brains of depressed people might be different from the brains of normal people. For example, finding that a treatment for depression increases the concentration of a transmitter in the synaptic cleft predicts that depressed people will have an abnormally low concentration of that transmitter. Unfortunately, many of these predictions have turned out to be incorrect, and the interpretation of the original experiments has become increasingly complex. In the next few sections we trace the development of the original hypotheses and how they were modified by later experiments.

The Reuptake Hypothesis

Reserpine, a drug that was formerly used to treat high blood pressure, sometimes causes depression. It causes norepinephrine and serotonin[1] to leak out of synaptic vesicles into the interior of the synaptic terminal where they are destroyed by enzymes. Because nerve impulses can release only transmitter that is inside vesicles, reserpine treatment depletes the transmitter available for release. The fact that reserpine can cause depression suggested that depression might result from a deficiency of norepinephrine and/or serotonin. This notion is called the norepinephrine/serotonin theory of depression.

This hypothesis was supported and expanded by studies of the cellular effects of drugs that ameliorate depression. Iproniazid, the first MAOI, was originally used to treat tuberculosis. Physicians noticed that it also improved the depression that frequently accompanies chronic illness. This drug increases the amount of norephinephrine and serotonin in the synaptic cleft because it inhibits monoamine oxidases, the enzymes that destroy these transmitters inside the presynaptic terminals. Treating a patient with an MAOI increases the amount of transmitter released in response to a presynaptic nerve impulse. According to the norepinephrine/serotonin theory of depression, the increased transmitter release is the basis of the antidepressant action of MAOIs. After the discovery that iproniazid had antidepressant effects, a number of other MAOIs were shown to be effective antidepressants.

The discovery of tricyclic antidepressants provided additional evidence for the norepinephrine/serotonin theory of depression. The first tricyclic was imipramine, originally studied during a search for new antipsychotic drugs. It was not effective as an antipsychotic, but it did lighten the mood of many patients who had depressive symptoms in addition to schizophrenia.[2]

The Nobel Prize – winning biochemist Julius Axelrod and his colleague Jacques Glowinski showed that imipramine increased transmission at norepinephrine synapses by blocking the reuptake of norepinephrine into presynaptic endings. As a consequence, the transmitter was available for binding to postsynaptic receptors for a longer time.[3]

In their experiments Glowinski and Axelrod compared the reuptake of norepinephrine in the absence of the drug with reuptake in the presence of the drug. In their first experiment, they injected radioactive norepinephrine into the ventricles (fluid-filled spaces) of a rat's brain. Next, they removed portions of brain and washed it to remove any radioactive norepinephrine that was not taken up by the presynaptic endings. Finally, they measured the amount of radioactivity in the washed brain to discover how much radioactive norepinephrine had been taken up. In the second experiment, Glowinski and Axelrod measured the effect of imipramine on norepinephrine uptake. They repeated the initial experiment, but one hour before injecting the radioactive norepinephrine, they treated the rat with imipramine. The imipramine decreased the amount of radioactive norepinephrine taken up by the presynaptic endings. This finding indicated that imipramine increased the amount of time that norepinephrine is available to the postsynaptic receptor before it is taken up by the presynaptic ending.

Later experiments in which a variety of tricyclic antidepressants were used showed that these drugs inhibited the reuptake of norepinephrine and serotonin but not that of dopamine.[4] Antidepressants differ from each other in their relative abilities to block norepinephrine and serotonin reuptake. Some, like amitriptyline, have their greatest effect on serotonin reuptake. Others, like desipramine, have their greatest effect on norepinephrine reuptake. Still others, like imipramine, effectively block the reuptake of both transmitters.[5]

In summary, reserpine depletes norepinephrine and serotonin and causes depression. MAOIs and tricyclics increase norepinephrine and serotonin at the synapse and improve depression. These facts support the norepinephrine/serotonin theory of depression. Nevertheless, we cannot make as powerful an argument for the norepinephrine/serotonin theory of depression as we made for the dopamine theory of schizophrenia. We cannot state that the clinical potency of an antidepressant is related to its ability to block transmitter reuptake, because the various tricyclics are not very different from each other in potency, and therefore we cannot compare high- and low-potency drugs.

Unfortunately, other facts contradict the simple notion that a deficiency in norepinephrine and/or serotonin causes depression. First, reuptake inhibition begins as soon as the drug is absorbed into the blood, but relief from depression takes from 7 to 14 days. This time lag reveals that increasing norepinephrine or serotonin cannot, by itself, decrease depression. At most, it is only the first step. In addition, some very effective antidepressants, such as iprindole and mianserin, do not inhibit reuptake.

Receptor Sensitivity Hypothesis

Because an increase in the amount of transmitter in the cleft cannot completely account for the clinical effects of antidepressants, scientists have been looking for other possible effects of drugs on transmitters and receptors. Studies of the binding of transmitter to receptor show that about 10 days after beginning antidepressant treatment, the density of one type of norepinephrine receptor (the beta adrenergic receptor) and one type of serotonin receptor (the 5-HT2 receptor) decreases.[6] (By receptor density we mean the number of receptors per gram of brain protein.) This decrease in receptor density is called receptor subsensitivity. When a class of receptors becomes subsensitive, there are fewer sites where transmitter can bind to receptor. Most of the effective treatments for depression, including tricyclics, MAOIs, and electroconvulsive therapy, cause subsensitivity of one or both of these types of receptor. (It is not possible to test the effect of psychotherapeutic treatments on receptor density because psychotherapy cannot be done on animals and the measurement of receptor density requires removal of brain tissue.)

Mianserin at first appears to be an exception to this rule. This drug is an effective antidepressant but does not decrease receptor density. It does, however, decrease the postsynaptic biochemical effects of binding norepinephrine to its receptor.[7] Thus mianserin has the same ultimate biochemical effect as antidepressants that decrease beta receptor density.

The experiments on subsensitivity led to a second hypothesis for the cause of depression: Depression is caused by an excess of norepinephrine and serotonin receptors. We call this the receptor supersensitivity hypothesis of depression. The major evidence for this hypothesis is that the decrease in receptor sensitivity occurs at just about the time that antidepressants begin to alleviate depression.[8] But even this second hypothesis does not fit all the data. First, some new antidepressants that are extremely specific serotonin reuptake blockers may not decrease beta receptor density or the biochemical effects of norepinephrine receptor activation; this point is, however, controversial.[9] Second, electroconvulsive therapy increases sensitivity of one type of serotonin receptor, while all other treatments decrease it.[10]

Both the norepinephrine/serotonin deficiency hypothesis and the supersensitivity hypothesis make predictions about how the brains of untreated depressed people might be different from the brains of normal people. The deficiency hypothesis predicts that depressed people should have a lower concentration of norepinephrine or serotonin metabolites in their blood than do normal people. Metabolites of a compound are the molecules formed when a compound is broken down (metabolized) by the body. This prediction is difficult to test because scientists cannot directly measure transmitters in the human brain. However, they can estimate the total rate of transmitter synthesis by adding together the concentration of a transmitter and all of its metabolites in blood, urine, or cerebrospinal fluid. Recent measurements using this method suggest that at least some depressed people have too much, rather than too little, norepinephrine.[11] This is just the opposite of the result predicted by the transmitter deficiency theory.

Like the deficiency hypothesis, the receptor supersensitivity hypothesis has not been tested directly because receptor sensitivity cannot be measured in the brains of live humans. (PET scanning may make this possible in the future.) Scientists have substituted measurements of receptor sensitivity in a type of blood cell that has norepinephrine receptors. Unfortunately, the results of different investigators are inconsistent with each other. Surprisingly, the weight of the evidence is that depressed people have a decrease, rather than the expected increase, in norepinephrine receptor sensitivity.[12] Furthermore, depressed people amplify the effect of their decreased receptor sensitivity because their norepinephrine receptors have a decreased ability to promote biochemical responses.[13]

An added cautionary note: For simplicity we have been discussing brain abnormalities in depression as if only the beta type of norepinephrine receptors and the 5-HT2 type of serotonin receptors were involved. Other receptors for norepinephrine and serotonin and other transmitters, such as acetylcholine, GABA, and dopamine, may play a role.

Dysregulation of Transmitter Release Hypothesis

The transmitter deficiency hypothesis is inconsistent with the evidence that some depressed people have abnormally high levels of norepinephrine and its metabolites. The receptor supersensitivity hypothesis is inconsistent with the finding that depressed people already have subsensitive receptors. These paradoxes may indicate that we should not think about depression in terms of too much or too little of a particular transmitter or receptor. Rather, the regulation of norepinephrine release may be faulty. Many factors control norepinephrine release. Norepinephrine release depends on the release of a multitude of transmitters onto norepinephrine-releasing cells. The amount of norepinephrine released by an action potential changes with the state of the presynaptic terminal which controls release. The postsynaptic effect of the transmitter is also variable, depending on receptor sensitivity and the activity of postsynaptic enzymes associated with the receptors. In the depressed person any of these synaptic functions may be abnormal, such that the brain responds abnormally to the input provided by life events.

Some evidence for the notion that the depressed brain does not regulate transmitter release properly comes from an experiment measuring the increase in norepinephrine in the blood plasma when a person stands up from a lying position. This increase is much greater in depressed patients than in normal patients, suggesting that the norepinephrine system is overresponding to an environmental change requiring a change in norepinephrine release.[14] In thinking about how antidepressants might work, we emphasize the regulation of the transmitter receptor system. By increasing the amount of transmitter in the cleft and by decreasing receptor sensitivity, an antidepressant may increase the percentage of receptors normally occupied by transmitter. Thus an environmental stimulus will cause a smaller change in receptor occupancy, and the system will be more stable. In addition, the increased amount of transmitter in the cleft may stimulate presynaptic receptors and decrease the release of new transmitter, thus decreasing the amount released in response to an environmental stimulus. This, too, would increase the stability of the system.

It seems paradoxical that the antidepressants seem to amplify abnormalities in transmitter concentration and receptor sensitivity already present in depressed patients. Perhaps the abnormalities are the brain's inadequate attempt to compensate for a poorly regulated norepinephrine system. Antidepressants improve on this attempt.

Further evidence comes from studies relating the release of norepinephrine to corticotropin releasing factor (CRF). CRF is a hormone that indirectly stimulates the release of cortisol from the adrenal gland. In addition, CRF is a neurotransmitter. Acting as a hormone, CRF helps the body prepare for stress by causing cortisol release; acting as a neurotransmitter, it may help the brain prepare for stress. As known from the dexamethasone suppression test (see Chapter 3), many depressed patients have abnormal cortisol secretion. In response to a dose of dexamethasone, most normal people suppress the secretion of cortisol, but many depressed patients fail to do so.

Recent research by C. B. Nemeroff and his colleagues at Duke University suggests that high levels of CRF, which might be a response to real or imagined stress, may cause depression. They have two pieces of evidence for this. First, they find that CRF levels are abnormally high in many depressed patients.[15] Second, rats show many symptoms of depression, such as loss of appetite and decreased sexual behavior, when CRF is infused into their brains.[16]

Several types of experiments show that CRF is intimately involved with the norepinephrine system and that this relationship is disrupted by depression. First, norepinephrine-releasing cells in rats normally respond to stress like the stimulation of a nerve in the leg with excitation followed by inhibition; these responses are decreased if the rats are given CRF.[17] Second, normal people show an orderly correlation between the concentration of CRF and the concentrations of norepinephrine and serotonin metabolites in their cerebrospinal fluid. In many depressed people this correlation is absent.[18]

These results suggest the following scheme. CRF increases in depression. The increased CRF, acting as a hormone, prevents suppression of cortisol secretion in response to dexamethasone. The increased CRF, acting as a transmitter, causes abnormal responses in norepinephrine-producing cells. Thus, these cells lose their ability to respond appropriately to stress. In other words, norepinephrine release is improperly regulated.

SIDE EFFECTS OF ANTIDEPRESSANTS

Antidepressants are no exception to the dictum that all drugs have unwanted side effects.[19] Many of the side effects are transient; they are the worst during the first one to two weeks of therapy and tend to decrease thereafter. A few cause continuing medical problems. Here we discuss some of the most common side effects. Some of them can be understood from the effects of antidepressants on synapses. The biological bases of others, particularly those affecting complex brain functions, are unknown.

Anticholinergic Side Effects

Modifying norepinephrine receptor sensitivity and inhibiting norepinephrine and serotonin reuptake are not the only ways that antidepressants alter synaptic function. Blockade of certain acetylcholine synapses is responsible for the anticholinergic side effects—dry mouth, blurred vision, urinary retention, sexual dysfunction, and constipation.[20] These side effects are both more common and more severe in patients taking antidepressants than in patients taking antipsychotics, and tricyclics are worse offenders than are MAOIs. Most anticholinergic side effects are not serious, but urinary retention and severe constipation can be. Should either of these occur, the patient should alert his or her physician immediately. Anticholinergic side effects are particularly likely to occur with a sudden increase in dosage. For this reason, most physicians start the patient on a small dose and increase it gradually.

Patients requiring both antidepressants and antipsychotics must contend with more severe side effects. These patients include people with both schizophrenic and depressive symptoms, as well as delusional depressed patients. The two types of drug should be used together only with extreme caution because the anticholinergic effects of one can add to the anticholinergic effects of the other.[21]

Interactions with Norepinephrine and Dopamine Receptors

Fortunately, tricyclics do seem to distinguish between norepinephrine and dopamine synapses. Because these drugs do not block dopamine synapses, they do not cause the motor side effects that are so often troublesome to patients taking antipsychotics. In particular, tricyclics do not cause tardive dyskinesia. In high doses tricyclic antidepressants can block norepinephrine receptors. Scientists do not know whether this action is significant in humans at therapeutic doses.

Cardiovascular Side Effects

Tricyclics effect the cardiovascular system.[22] Some of these effects may be due to effects on norepinephrine and acetylcholine synapses, but others may be direct effects on the heart. Tricyclics can cause the heart to exhibit abnormal electrical activity and arrhythmias. Orthostatic hypotension, dizziness due to low blood pressure in the brain (see Chapter 8), is common in patients taking tricyclics. Occasionally, there is a decrease in the ability of the heart to pump blood, leading to cardiac failure. Rapid changes in blood pressure can also precipitate stroke. If elderly patients fall as result of orthostatic hypotension, hip fractures can occur. Most of these cardiovascular side effects are not problematic in healthy people, but they can be serious in patients with preexisting cardiac disease. Therefore, tricyclics must be prescribed with extreme caution for such patients.

Miscellaneous Side Effects[23]

Tricyclics can cause a variety of other side effects, some trivial and some serious. One is fatigue in a variety of forms: decreased energy, excessive sleep, lassitude. These effects are potentiated by alcohol. They are not serious unless the patient is driving a car or operating machinery. Other less serious side effects include weight gain, tremor, and tinnitus, a ringing in the ears. Seizures are a more serious consequence, and their likelihood is increased in alcoholics.

Cognitive Side Effects

When healthy people take any of the tricyclic antidepressants that have sedative side effects, such as imipramine and amitriptyline, their cognitive abilities decrease. The decrease occurs for intellectual tasks, such as memory, and for psychomotor tasks, such as performance in a driving simulator. The decrease is not just due to short-term sedation, which disappears with continued drug use; it is present even when healthy people take the drug for several weeks.[24] On the other hand, antidepressants that are not sedative, such as fluoxetine, do not cause cognitive or psychomotor impairments.[25] The fact that some antidepressants do not cause cognitive impairments implies that antidepressants do not work simply by dulling the mind or making one forget about the problems that "caused" the depression. Practically, these findings mean that nonsedating antidepressants should be used for patients who must operate machinery or do intellectual work.

The effects of tricyclics on cognition in depressed people is harder to assess because depressed people have cognitive deficits in the absence of medication. On the one hand, we would expect a sedating antidepressant to make matters worse. The actual data suggest that the net effect depends on the task. Memory probably improves in response to treatment with both sedating and nonsedating antidepressants.[26] Sedating antidepressants worsen performance on psychomotor tasks, while nonsedating drugs cause either no change or slight improvement.[27] Unfortunately, the lifting of depression in response to a sedating antidepressant may not make a person a safer driver.

Sexual Side Effects

Recent research has revealed that antidepressants and MAOIs alter sexual function. Getting reliable information about these effects can be difficult partly because many depressed patients have sexual dysfunctions prior to treatment and partly because patients do not bring up sexual side effects unless asked. When patients are asked about sexual functioning before and after treatment with tricyclics or MAOIs, more than half report impairments after drug treatment. The exact percentage varies with sex and the specific drug used. The changes include both decreases in motivation and impaired performance. Both men and women report a decreased ability to experience orgasm. Erectile function is less likely to be affected.[28] The effect is clearly drug related because placebo patients do not report significant changes in sexual functioning.[29]

To separate pure drug effects from psychosocial effects, a team of psychiatrists measured nocturnal erections on a group of normal men who were taking either antidepressants or placebo. Each man took each drug for two weeks, with a two-week washout period between drugs. Nocturnal erections decreased in both size and duration during antidepressant treatment.[30]

Physicians should query their patients about sexual changes during antidepressant treatment. If decreases in sexual function are distressing, they may cause treatment noncompliance. In such a case, perhaps the patient and physician should try another antidepressant. Unfortunately, we do not have data on sexual side effects for all antidepressants and so do not know with certainty which to recommend if sexual dysfunction is a distressing problem. Animal data suggest that increasing brain serotonin decreases sexual behavior, while increasing brain norepinephrine has more complex effects.[31] Therefore, a tricyclic like desipramine, which decreases norepinephrine but not serotonin reuptake, might have fewer sexual side effects than antidepressants that decrease serotonin reuptake. A few case reports suggest that this is, in fact, the case.[32]

Side Effects Peculiar to MAOIs

Because inhibition of monoamine oxidase prevents the normal metabolism of many foods and drugs, people taking MAOIs must avoid foods containing compounds that are rapidly metabolized by the liver of a normal person. For example, a patient taking MAOIs must avoid foods containing the amino acid tyramine. Since the patient's liver cannot efficiently metabolize tyramine, it enters the circulation. Tyramine releases norepinephrine from the nerve terminals that regulate blood pressure, causing a sudden increase in blood pressure and occasionally even a stroke. Smaller amounts of tyramine cause milder increases in blood pressure and a variety of unpleasant symptoms, such as a throbbing headache, nausea, and vomiting. Unfortunately, a wide variety of foods contain enough tyramine to be dangerous. Aged cheese is a major culprit, but many other foods, such as beer, wine, chocolate, and liver, are also hazardous.[33]

Likewise, patients taking MAOIs probably should not use nose drops or cold remedies that shrink mucous membranes. These drugs are chemically similar to catecholamines and are normally metabolized by monoamine oxidases. When MAOIs prevent the metabolism of these drugs, their concentration in the blood may become sufficient to cause dangerous increases in blood pressure.

Patients taking MAOIs must use many other drugs very cautiously and must take smaller doses than typically prescribed.[34] These drugs include alcohol, barbiturates, opiates, and tricyclic antidepressants. Because of the inhibition of monoamine oxidase, drugs metabolized in the liver remain in the blood and in the brain longer than they normally would. If a second dose is taken at the usual interval, drug concentration may become dangerously high. In addition, the combination of MAOIs and tricyclics poses a special risk. It can cause high fever, convulsions, and death. Some psychiatrists, however, believe that the combination can be used safely if the patient is monitored carefully so that any problem can be treated before it becomes serious.

Even a clear-thinking and conscientious person who is not depressed might have difficulty remembering all the prohibitions, from cheese to nose drops, that accompany MAOIs. Following complex instructions becomes more difficult when depression causes cognitive problems. The patient may eat dangerous foods inadvertently in a restaurant or when visiting family or friends. Furthermore, the suicidal patient can use the prohibited foods to serve his or her suicidal intentions.

Although the dangers are real, they should not preclude the prescription of MAOIs. For many patients, the benefits of MAOIs outweigh their risks. Fatalities are rare, about 0.4 per 100,000 patients.

Side Effects of Fluoxetine

The newer antidepressants differ from the tricyclics primarily in their side effects, and these are different for each drug. Fluoxetine (see Chapter 12) has no cardiac side effects or anticholinergic side effects, and it does not cause orthostatic hypotension,[35] so it is a very safe drug. Its main side effects are "nuisances," such as nausea, headache, insomnia, and nervousness. All of these except for insomnia decrease dramatically with time. After four to five months, only about 4 percent still have these side effects.[36]

CLINICAL DECISIONS

The physician may be uncertain about how to respond when a patient reports side effects from antidepressants. These side effects, like those of antipsychotics, are often similar to symptoms of the original disease; common symptoms of untreated depression and anxiety, such as fatigue, constipation, sweating, dry mouth, and palpitations, can also be side effects of antidepressant drugs. When a patient complains about side effects and the symptoms are merely annoying, the physician might (1) decrease the medication if he or she thinks the symptoms are due to overdose, (2) increase the medication if he or she thinks the symptoms are due to depression, or (3) keep the dose the same if he or she thinks the symptoms are normal side effects that will decrease with time. Of course, if the side effects are medically dangerous (for example, severe constipation or inability to urinate), the patient must cease taking the drug and be treated for the side effect.

There is no convincing evidence that one antidepressant is more effective than any other. Physicians frequently choose an antidepressant based on the patient's symptoms. It is a common belief that sedating antidepressants are the best choice for agitated patients and nonsedating drugs are best for those with psychomotor retardation. This method of selection is a commonsense approach, but research has not supported it. The antidepressant effect of a drug is unrelated to its sedative properties. Often, the choice of a particular antidepressant, like the choice of a particular antipsychotic, is dictated by its side effects. A person who must be alert on the job (for instance, someone operating heavy machinery) is usually given a nonsedating antidepressant. A person who has trouble falling asleep may be given a sedating antidepressant, with instructions to take the entire daily dose at bedtime.

LITHIUM AND
BIPOLAR DISORDER

—

We begin this chapter with the history of lithium treatment. We then provide a case study of a bipolar patient who was helped by lithium. Next we provide the actual evidence that lithium helps most bipolar patients. This is followed by a discussion of the controversial issue of treatment for mild mania. Lithium is used to treat depression as well as mania, and treating depression with lithium is discussed next. Sections dealing with the biology of lithium and lithium's side effects follow. Finally, we discuss alternative treatments that might be tried when lithium fails to work.

Bipolar disorder is much less common than major depression, but it is not a rare disease.[1] In fact, it is about as common as schizophrenia. The lifetime prevalence of bipolar disorder is between 0.5 and 2.0 percent, about one-tenth that of major depression. Bipolar illness is about equally common in men and women.[2] It usually begins in young adulthood, typically in the late twenties or early thirties. It is no respecter of social class or upbringing. Stress and loss, whether occurring in childhood or near the time of illness, cannot account for it.[3] The adoption study described in Chapter 10 suggests that genes play a major role.[4] Some studies found that the families of bipolar patients tend to be unstable, but this finding does not demonstrate that unstable families cause bipolar illness.[5] Another possibility is that the genes that afflict the children with bipolar disorder are also present in the parents, thus producing unstable families.

ENTRY OF LITHIUM INTO PSYCHIATRY

Lithium carbonate is a very effective treatment for bipolar disorder. Unlike antipsychotics and antidepressants, lithium carbonate is not a complex organic molecule; it is a simple metallic ion administered as a salt. Lithium was introduced into psychiatry in 1949 by John Cade, an Australian psychiatrist and researcher who was testing the hypothesis that uric acid caused excited behavior. When he injected the lithium salt of uric acid, lithium urate, into guinea pigs, they became calm and unresponsive instead of excited. When he put them on their backs, they lay quietly instead of trying to scramble to their feet. When he poked or prodded them, they did not scamper away. Cade concluded that lithium was a calming drug. In another of those leaps of faith that are possible only outside the jurisdiction of a strict drug regulatory agency, Cade tried lithium carbonate on ten patients with mania, on six with schizophrenia, and on three with depression. Only the manic patients were helped, but these improved dramatically.[6]

Although Cade's clinical trial was successful, his report generated very little interest among psychiatrists.[7] Maybe the psychiatrists just could not believe that a simple salt could treat a disease as complex as bipolar disorder, or perhaps they could not believe that a single drug could protect against both mania and depression. If either of those was the case, they were espousing the fallacy that causes many laypersons to reject all psychiatric drugs, that is, that drugs can only suppress, that they cannot normalize. Perhaps the psychiatrists were not excited because the drug companies had no interest in promoting a drug on which they could not make huge profits. Because the chemical is a natural mineral, it could not be patented and given a fancy name and an accompanying fancy price.

Until the middle 1960s lithium treatment and research were kept alive primarily by the Danish psychiatrist Mogens Schou, who firmly established the effectiveness of lithium. Schou's research persuaded most psychiatrists that lithium was an effective treatment for mania, but it was not approved by the U.S. Food and Drug Administration (FDA) until 1970.[8] The FDA held back out of concern that lithium was dangerous. In the 1940s lithium had been widely used as a salt substitute for cardiac patients. Dosage was not monitored, and consumption of toxic quantities led to coma and death in a few patients. The FDA scientists insisted on extensive testing before they were persuaded that, properly monitored, lithium treatment was safe. Finally, it was approved for treatment of bipolar disorder, but not for any other diagnoses.[9]

LITHIUM TREATMENT FOR MANIA

Lithium calms manic patients. Continued lithium therapy protects them against future manic and future depressive episodes. The drug's effects can be astounding. When it removes the wraps of mania, it often reveals a healthy person, one very different from the bipolar patient.

Anna's story illustrates the change lithium can bring about in the life of a bipolar patient. (Anna's story is elaborated from a case described by a team of well-known psychiatrists at the NIMH and the Illinois State Psychiatric Unit.[10]) Anna was a 21-year-old college senior. Before she became ill, Anna was sedate and polite, perhaps even a bit prim. During the fall of her sophomore year at college, she had an episode of mild depression that began when she received a C on a history paper she had worked quite hard on. The same day she received a sanctimonious letter from her father reminding her of the financial hardships he was undergoing to send her to college; he warned her to stick to her books and not to play around with men. Anna became discouraged; she doubted that she deserved her parents' sacrifice. Her depression did not seem unusual to her roommate, to her other friends, or even to Anna herself. It seemed a natural reaction to her father's unreasonable letter and her fear that she could not live up to the standards he set. In retrospect, this mild depression was the first episode of her bipolar illness.

Several months later, Anna became restless, angry, and obnoxious. She talked continuously and rapidly, jumping from one idea to another. Her speech was filled with rhymes, puns, and sexual innuendoes. During Christmas vacation, she made frequent and unwelcome sexual overtures to a friend of her brother's in the presence of her entire family. When Anna's mother asked her to behave more politely, Anna began to cry and then slapped her mother across the mouth. Anna did not sleep that night; she sobbed. Between sobs she screamed that no one understood her problems and no one would even try. The next day, Anna's family took her to the hospital. She was given chlorpromazine, which calmed her. When she was discharged two weeks later, she was less angry and no longer assaultive, but she was not well and did not go back to school. Her thought and speech were still hypomanic (slightly manic); she had an exaggerated idea of her attractiveness, expected men to fall for her at the first smile, and was irritated when they ignored her attentions. Depressive symptoms were still mixed with the manic ones. She often cried when her bids for attention were not successful or when her parents criticized her dress or behavior.

Anna returned to school the following fall but suffered another depressive episode, followed by another attack of mania within seven months. She had to withdraw from school and enter the hospital. This time, Anna was fortunate to enter a research unit that was authorized to use lithium. The psychiatrists diagnosed her illness as bipolar disorder. Because she was so agitated, they began treatment with chlorpromazine as well as lithium. The initial sedative action of the chlorpromazine rapidly calmed her agitation, and this drug was discontinued after only a few days. As the effects of the chlorpromazine subsided, the lithium began to take effect. After 17 days on lithium, Anna's behavior was quite normal. She was attractively and modestly dressed for her psychiatric interviews. Earlier, she had been sloppily seductive: hair in disarray, half-open blouse, smeared lipstick, bright pink rouge on her cheeks, and bright green makeup on her eyelids. With the help of lithium, she gained some ability to tolerate frustration. During the first week of her hospital stay, she had screamed at a nurse who would not permit her to read late into the night in violation of the ward's 11:00 P.M. lights-out policy. On lithium Anna was still annoyed by this "juvenile" rule, but she controlled her anger. She gained some insight into her illness, recognizing that her manic behavior was destructive to herself and others. She also recognized the depression that was often mixed with her mania. Anna speculated that the mania was an attempt to cover up depression; she admitted, "Actually, when I'm high, I'm really feeling low. I need to exaggerate in order to feel more important."

Because Anna was on a research ward, the effectiveness of lithium had to be verified by removal of the drug. When she had been off lithium for four to five days, Anna began to show symptoms of both mania and depression. She threatened her psychiatrist, and as before, the threats were grandiose, with sexual overtones. In a slinky voice, she warned, "I have ways to put the director of this hospital in my debt. He crawled for me before and he'll do it again. When I snap my fingers, he'll come down to this ward and squash you under his foot." Soon afterward, she threatened suicide. She later explained, "I felt so low last night that if someone had given me a knife or gun, POW." By the ninth day off lithium, Anna's speech was almost incomprehensible: "It's sad to be so putty, pretty, so much like water dripping from a faucet. . . ." (Is it surprising that distinguishing a hostile manic patient from a schizophrenia patient is so difficult, that mistakes are often made?) Lithium therapy was reinstituted, and within about 16 days, Anna again recovered and was discharged on lithium.

HOW EFFECTIVE IS LITHIUM?

Anna's recovery is typical. Within one to two weeks of beginning lithium therapy, most manic patients are well on their way to recovery. Because lithium produces no enduring sedative effects, it does not slow down patients' thoughts or subdue their feelings. Thus, college students can return to school and work normally. Managers, executives, and writers can perform as well as they did before they became ill. Lithium patients feel the normal range of human emotions. Mania is prevented, but happiness is not. These patients experience love, sexuality, pride, friendship, and compassion just as normal people do. Likewise, the depression that may have been mixed with the mania is gone, but the ability to feel sadness is not.

Lithium patients are disappointed by failure, and they grieve at the loss of a loved one. Indeed, normal people who take lithium for a few days or weeks experience its side effects but do not detect any dramatic psychological changes. Some experience a slight feeling of detachment, as if they were viewing the world from behind a glass wall. Most notice no change in mood or alertness.[11] The normalizing effects of lithium on mood have been likened to the normalizing effects of aspirin on temperature: Aspirin brings down a fever but does not change the temperature of a healthy person.

Lithium does not work for all bipolar patients. Although the results of research studies vary, it is fair to say that about 80 percent of all manic patients respond to lithium.[12] Psychiatrists do not know how to explain the failures. Improper diagnosis is always a possible explanation, but we have no direct evidence to support it. Another possible explanation is that there are several biologically different categories of bipolar patients, that one category includes those who are responsive to lithium and another includes those who are nonresponsive. This hypothesis is supported by the fact that lithium responders are more likely than nonresponders to have bipolar patients in their immediate families.[13] Still another possibility is that the nonresponders have not received an adequate dose of lithium, that some might respond to a higher dose. Lithium is effective only if its concentration in the blood is maintained within narrow limits: Too little is ineffective; too much is toxic.

Lithium's ability to protect patients against relapse is so dramatic that the effect of placebo is inconsequential by comparison. Schou compared the relapse rate when patients and doctors knew that placebo had been substituted for lithium with the relapse rate when patients and doctors were blind to placebo substitution; the two relapse rates were not different.[14]

Like other psychiatric drugs, lithium is not a permanent cure. If patients stop taking it, they are likely to relapse into mania or depression. Double-blind studies prove unequivocally that lithium protects bipolar patients against both mania and depression. Without lithium, typical bipolar patients have about one manic episode every 14 months and about one depressive episode every 17 months. With lithium maintenance, their manic episodes occur only once every nine years and their depressive episodes only once every four years. Without lithium, they spend an average of 8 to 13 weeks per year in the hospital. If they take lithium, they are hospitalized for less than two weeks per year.[15]

One group of psychiatrists tried to estimate the economic benefits of lithium treatment. Lithium capsules, accompanied by a monthly or bimonthly blood test and a brief psychiatric interview, are obviously much cheaper than intensive psychotherapy and eight weeks of hospitalization per year. Lithium has cut in half the cost of treating bipolar disorder; in the United States this savings represents approximately $270 million per year. The patients and their families are not the only people to benefit from these savings; anyone who buys medical insurance benefits, too. Lithium also permits bipolar patients to be economically productive: Before lithium, bipolar illness caused a loss in work productivity equaling about $152 million per year; lithium has decreased this yearly loss to about $40 million. Again, this savings benefits everyone, not just the patients and their relatives.[16]

SHOULD HYPOMANIA BE TREATED?

When depressed people refuse maintenance drug treatment, they are often expressing an opinion about antidepressant drugs and making inferences about long-term drug use. For instance, they may not like the idea that their mental health depends on a drug, they may not want to admit that they have a chronic illness, and they may not be willing to tolerate the side effects. Although they reject drug treatment, these depressed people are not choosing illness over health. Some bipolar patients may refuse lithium maintenance for these same reasons. Others, however, refuse lithium because they do not want to be cured. They enjoy their hypomanic periods and are loath to give them up. Artists may feel that they are most creative when hypomanic; business people may feel most enterprising; home-makers may feel most efficient.

In *Moodswing*, Ronald R. Fieve told the story of a well-known modern painter who suffered from a bipolar illness that threatened to destroy his life. During his hypomanic periods, the artist was enormously productive; his canvases were bright and showed a creative use of color. The work he produced during these periods had gained him considerable critical acclaim. Unfortunately, his moods and hence his work were not consistent; hypomania inevitably gave way to depression. During his depressed periods, the artist not only refused to paint, but refused to eat. He would not see his friends. He slept 16 hours out of 24.

In spite of his debilitating depressions, the artist was reluctant to take lithium. He feared that, without hypomania, he would lose his creativity, and without his hypomanic passions and generosity, his family and friends might cease to love him. The risks were too great; he would not give up hypomania merely to escape the depression that inexorably followed.

Fieve comments that a patient who is merely hypomanic should not be pressured into taking lithium. However, when hypomania becomes mania, treatment must be initiated. Late one night, a 747 flying from New York to San Francisco made an unscheduled stop in Chicago so that the artist could be taken off the airplane and hospitalized. He had adamantly insisted on holding a prayer meeting in the aisles, and the flight attendants could not control him. During another manic period, he squandered all his family's resources on a trip to Hawaii that he was certain would put him in contact with influential art dealers. In fact, the artist could not negotiate with art dealers while in a manic state. His demanding and arrogant tone antagonized them. The manic artist nonetheless painted energetically, convinced that his work was inspired. In reality, it was merely disorganized. After his manic high receded, he realized that his "inspiration was ridiculous."

After the manic episode on the 747, Fieve, feeling that the artist needed continuous lithium therapy, persuaded him to examine the havoc left in the wake of his mania. Realizing that another episode might destroy his family, the artist decided, despite his fears, to take lithium. As it turned out, his fears had been unfounded: He did not need hypomania to paint, and his paintings continued to be well received. Fieve does not describe the effect of lithium on the artist's relationships with his family, but we suspect that the family loved him more in a normal mood state. Normal hugs and thoughtful small gifts probably made his family happier than did explosive bear hugs and extravagant purchases he could ill afford.[17]

LITHIUM TREATMENT FOR DEPRESSION

Once a bipolar patient has responded to treatment, lithium prevents relapses of both depression and mania, just as it did for Anna. Might lithium also be an effective treatment for depressive episodes in bipolar patients or in patients suffering from major depression? The research data on lithium as a treatment for depression are not very encouraging. Some depressed patients respond to lithium, and the drug is more likely to succeed with bipolar patients than with unipolar patients. But a tricyclic is more likely to produce results if a person begins treatment in a depressed episode.[18] Unfortunately, some bipolar patients do not respond well to tricyclics. There is some, but not conclusive evidence that instead of restoring the normal mood, a tricyclic may precipitate a switch from depression to mania. A psychiatrist who prescribes an antidepressant for a bipolar patient should observe the patient very carefully. If manic symptoms develop, the patient must cease taking the tricyclic.[19]

Although lithium is not an effective drug for terminating an episode of depression that is already in progress, it does prevent depressive relapses both in patients who have major depression without mania and in those who have bipolar disorder.[20] Twenty to 30 percent of depressed patients taking lithium relapse in a year, about the same percentage that relapses on tricyclics. The fact that 70 percent would relapse on placebo shows that both treatments are effective.

When a patient suffers from recurrent depression, the psychiatrist, in consultation with the patient, must decide whether the patient should take preventive medicine and, if so, whether it should be lithium, an antidepressant, or both. If the symptoms are primarily depressive, but there are also hints of mania (for example, irritability or restlessness), lithium may be the best choice. If the patient suffers frequent depressive episodes on lithium, a combination of lithium and a tricyclic is likely to be the best treatment.[21] However, if adding the tricyclic provokes mania, lithium alone may be the only practical approach. A recent study suggests that the type of episode that caused the patient to seek treatment (the index episode) may provide some useful information. If the index episode was manic, lithium is required, and there is probably nothing to be gained by adding a tricyclic. If the index episode was depressive, a combination of lithium and a tricyclic is probably the most effective treatment.[22]

Of course, side effects are also a major consideration in drug selection. If the patient cannot tolerate anticholinergic side effects, perhaps lithium is the better choice. A patient whose work requires delicate coordination may not tolerate the lithium tremor. (We discuss lithium side effects in detail later in this chapter.)

THE BIOLOGY OF LITHIUM

Any attempt to explain how lithium works must explain how it can protect against both mania and depression. Earlier explanations were speculative and focused on lithium's ability to moderate receptor sensitivity,[23] but recent work has suggested a quite different type of explanation. The clinically relevant effect of lithium may not be an alteration of transmitter–receptor interactions, but a change in the biochemical consequences of transmitter–receptor interactions.

The newest theory is based on the finding that many transmitter–receptor interactions cause the postsynaptic cells to synthesize molecules called second messengers. These second messengers activate enzymes that alter neuronal function. For example, these enzymes can alter transmitter release, receptor sensitivity, or the electrical activity of postsynaptic neurons.[24] A variety of neuronal circuits and a variety of transmitters may cause synthesis of the same second messenger.[25] Scientists now hypothesize that lithium prevents the synthesis of a second messenger called phosphatidyl-insitol-bis-phosphate (PIP_2), thus preventing a cell from responding biochemically to transmitter inputs.[26]

How does this explain lithium's ability to protect against both mania and depression? Suppose that a cell is driven by inputs that are overactive in mania. Lithium treatment would prevent that cell from synthesizing PIP_2, and the decreased supply of PIP_2 would dampen our cell's response to the "manic input" and prevent it from transmitting the "manic signal" any further. Similarly if a different cell were being driven by inputs that were overactive in depression, lithium treatment of that cell would dampen the response to the "depressed" input. Thus lithium would dampen all postsynaptic activity dependent on PIP_2 regardless of whether the presynaptic input was signaling mania or depression.

Evidence for this theory is gradually accumulating; most of it is biochemical, however, and beyond the scope of this book. There is good biochemical evidence, for example, that lithium does actually block the synthesis of PIP_2.[27] This block affects the function of nerve cells, and some of these effects have been measured experimentally. For example, the activation of one type of acetylcholine receptor causes synthesis of PIP_2. This synthesis is impaired by lithium, and without the second messenger, the cells can no longer respond to acetylcholine.[28] More evidence is needed, but so far most of the available biochemistry supports the theory.

SIDE EFFECTS

Lithium can produce many unpleasant side effects, but fortunately, most patients experience only a few, and even these usually disappear in one to four weeks. The most common side effects are weakness, tremor, fatigue, nausea, abdominal cramps, diarrhea, weight gain, lethargy, and increased thirst and urination.[29] The psychiatrist should warn patients of these temporary side effects and encourage them to persist with lithium therapy until they have had a chance to reap its benefits. A fine tremor is the only neurological effect that is likely to remain beyond the first month of therapy.[30] The tremor will not bother most patients, but it may disturb those whose livelihoods depend on precise coordination; for instance, surgeons, dancers, jewelers, violinists, and athletes may be unwilling to tolerate the lithium tremor. Fortunately, it can frequently be alleviated by propanalol, a drug that blocks certain norepinephrine receptors.[31]

Lithium Toxicity

The major danger in lithium therapy is that the prescribed dose will be too high, resulting in lithium poisoning. The psychiatrist cannot know the correct dose in advance because each patient's body eliminates lithium at a different rate. Determination of the correct dose requires measurement of lithium concentration in the blood. During the first few weeks of treatment, the amount of lithium in the patient's blood changes rapidly. Therefore, lithium concentration must be measured frequently. After the proper dosage has been established and the lithium concentration stabilized, blood concentration needs to be measured only 3 to 12 times per year. Reasonably frequent measurements are important because changes in diet, health, and activity can cause marked changes in lithium concentration even though the patient is taking the lithium precisely as directed. Failure to adjust lithium intake can cause relapse when the lithium level is too low or toxicity when it is too high.[32]

Lithium toxicity primarily affects the brain. Its symptoms are confusion, slurred speech, drowsiness, loss of balance, tremor, vomiting, diarrhea, and eventually coma and death.[33] Some of these symptoms, such as drowsiness and diarrhea, are similar to those occurring at the beginning of lithium therapy. If these symptoms occur in a patient who has been taking lithium for some time, the drug should be stopped, and the patient should receive immediate medical attention.

Cognitive Effects

Although lithium patients, such as the artist discussed earlier, continue to be competent and creative, lithium can have some subtle effects on cognitive processes. Bipolar patients taking lithium perform slightly more poorly on a variety of memory, word association, and motor tasks than do bipolar patients not taking lithium.[34] A slowing of motor behavior or decrease in word associations might be ascribed to control of hypomania, but a decrease in verbal short-term memory probably does not signal a therapeutic effect. However, the cognitive effects of lithium are reversible: If the performance of the same patients is compared on and off lithium, performance improves when lithium is removed.[35] The significance of these deficits is hard to evaluate. Perhaps lithium patients think slightly more slowly than they would if they were not taking lithium, but this is a small price to pay for the relief of bipolar disorder. Furthermore, there is no evidence that overall intellectual achievement is impaired.

Lithium and the Kidney

Lithium sometimes affects the kidneys.[36] The kidney concentrates waste molecules so that they can be excreted in the urine with minimal loss of water. In about 7 to 13 percent of lithium patients, the kidney's ability to concentrate urine is decreased. Thus, these patients drink large quantities of water and excrete large quantities of dilute urine. Although frequent urination is a nuisance, it probably does not indicate any significant kidney damage because the results of tests that predict kidney problems are normal in lithium patients. Furthermore, 35 years of lithium treatment has not produced a single documented cases of kidney failure associated with lithium therapy.[37]

When lithium was first introduced, research indicating that lithium caused changes in the microscopic anatomy of the kidney caused some concern. These early reports compared the kidneys of lithium patients with the kidneys of normal people, not with the kidneys of bipolar patients not taking lithium. This distinction turns out to be important because bipolar patients who are not taking lithium have more kidney damage than do healthy people. In fact, the changes that might signify kidney damage are not specific to lithium and can be seen in the kidneys of patients about to start lithium therapy.[38] While other changes in kidney anatomy are associated with lithium, these are reversible and do not signify loss of kidney function.[39]

In summary, there is no evidence that the changes lithium causes in kidney anatomy indicate health-threatening kidney damage. We think that for people with a severe affective disorder, the benefits of lithium maintenance are greater than the risks. We suggest that a patient taking lithium, or a relative of that patient, ask the prescribing doctor for current information about the effects of lithium on the kidney.

OTHER DRUG TREATMENTS FOR BIPOLAR DISORDER

Antipsychotics

Some psychiatrists, like Anna's, recommend a few days of antipsychotic treatment at the beginning of lithium therapy. Antipsychotics, because of their initial sedative effect, act more promptly than does lithium to slow speech, inhibit aggressiveness, and decrease rapid-fire activity. Lithium works only gradually and does not decrease manic symptoms for 7 to 14 days. After this time has elapsed, most psychiatrists discontinue the antipsychotic. Some psychiatrists believe, however, that antipsychotics are as effective as lithium in the long-term treatment of mania. Research has not yet definitively resolved the issue.[40]

Manic patients receiving only antipsychotics and those receiving only lithium score very similarly on psychiatric rating scales that measure mania, but more lithium patients become well enough to leave the hospital. Some psychiatrists suggest that this discrepancy between the measurements on rating scales and hospital release rates exists because the rating scales are insensitive to the differences between the two drugs. They believe that antipsychotics subdue manic patients, whereas lithium normalizes them. Obviously, this hypothesis cannot be substantiated until improved rating scales are developed.

Anticonvulsants

If lithium controlled mania and prevented relapses in all bipolar patients, researchers would not be experimenting with alternative treatments. Unfortunately, about 20 to 25 percent of manic patients fail to respond to lithium, and about 33 percent will have some recurrences in spite of continued treatment.[41] Lithium seems to be particularly ineffective for rapid-cycling patients, that is, patients who have four or more episodes per year, and for patients with simultaneous manic and depressed symptoms.[42] Several experimental alternative treatments for these patients are promising, but none has proven effectiveness. The best studied is carbamazepine, a drug that has been used for a long time to prevent convulsions.

No large-scale controlled trials have compared carbamezepine to lithium or to placebo. A study similar to the NIMH study of antipsychotics could tell us unequivocally whether these drugs were effective in the treatment of mania. The available data only permit some encouraging guesses.

Two studies have compared carbamazepine to placebo. Both of these examined the ability of carbamazepine to prevent relapse. Only one found a statistically significant difference between carbamazepine and placebo.[43] Two studies compared carbamazepine to lithium; one examined the response of acute mania and the other examined the ability of each drug to prevent relapse. Both found that lithium was more effective than carbamazepine.[44]

The studies described so far used a random selection of manic patients, but this is not the best population of patients for testing the hypothesis that lithium nonresponders are the ones who will respond to carbamazepine. To test this hypothesis, Post and his colleagues selected lithium nonresponders for their studies. Rather than comparing a carbamazepine group to a placebo group, they compared the behavior of each patient while taking carbamazepine and while taking placebo. Many patients had significantly fewer manic and depressive episodes on carbamazepine than on placebo. Some severely incapacitated patients who had been hospitalized for many years were released with carbamazepine treatment.[45] Some manic patients fail to respond to either lithium or carbamazepine alone. Post and his colleagues experimented with giving both drugs to a small group of patients of this type; six out of seven responded.[46] Carbamazepine, with or without lithium, seems to offer real hope to bipolar patients refractory to lithium alone.

Valproate is another anticonvulsant that may bring relief to bipolar patients who fail to respond to lithium, but even less data support its effectiveness. Two double-blind trials using small numbers of patients found that valproate controlled mania in about two-thirds of the patients.[47] This conclusion is supported by a larger number of studies that lacked placebo control.[48] The available evidence suggests but does not prove that valproate is probably effective for both acute treatment of mania and for prevention of relapse.[49]

THE ROLE OF PSYCHOTHERAPY

We were unable to find a single controlled study on the effectiveness of psychotherapy in treating mania. However, Ronald R. Fieve discusses psychotherapy for bipolar patients in his book *Moodswing*. Fieve, one of the foremost authorities on lithium in the United States, was trained in the psychoanalytic tradition. He describes the frustrations of the early years of his career, which he devoted to treating depressed and manic patients with psychotherapy; he does not think he accomplished very much. When a manic patient improved after months of therapy, he was never certain that psychotherapy had played a role. The improvement was usually a spontaneous mood swing and did not last very long. When he began to treat patients with antidepressants and lithium, he saw dramatic improvement in just a few weeks, and with lithium maintenance therapy, the improvement was permanent.[50]

Fieve's observations are, of course, only anecdotal; they are not scientific evidence. Yet there seems to be no experimental evidence for or against the effectiveness of psychotherapy for mania. We surmise that research psychiatrists do not want to waste their time proving what seems obvious from clinical experience, that psycho-therapy is not an effective treatment for mania. Moreover, because the evidence for the effectiveness of lithium is so strong, withholding lithium from the psychotherapy group would be unethical.

Fieve's view of the appropriate uses of psychotherapy is similar to that of Gerald Klerman and Myrna Weissman at the NIMH. He recognizes that problems in living often result from prolonged affec-tive illness. Psychotherapy is often helpful in solving these problems once the underlying mania and depression have been relieved.

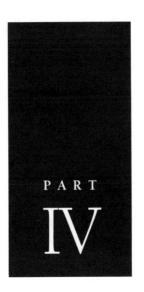

PART

IV

ANXIETY DISORDERS

15

DIAGNOSING ANXIETY
DISORDERS

—

T his chapter opens with a discussion of how we know when
anxiety can be considered a disorder and when it can be
properly treated with drugs. Next, we describe the symptoms and provide examples of anxiety disorders that are defined in
the *DSM-III-R*, giving special attention to those disorders that benefit
from drug treatment. Finally, we discuss the relationship between
anxiety disorders and two categories of mental illness that often
accompany anxiety disorders; depression and substance abuse.

WHEN IS ANXIETY A DISORDER?

Anxiety is fearful anticipation. It is an unpleasant necessity of life.
Anxiety inhibits procrastination, combats carelessness, and subdues
overagressiveness. Without anxiety, people would play the first little

pig, lazing the time away while the wolf sneaks up. Students would party all night and seldom study. Everyone would drive too fast. Workers would insult the boss. The beauty of anxiety is that it is intolerable. It forces us to do what has to be done in order to avoid even greater unpleasantness in the future. Let no one say that he or she wishes to be totally free of anxiety.

The signs of anxiety are indeed intolerable. Anxious people are consciously fearful that something terrible is about to happen. They can think of nothing else. They are unable to sleep. Their muscles shake and ache; relaxation is impossible. Strain is visible on their anxious faces. Anxious people may experience sweating, a pounding and racing heart, cold and clammy hands, dry mouth, dizziness, light-headedness, tingling of the hands and feet, hot and cold spells, upset stomach, urge to urinate, diarrhea, a lump in the throat, butterflies in the stomach, belching, gasping, and difficult breathing.[1] If someone has these symptoms in the absence of actual danger, an illness is present. Because the symptoms involve bodily organs so extensively, patients may believe — incorrectly — that they are suffering from a life-threatening disease.

Harmful anxiety is not always a mental disorder. Sometimes it occurs uselessly in situations where it would be mentally disordered not to be anxious. John Smith, for example, has acute appendicitis, he is anxious that he will die if he doesn't have surgical treatment, but if he does have surgery, he must delegate responsibility for his body to another person who will cut open his abdomen and remove an internal organ. Anxiety in this situation is hardly irrational. But once the illness has been diagnosed and the treatment plan established, anxiety would be useless and might actually harm John by causing him to forego treatment. This example illustrates the point that anxiety is a universal accompaniment of bodily illness and injury. Such anxiety contributes little to recovery or to the patient's long-term well-being. Even though such anxiety is not itself an illness, it would be appropriate to relieve suffering with antianxiety drugs.

Anxiety is a mental disorder when it is more intense than is justified by actual threat. Aaron Able, for example, was an intelligent, hardworking college freshman. His grades were adequate, but his excessive anxiety prevented them from being even better. The trouble was that he became desperately anxious at exam time. Before his first math exam, his heart started pounding, and he broke out in a sweat and vomited. During the exam itself, his mind was so over-whelmed with anxiety that the whole classroom felt unreal. He could not think about the problems even though they were just like the ones he had easily solved in optional homework assignments. In a situation where some anxiety was justified, Aaron panicked. He was frustrated by his inability to perform up to his potential.

Anxiety is a mental disorder when it occurs without any justification whatsoever. Alison, for example, was a homemaker with three children. She was 28 when she first sought help from a psychiatrist. At that time she and her husband had just canceled their annual vacation at the shore because she was afraid that being away from home would make her a nervous wreck. Over the preceding year she had had a number of nervous spells in which she had experienced dizziness, trembling, shortness of breath, and a pounding heart. These experiences had been very frightening, and after a few of them she had become preoccupied with fear that one of her attacks would occur in a situation where no one could help her. Her doctor found no somatic health problems. About six months before she sought professional help, Alison's fears had developed to the point that she was afraid leave the house without her husband beside her to help in case of an attack. As a result it was hard for her to go shopping or to enter any public place. When she did enter a public place she constantly checked for doors and windows through which she could rapidly escape. When she went out to sweep the walk in front of her house, she left the door open so that she could run back in if something bad happened. Alison tried to persuade her mother to stay with her in order to take care of the children in case she became incapacitated. Neither Alison nor her family could understand what had happened. Alison had been a sociable and outgoing person.

For Aaron and Alison anxiety was the problem, not a part of the solution. In these examples, which represent typical cases, excessive anxiety can accurately be called an illness. It causes suffering and distress. It causes social and occupational impairment. It reduces human potential. For people like Aaron and Alison life would be happier, more free, and more dignified if, through treatment, the anxiety could be reduced — provided, of course, that the treatment is not worse than the anxiety that it eliminates.

Anxiety is present in many psychiatric illnesses that are not referred to as anxiety disorders. For example, in major depression, anxiety can be intense, and it may be the most prominent form of suffering. Other symptoms, such as hopelessness, guilt, weight loss, and sleep disturbance, may be present but less salient by comparison.

Many people are reluctant to take pills to reduce anxiety even though they understand that the anxiety is a mental disorder. They may be fearful that they will become addicted to tranquilizers, or they may believe that pills will not provide relief from illness but relief from responsibility. Psychiatric Calvinists are common. They believe that proper treatment requires hard work and that taking pills is just a cheap escape. In some cases they are right; psychotherapy is an effective treatment for some types of anxiety. But in some cases excessive anxiety is nearly impossible to control with known psychological methods, and in these cases anxiety-relieving pills are justified. A basic problem, therefore, is how to distinguish among rational anxiety, anxiety that can benefit from psychotherapy, and anxiety that requires drug treatment.

Decisions about when to seek treatment for anxiety would be vastly simplified and drug abuse could be avoided if we had clear and valid diagnostic procedures for distinguishing between helpful and harmful anxiety. The *DSM-III-R* attempts to provide such procedures. Since harmful anxiety can occur in many situations outside the scope of psychiatry, however, the *DSM-III-R* does not specify all the situations in which anxiety should be treated. Also, as we have emphasized in Chapter 3, the *DSM-III-R* is a single still frame in the scientific evolution of diagnostic practices in psychiatry. We should expect the diagnostic categories of the *DSM-III-R* to undergo revision as knowledge accumulates in the 1990s.

ANXIETY DISORDERS DEFINED IN THE *DSM-III-R*

The *DSM-III-R* defines seven types of anxiety disorders. These are panic disorder, agoraphobia, social phobia, simple phobia, obsessive compulsive disorder, post-traumatic stress disorder, and generalized anxiety disorder.[2]

Anxiety disorders are very common in the general population. Data from the NIMH Epidemiological Catchment Area study (see Chapter 9) indicate that about 10 percent of Americans have suffered from an anxiety disorder, as defined in the *DSM-III*, during the past six months. If the time window is enlarged to include the entire life prior to the interview, then the percentage rises to about 13 percent. These percentages do not include cases of post-traumatic stress disorder or generalized anxiety disorder. It is believed that these two disorders, as defined by the *DSM-III-R*, are rather rare, so their inclusion would probably not increase the apparent prevalence of anxiety disorders by more than 1 or 2 percent.

Different anxiety disorders respond to different forms of treatment. This is an important justification for considering the various types of anxiety disorder to be distinct and not just several different faces of the same underlying disorder.

It is now generally agreed that drugs can contribute to the proper treatment of panic disorder (with or without agoraphobia), obsessive compulsive disorder, generalized anxiety disorder, and excessive anxiety in response to stressful events. We will pay most attention to these disorders. Research has not yet provided a well-defined beneficial role for drugs in the treatment of agoraphobia without panic, social phobia, simple phobia and post-traumatic stress disorder. Therefore we will discuss diagnosis of these disorders only briefly, saving most of our space for panic disorder (with and without agoraphobia), obsessive compulsive disorder, and generalized anxiety disorder.

Social Phobia, Simple Phobia and Post-traumatic Stress Disorder

Social phobia is an intense fear of being scrutinized or evaluated by others. The afflicted person is excessively concerned about doing something embarrassing or humiliating. An example would be extreme fear of public speaking or performance or, going further, fear of eating in public because of possible display of bad manners. Aaron Able, who was afraid of exams, possibly had social phobia. A person with social phobia might refuse to go to parties for fear of saying something foolish or being unable to think of an answer when asked a question. With proper psychotherapy, many people can learn to overcome social phobia. The criteria for diagnosing social phobia can be found in the *DSM-III-R*.[3]

Simple phobia is an intense fear of a particular object or situation. The fear is absent unless the person actually has to confront the feared object. It is common for the feared object to be an animal. Helen, a family friend of ours, is deathly afraid of cats. If she gets close to a cat, she panics, just as Aaron Able does at exam time. The phobia is only a minor handicap as Helen can easily avoid getting close to a cat. The criteria for diagnosing simple phobia are also stated in the *DSM-III-R*.[4] Simple phobias can often be overcome with the aid of psychotherapy.

Post-traumatic stress disorder, by definition, occurs following an intense experience that is outside the normal range of stress encountered in everyday life. An example of such a stress would be seeing your friends killed on a battlefield or seeing your child die in a fire. Following such stress, the afflicted person may reexperience the traumatic event in such a way that it interferes with his or her life. The person may seek to avoid any situation that might set off memories of the event, and the undesired recollection of the event may induce chronic anxiety, sleep disturbance, difficulty concentrating, outbursts of anger, and other evidences of emotional distress. The criteria for post-traumatic stress disorder are also found in *DSM-III-R*.[5]

Panic Disorder

For many decades it has been known that some psychiatric patients experience periodic bouts of intense anxiety, called panic attacks. These attacks involve intense subjective fear and dread. Victims may believe they are dying of a heart attack or going crazy. The fear may become so intense that the patients feel faint, vomit, have diarrhea and a racing and pounding heart. Alison, the fearful homemaker, had panic attacks.

A time-honored view of panic attacks is that they are very intense episodes of anxiety that are not qualitatively different from less intense anxiety experienced as, say, stage fright or a fear of flying. This view is challenged, however, by the observations of Donald Klein of the Hillside Hospital, Glen Oaks, New York. Klein found that the tricyclic antidepressant imipramine would specifically relieve panic attacks while leaving other forms of anxiety unimproved. His observations were made on a group of patients who, like Alison, experienced frequent panic attacks and were also routinely anxious in many different kinds of situations. Most of them had agoraphobia, a fear of being in public places. Imipramine relieved the panic attacks but did not relieve the agoraphobia.[6] Imipramine also fails to relieve simple phobias.[7]

A drug that relieves severe anxiety should also relieve mild anxiety, provided that severe and mild anxiety do not differ in quality but only in degree. The action of imipramine suggests, then, that panic attacks differ in quality from at least some other forms of anxiety. Supporting this view are data showing that the bodily symptoms experienced by people with panic attacks are somewhat different than those experienced by people with social phobia.[8]

Armed with this and other evidence that panic attacks are distinct from intense anxiety, the *DSM-III-R* advisory committee on anxiety disorders defined panic disorder as a condition whose definitive symptom is the repeated and frequent experience of panic attacks. No other type of anxiety need be present. The attacks occur at unpredictable times and do not invariably occur when the patient confronts a fearful situation. For example, Klein's patients, like Alison, were typically afraid to go into public places without a companion, but when they did leave home alone, they did not always experience a panic attack. Panic disorder patients have even been known to be awakened from sleep by a panic attack.[9] This unpredictability of the attacks contrasts with anxiety attacks experienced as a part of simple phobia or social phobia. In the latter disorders the attack is reliably provoked by the feared stimulus and does not occur in the absence of the stimulus.

Panic disorder usually strikes in the late twenties and may last for years. During this time the frequency and intensity of attacks waxes and wanes. In some cases the person may be able to carry on his or her life fairly well between the attacks, which last only 10 to 30 minutes. In other cases, the person may become concerned and anxious about the possibility of having another attack or having an attack under circumstances in which help would be unavailable. When the person develops these associated fears (agoraphobia), panic disorder can be very debilitating indeed.

Panic disorder is not common, but neither is it rare. According to the NIMH Epidemiological Catchment Area study, about 0.8 percent of the population has suffered panic disorder during the past six months[10]; about 1.4 percent at some point during the lifetime.[11] Among those people who seek treatment for panic disorder, men and women are about equal in number. These frequencies are based on the *DSM-III* rather than the *DSM-III-R*, so they might be slightly modified if the study were repeated today.

The *DSM-III-R* lists five criteria, A to E, that must be satisfied for the diagnosis of panic disorder.

Criterion A

At some time during the disturbance, one or more panic attacks (discrete periods of intense fear or discomfort) have occurred that were (1) unexpected, i.e., did not occur immediately before or on exposure to a situation that almost always caused anxiety, and (2) not triggered by situations in which the person was the focus of other's attention.

This criterion rules out panic states that are a part of simple phobia and social phobia. Helen's panic reaction to cats would not count toward panic disorder because these reactions occur only in the presence of a cat. Aaron Able's attacks before exams are disqualified by item 2 of the criterion, which rules out fear of public scrutiny. Even though the attacks may be statistically associated with recognizable situations, such as driving on a bridge or being in a crowded elevator, the person is never sure when or where an attack will occur.

Criterion B

Either four attacks, as defined in criterion A, have occurred within a four-week period, or one or more attacks have been followed by a period of at least a month of persistent fear of having another attack.

This criterion establishes a minimum frequency of attacks. The minimum is arbitrary. Obviously, questions are raised about the diagnostic status of borderline cases. Should a patient who has three attacks in four weeks be regarded as having a mild form of panic disorder or no panic disorder at all? As mentioned above, people with agoraphobia commonly have panic attacks. Their attacks may vary in frequency from one attack per month to several per week. Is it correct to say that those patients who have only infrequent attacks have only agoraphobia, while those with frequent attacks have panic disorder and agoraphobia? This question is not settled at the present time.

Criterion C

At least four of the following symptoms developed during at least one of the attacks:

1. shortness of breath (dyspnea) or smothering sensations
2. dizziness, unsteady feelings, or faintness
3. palpitations (pounding heart) or accelerated heart rate (tachycardia)
4. trembling or shaking
5. sweating
6. choking
7. nausea or abdominal distress
8. depersonalization or derealization
9. numbness or tingling sensations (paresthesias)
10. flushes (hot flashes) or chills
11. chest pain or discomfort
12. fear of dying
13. fear of going crazy

Although a full-blown panic attack requires four items from this list, an attack involving fewer symptoms can be called a limited symptom attack. By providing a name for attacks with fewer symptoms, the committee honored the probability that there are attacks of lesser intensity that represent a milder form of panic disorder.

Most of the symptoms are self-explanatory. Depersonalization (symptom 8) is a dreamlike state that is difficult to explain to someone who has not experienced it. You feel detached from events, as if you are not actually present but are having a dream. Your body may seem like a robot that is doing things that you are watching but are not involved in. Derealization is a feeling that your environment is not real. Other people may seem like robots; strange changes in the perception of the size and shape of objects may occur. This sounds like some kind of mystical or psychedelic experience, and perhaps there is some similarity. Depersonalization and derealization when experienced as a part of a panic attack are not pleasant experiences, however.

Criterion D

During at least some of the attacks, at least four of the C symptoms developed suddenly and increased in intensity within ten minutes of the beginning of the first C symptom noticed in the attack.

Once the first symptom occurs, the others follow within a few minutes. The symptoms do not build up gradually over hours or days.

Criterion E

It cannot be established that an organic factor initiated and maintained the disturbance; e.g., Amphetamine or Caffeine Intoxication, hyperthyroidism.

There are many organic conditions that are expressed in symptoms resembling panic attacks. Although it usually does not present any diagnostic uncertainty, a genuine heart attack would easily satisfy criterion C. Dr. John Feighner, a research psychiatrist well known for his studies of diagnosis, warns psychiatrists and psychologists not to confuse panic attacks with deficient blood sugar, epilepsy, brain cancer, or abnormal hormonal activity. Drug intoxication with amphetamine or cocaine can resemble a panic attack. It is especially noteworthy that in susceptible individuals, caffeine can cause panic attacks or make the attacks worse. People who do not suffer from panic attacks are apparently much less sensitive to caffeine.[12] The drug withdrawal syndrome experienced by people who are dependent on alcohol and other anxiety-relieving drugs can easily be confused with panic attacks. Indeed, all 13 symptoms listed in criterion C are symptoms of alcohol withdrawal.

Agoraphobia

Agoraphobia is an illness whose dominant feature is fear of being unprotected in a public place. Translated from its Greek roots, *agoraphobia* means "fear of the marketplace." And indeed, many people with agoraphobia are afraid to go shopping by themselves; they may also be afraid of other crowded public places, such as elevators or subways. The degree of impairment is varied. Some are so severely afflicted that they literally will not leave home and thus become unable to work or go shopping. Others can muster enough courage to leave home but suffer intense anxiety until back in their safe place. It is typical for people with agoraphobia to become emotionally dependent on their family members for help in overcoming their multiple fears. Agoraphobia usually strikes people who are in their late twenties or thirties, and it lasts for years. It is more common in women than in men. Alison, whose case we described at the beginning of the chapter, had agoraphobia.

The *DSM-III-R* gives only one criterion for agoraphobia that simply describes a fear of being in unsafe places. The wording is as follows:

> Agoraphobia: Fear of being in places or situations from which escape might be difficult (or embarrassing) or in which help might not be available in the event of suddenly developing a symptom(s) that could be incapacitating or extremely embarrassing. Examples include: dizziness or falling, depersonalization or derealization, loss of bladder or bowel control, vomiting, or heart pounding. As a result of this fear, the person either restricts travel or needs a companion when away from home, or else endures agoraphobic situations despite intense anxiety. Common agoraphobic situations include being outside the home alone, being in a crowd or standing in a line, being on a bridge.

Fear of being away from home is sometimes entirely justified, and in these cases the person does not have agoraphobia. For example, we know an elderly man who recently suffered a heart attack. As an aftermath of the attack and bypass surgery, he no longer has control of his bladder and has to run to the toilet about 30 times a day; his incontinence has prevented him from attending church or his service club because he is afraid he will be embarrassed. This is not agoraphobia. Neither is it agoraphobia when a woman fears to walk on the street at night in a rough neighborhood. The fact that fears similar to agoraphobia also occur in normal people suggests that the disorder may represent a normal fear that has escaped from adaptive control. The brain may have lost its ability to inhibit fear when fear is unjustified.

Agoraphobia frequently occurs in conjunction with panic disorder, panic attacks, or less severe limited symptom attacks. Alison had both agoraphobia and panic attacks. Psychologists and psychiatrists see agoraphobia and panic disorder together so frequently that many think the two disorders are not separate illnesses, but two parts of a single illness.

Donald Klein has suggested that agoraphobia may be an expression of anxiety about the unpredictable occurrence of another panic attack.[13] This hypothesis proposes that in agoraphobia the only thing to fear is fear itself. Klein's hypothesis is consistent with the fact that many cases of agoraphobia also involve panic attacks or limited symptom attacks. It is also supported by the fact that panic attacks usually strike first, with agoraphobia developing later.[14] Most people with agoraphobia say that they consciously fear having an attack, becoming embarrassed, or becoming helpless. Since panic attacks occur at unpredictable times and may involve uncontrollable diarrhea, voluminous sweating, fainting, or other signs of catastrophic illness, it would indeed be terrible to have a panic attack on the way to the forum. Viewed in this light, agoraphobia is not a disorder, but rational anxiety. The rational approach to treatment is to eliminate the panic attacks if possible, then help the patient learn that it is safe to venture into the market place.

Despite its plausibility, Klein's hypothesis is far from proved. Several different types of evidence indicate that agoraphobia is not always caused by fear of panic attacks. First, psychiatrists occasionally see cases in which agoraphobia occurs without accompanying panic attacks or limited symptom attacks.[15] Second, a small number of agoraphobia patients are afraid of an attack when none has actually occurred.[16] An additional small number of agoraphobia patients have a vague fear that something terrible (not specifically a panic attack) will happen if they go out. Third, full-blown panic attacks do not invariably lead to agoraphobia.[17] Fourth, patients with agoraphobia usually have multiple fears in addition to the fear of leaving home. They may also be anxious about their health, their children's health, prospects of poverty, and so on. To use the technical term, patients with agoraphobia often have "generalized anxiety."

Household survey data also support the notion that agoraphobia and panic occur separately. Preliminary data from the NIMH Catchment Area Epidemiological survey find that about 1.5 percent of the population has experienced agoraphobia within the past year but has never experienced symptoms of panic attacks. About 1 percent suffers from panic disorder with agoraphobia, and about 0.3 percent suffers from the combined disorder. Among those who have agoraphobia alone or panic disorder with agoraphobia, there are about twice as many women as men. Men and women are about equally represented among those who suffer from panic disorder without agoraphobia.[18]

Obsessive Compulsive Disorder

In obsessive compulsive disorder, which we will abbreviate OCD, the patient is plagued with unwanted, time-wasting, emotionally distressing obsessions and compulsions. An obsession is a pattern of thoughts that runs through the patient's mind repetitively and unstoppably even though the patient wants to think about something else. A compulsion is a purposeful behavioral routine or ritual that the patient feels compelled to perform repetitively despite the desire to stop or do something else. If the patient resists the urge to perform the ritual, anxiety results. The longer the patient resists, the greater the anxiety. Many interesting cases of obsessive compulsive disorder are described by Judith L. Rapoport in *The Boy Who Couldn't Stop Washing*.

A common obsession is to be overcome with doubt about whether one's hands and body are clean enough. The idea of contamination takes control of the mind. The patient may worry that touching a common object like a doorknob has soiled his or her hands. An encounter with the bathroom, house dust, a pet animal, or a person may launch a storm of anxiety that can only be pacified by a session of washing and scrubbing. The patient may spend many hours a day washing and grooming. Obsessions can also take the form of images in the mind or impulses to commit some terrible act.

A mother might uncontrollably imagine the sight of her child being hit by a car or feel an impulse to kill her child by throwing him or her into the river.

The patient usually realizes that these obsessions, images, and impulses are utterly absurd and sincerely wishes to stop thinking in such unproductive or reprehensible ways. But will power is weaker than the obsession. Even though a person knows his hands are clean, obsessional doubt gnaws and intensifies. Finally he gives in and washes his hands, again. After many years or trying to resist he may become demoralized and give up his efforts to resist the obsessions and compulsions.

Rituals are often performed according to exact rules of procedure. For example, in preparing for school in the morning, an afflicted student might first have to wash her hands, then shake the germs off her clothes, then wash her hands again, then brush her teeth. If she is distracted before completing brushing her teeth (which may take a long time), she may have to start the sequence over again with the first round of hand washing.

Obsessions and compulsions can be mild enough for the patient to cover up, or they can interfere grossly with normal life. A teenager with a serious case was known to spend six hours a day washing her hands and scrubbing them with alcohol until they bled. She would then be embarrassed when others asked what was wrong with her hands.[20] A mother who obsesses about killing her child may then be incapacitated with guilt for having such horrible thoughts. The disorder is obviously an obstacle to courtship and marriage. People with the disorder are less likely than people not so afflicted to have children.[21]

Howard Hughes, the famous moviemaker, ladies' man, aviator, and industrialist had OCD. He obsessed about contamination and compulsively washed. During the later part of his life the affliction became so severe that he could no longer suppress his compulsions long enough to make public appearances. As a result he became a recluse, which aroused the suspicion of fellow business people and financiers. Toward the end of his life his obsessions became so intense that it became humanly impossible for him to wash enough to satisfy the obsessive need. At this point, it is believed, he simply gave up and stopped washing and grooming altogether. His fingernails, hair, and beard simply grew uncontrollably as he flew around the country in one of his airplanes attended by employees.[22]

The *DSM-III-R* gives two criteria for the diagnosis of OCD:

A. Either obsessions or compulsions:

Obsessions: 1, 2, 3, and 4.
1. recurrent and persistent ideas, thoughts, impulses, or images that are experienced, at least initially, as intrusive and senseless, e.g., a parent's having repeated impulses to kill a loved child, a religious person's having recurrent blasphemous thoughts
2. the person attempts to ignore or suppress such thoughts or impulses or to neutralize them with some other thought or action.
3. the person recognizes that the obsessions are the product of his or her own mind, not imposed from without (as in thought insertion).
4. if another . . . disorder is present, the content of the obsession is unrelated to it, e.g., the ideas, thoughts, impulses, or images are not about food in the presence of an Eating Disorder, about drugs in the presence of a Psychoactive Substance Use Disorder, or guilty thoughts in the presence of Major Depression.

Compulsions: 1., 2., 3.
1. repetitive, purposeful, and intentional behaviors that are performed in response to an obsession, or according to certain rules or in a stereotyped fashion.
2. the behavior is designed to neutralize or to prevent discomfort or some dreaded event or situation; however, either the activity is not connected in a realistic way with what it is designed to neutralize or prevent, or it is clearly excessive.
3. the person recognizes that his or her behavior is excessive or unreasonable (this may not be true for young children; it may no longer be true for people whose obsessions have evolved into overvalued ideas)

B. The obsessions or compulsions cause marked distress, are time-consuming (take more than an hour a day), or significantly interfere with the person's normal routine, occupational functioning, or usual social activities or relationships with others.[23]

These criteria are fairly self-explanatory. Criterion A defines obsessions and compulsions. Criterion B specifies that the obsessions and compulsions have a negative impact on the patient's life.

In the definition of obsessions, item 2 of criterion A distinguishes obsessions from the delusions of schizophrenia. In schizophrenia the patient believes from the beginning that the thoughts are correct, important, and brilliant; there is no attempt to suppress, or substitute for the thoughts. In item 4 of the definition of obsessions, diagnosis of OCD is ruled out when the thoughts are the product of some other disorder that is diagnosed according to *DSM-III-R* criteria. Of particular interest here are obsessions of guilt. Guilt is an emotion and thought pattern that is common in depression. If the patient otherwise satisfies the criteria for major depression, the obsessions of guilt do not count toward the additional diagnosis of OCD.

The definition of compulsions requires that the patient be aware that the rituals are counterproductive and undesirable (an exception is made for young children, who may think they are accomplishing some objective through magic). Sometimes, however, after many years of suffering, an adult patient may develop what is called an overvalued idea, which justifies the ritual. A homemaker might have the overvalued idea that her excessive washing and cleaning was protecting the family from an incurable disease that had afflicted here sister.

OCD had been suffered at some point during the lifetime of about 2.5 percent of the 10,000 Americans sampled in the NIMH Epidemiological Catchment Area Study; about 1.6 percent of the same group had suffered from the disorder during the six months prior to the diagnostic interview.[24] The illness usually begins in adolescence, although it can begin in childhood. Once it begins, it usually does not go away, but waxes and wanes in severity. OCD was about 1.5 times as frequent in women as in men in the Epidemiological Catchment Area sample. According to Susan Swedo and colleagues, however, there is a three to one preponderance of males among patients in whom the disorder begins in childhood.[25] Childhood onset cases are usually more serious than adult onset cases.

Generalized Anxiety Disorder

As conceived by the *DSM-III-R* advisory committee, generalized anxiety disorder, which we will abbreviate as GAD, is a condition in which excessive anxiety is generalized. That is, anxiety is not evoked by a particular situation or stimulus, but instead occurs in almost any situation and in response to almost any stimulus. The person may be anxious at work, at home, at a party, or in church. In extreme cases, nervous tension indiscriminately pervades nearly all activities. Patients are excessively vigilant about the possible occurrence of disasters. They constantly scan the environment for signals of danger. Bodily symptoms of arousal are present, as in all anxiety disorders. It is as if the brain were continuously doing the night watch at the battlefront.

GAD is not a reaction to stressful experience. Rather, it is conceived to arise within the brain in the absence of convincing environmental provocation. In the *DSM-III-R*, excessive anxiety in response to stressful experience is called adjustment disorder with anxious mood.

Annette, whose daughter calls her a nervous wreck, has GAD. She constantly worries about the possibility that her daughter and granddaughter, who live in the San Francisco Bay area, will die in an earthquake. Reassurances that her daughter's house is built to withstand even a maximal earthquake help only slightly. Annette is anxious because her husband smokes and is overweight. The likelihood that he might have a heart attack seems intolerably high to her. When he goes hunting, she is anxious that he will be shot accidentally. Driving with Annette is an ordeal. She herself will not drive for fear of having an accident, and when riding in the car, she constantly irritates the driver with unnecessary warnings. Money is a relentless concern. Will there be enough to cover medical emergencies? What if she or her husband has an extended illness? What is there isn't enough for her granddaughter's college education? What if . . . ? What if . . . ?

Annette also has bodily symptoms. She frequently feels shaky and has muscle twitches. Backaches and restlessness leave her feeling exhausted when she has actually done little work. She also has trouble falling asleep and staying asleep. Annette has been to the doctor several times in the past three months, seeking relief from her symptoms. The doctor prescribed Xanax (alprazolam), which helped a lot. Annette is concerned about taking alprazolam for more than a week or two, because she knows that drug dependence is a risk. Therefore she reserves the pills for occasions when the anxiety becomes unbearable or when it is absolutely necessary for her to appear relaxed.

The *DSM-III-R* lists five criteria for diagnosing GAD, which we paraphrase here. The first criterion states that the person must experience the disorder for a period of six months or longer. During this time the anxiety must be present more often than not. The worry and anxiety must be concerned with at least two different life circumstances; that is, the anxiety is generalized and not a fear of a particular stimulus, such as fear of flying.

The second criterion states that the anxiety is not the expression of other mental disorders defined in the *DSM-III-R*. For example if a young woman suffered from anorexia nervosa and worried constantly that she was too fat, this would not count toward the diagnosis of GAD. Likewise, worry about procuring a supply of alcohol in a man suffering from alcoholism would not count. It is not GAD if the anxiety is an expression of panic disorder, agoraphobia, social phobia, simple phobia, or OCD.

The third criterion specifies that the anxiety is not a symptom of a mood disorder or a psychotic disorder. As we have pointed out, mood disorders (e.g., depression) and psychotic disorders (e.g., schizophrenia) flood the patient with anxiety and worry. This worry does not justify the additional diagnosis of GAD. If, however, the anxiety occurs during times when the psychotic disorder or mood disorder is in remission, then it is permissible to give the additional diagnosis of GAD.

The fourth criterion is a list of 18 symptoms. The patient must experience at least six of these symptoms during periods of anxiety and worry. The symptoms are instructive:

Motor tension
1. trembling, twitching, or feeling shaky
2. muscle tension, aches, or soreness
3. restlessness
4. easy fatigability

Autonomic hyperactivity
5. shortness of breath or smothering sensations
6. palpitations or accelerated heart rate
7. sweating, or cold clammy hands
8. dry mouth
9. dizziness or lightheadedness
10. nausea, diarrhea, or other abdominal distress
11. flushes (hot flashes) or chills
12. frequent urination

13. trouble swallowing or "lump in throat"
Vigilance and scanning
  14. feeling keyed up or on edge
  15. exaggerated startle response
  16. difficulty concentrating or "mind going blank" because of anxiety
  17. trouble falling or staying asleep
  18. irritability

The fifth criterion rules out the diagnosis of GAD when the symptoms are due to some known organic cause. In individuals who are sensitive to caffeine, coffee can be the problem. Disturbances in the functioning of hormone systems can also cause symptoms resembling GAD.

There is a lack of precise information about the prevalence of GAD. Nearly all the information about prevalence has been obtained from surveys that were conducted before the publication of the *DSM-III-R*. The *DSM-III-R* defines GAD much more restrictively than the *DSM-III*, so we would expect to count many fewer cases under the *DSM-III-R* criteria than under the older criteria. A reasonable guess is that about 1 percent of the U.S. population has experienced GAD during the past year.[26] Many cases that formerly would have been counted as GAD are likely to be categorized as adjustment disorder with anxious mood in the *DSM-III-R*.

The *DSM-III-R* permits the simultaneous diagnosis of GAD along with other illnesses, if it is clear that the symptoms are neither related to nor caused by the other illness. Thus, a person with major depression could be diagnosed as having GAD as well, provided the GAD symptoms occurred at times when the patient was not depressed. A person with OCD who had trouble with hand washing could also have GAD if he or she experienced multiple fears unrelated to dirt.

GAD is unusual among the illnesses discussed in this book in that there is little evidence that it runs in families. Studies of twins indicate that the concordance for identical twins is no greater than that for fraternal twins. Thus it appears that GAD is not the expression of an inherited predisposition, nor is it the result of experience that is specific to style of childrearing practiced by a particular nuclear family.[27]

ANXIETY DISORDERS AND MAJOR DEPRESSION

At present there is uncertainty about the dividing line between anxiety disorders and mood disorders. Indeed, it is not certain that depression is different from anxiety disorders.[28] It is very common for people with anxiety disorders also to satisfy the criteria of major depression.[29] Conversely, about half of the people with depression have a coexisting anxiety disorder.[30]

Anxiety disorders can create depressive living conditions. The coexisting depression of some anxiety patients may be a response to these anxiety-provoked depressive conditions.[31] We would not be surprised to learn, for example, that Alison, who suffered from agoraphobia, became extremely demoralized in response to the fact that her life was being ruined by her fear of leaving home. A person with social phobia could be overcome with feelings of hopelessness and despair because anxiety turns him or her into a wallflower. To thicken the plot, our social phobic may find that drinking relieves anxiety at parties but causes him or her to use such bad judgment that he or she later becomes depressed about all the harmful things done while drunk.

There are also cases in which depression occurs prior to the onset of the anxiety disorder.[32] In these cases, obviously, the depression is not a response to the anxiety disorder. There is a possibility, however, that in at least some of these cases, the anxiety disorder and the major depression are actually two different manifestations of the same underlying disorder. There are numerous suggestions of physiological similarity between anxiety disorders and major depression. For example, results of the dexamethasone suppression test are similar in people with panic disorder, major depression, and OCD.[33] Further clarification of the relationships between depression and anxiety is a major goal of future research on mental illness.

ANXIETY DISORDERS, ALCOHOLISM, AND SEDATIVE DRUG ABUSE

Alcoholism and abuse of sedative drugs are also often present along with anxiety disorders. Among anxiety patients, the risk of alcoholism is about twice that of same sex-people who have no psychiatric disorder.[34] The converse is also true; those who suffer from alcoholism have a high risk of coexisting anxiety disorder. OCD is probably less frequently associated with alcoholism than are other anxiety disorders.[35]

Alcohol provides the special reward of relaxation and peace to people who are chronically anxious. It is plausible, therefore, that people who suffer from excessive anxiety might turn to alcohol as a self-medication.[36] In a study by Penelope Smail and colleagues, over half of a sample of alcoholics who also suffered from phobias said they found alcohol useful in controlling their fears. About 45 percent said that they used alcohol deliberately for this purpose.[37] Thus, anxiety disorders may be considered a risk factor for the development of dependence on alcohol and other anxiety-relieving drugs.

Another important fact is that withdrawal of alcohol or anxiety-relieving drugs in a person who has developed a drug dependence evokes anxiety states including panic. Thus drug dependence must be considered a risk factor for excessive anxiety. A drug-dependent person might try to procure a prescription for an abused drug (e.g., barbiturate, Valium, Xanax) by claiming that his or her withdrawal symptoms are actually symptoms of panic disorder. This person may not realize that his or her anxiety problems are actually drug withdrawal effects.

These possibilities suggest that a physician or psychologist should advise anxiety patients to stop using all drugs that evoke anxiety either directly or in withdrawal. Only when the state of the disorder is evaluated in the absence of pharmacologic provocation is it possible to plan an appropriate pharmacological and/or psychological treatment.

TREATING ANXIETY WITH
ANXIOLYTIC DRUGS

—

A *nxiolytics* are drugs that relieve anxiety. In this chapter we briefly review the situations in which anxiolytics are used. We then discuss four classes of anxiolytics: barbiturates, minor tranquilizers, benzodiazepines and buspirone. For each class we briefly describe the history of the drug, its benefits, and side effects. Since the benzodiazepines are the most widely used anxiolytics, we discuss them in the most detail, including a section comparing their mechanism of action with that of the barbiturates.

The majority of prescriptions for anxiolytics are not written by psychiatrists, but by physicians in family practice, internal medicine, and other nonpsychiatric specialties.[1] As we saw in Chapter 15, excessive anxiety causes many bodily symptoms, and these symptoms often lead patients to seek treatment for bodily illness. Such patients may be suffering from generalized anxiety disorder, atypical anxiety disorder, panic disorder, or post-traumatic stress disorder. Other patients may be suffering anxiety in association with mental illnesses that are not anxiety disorders, for example, somatization disorder or major depression. Still others may be experiencing bodily symptoms associated with anxiety about a stressful life event, such as a divorce, a financial reversal, or an impending death in the family.[2] Physicians frequently prescribe anxiolytics for medical patients who do not have psychiatric illnesses. Anxiolytics are very frequently prescribed to relieve anxiety prior to surgery. Patients with chronic diseases, such as cancer, arthritis, or back pain, often need anxiolytics to relieve the uneasiness and dread that accompanies their illness.[3]

In cases of anxiety that are not related to known organic illness, the patient and physician may find it difficult to decide whether the optimal treatment is an anxiolytic drug to relieve the symptoms directly or psychotherapy directed at suspected underlying problems. Indeed, talking to a friend, minister, or psychotherapist may be exactly what is needed in some cases. The best decisions about treatment strategy are based on sound knowledge of the causes of the symptoms. The causes of psychiatric anxiety are far from clear in many cases. It is wisest, therefore, to retain an open mind, acknowledging the fact that some educated guessing and trial and error may be required to discover an effective strategy for treating any particular case.

It is necessary to make a terminological point about the difference between anxiolytic drugs and sedative-hypnotic drugs. Most anxiolytic drugs also cause sedation (a slowing down of thought and behavior), and hypnosis (the production of sleep). A drug which causes sedation and hypnosis is called a sedative-hypnotic drug. Until recently all available drugs for combating anxiety also had significant sedative-hypnotic action. Indeed, it has been a common medical opinion that a certain amount of sedation and hypnosis is the price that must be paid for anxiety relief with a drug. An important question in psychopharmacology has been whether a drug can be found to relieve anxiety without the penalty of sedation and hypnosis.

The medical use of anxiolytics must be evaluated in light of the fact that nonprescription anxiolytics are readily available and widely used. Alcohol is an excellent anxiolytic, as well as a sedative-hypnotic. Many people drink without serious concern about its potential harms, which include increased risk of poor nutrition and obesity, several types of cancer, addiction, occupational and social incapacitation, and damage to many organs, including the liver, the cardiovascular system, the pancreas, the gastrointestinal tract, the immune system, the reproductive system, the blood-forming system, and the brain.[4] Since the late nineteenth century, an important goal of pharmacologists and medicinal chemists has been to discover and develop new drugs with anxiolytic efficacy equal or superior to alcohol's but with lower risks.

In the following pages we discuss four classes of synthetic anxiolytics; the barbiturates, the so-called minor tranquilizers, the benzodiazepines, and buspirone. Since the benzodiazepines are the most widely used, we discuss them in the most detail.

THE BARBITURATES

Barbital, the first medicinal barbiturate, was introduced in 1903.[5] It was thought to have lower addiction risk and fewer bad side effects than alcohol and other sedatives that were then available. A year later, however, it was reported that some people were becoming addicted to barbital.[6] Death by overdose also turned out to be a problem. A bottle of barbiturate pills was a convenient weapon in the hands of self-destructive patients. Nonetheless, the barbiturates were superior to alcohol because they had fewer side effects that were harmful to general health and their use could be supervised by physicians through the use of prescriptions. During the first half of the twentieth century, barbiturates were the dominant medicines for relieving excessive anxiety.

Barbiturates can produce all degrees of mental and behavioral depression, depending on dosage. At low doses, they reduce anxiety, slow down behavior, and encourage sleep. At somewhat higher doses they produce severe mental impairment, motor incoordination, and stuporousness similar to alcoholic drunkenness. At higher doses yet, barbiturates are suitable for use as anesthetics during major surgery. Still higher doses result in death due to blockade of the neural reflexes of respiration.[7] A difficulty with barbiturates as anxiolytics is that the dose required to relieve anxiety is also sufficient to cause drowsiness, accident proneness, and general dulling of the wits.

Another problem with barbiturates is their interference with drug metabolism. In the liver barbiturates induce activity in the enzyme system that transforms and deactivates toxins and foreign molecules in the blood. This abnormally fast detoxification may cause a reduction in the effectiveness of the barbiturates themselves and in the effectiveness of drugs that are being used to treat other illnesses. In addition, barbiturates interfere with the function of an important drug-metabolizing enzyme in the liver called cytochrome P-450. This enzyme blockade further disturbs the rate at which the liver degrades many compounds, including the steroid hormones. Hormone imbalances may result.[8]

THE MINOR TRANQUILIZERS

In 1955 Wallace Laboratories introduced a new nonbarbiturate anxiolytic called Miltown (generic name, meprobamate). Miltown was presented to the public as an improvement on the barbiturates.[9] At the time of its introduction, pharmacologists thought that Miltown carried less addiction risk than the older drugs, and this opinion was duly reported in advertising copy put out by Wallace Laboratories.[10] The new drug rapidly became popular with patients and physicians. Other drug companies, perceiving that North Americans and Western Europeans were ready to take more pills for the relief of anxiety, raced to capture a share of an expanding market. A parade of new drugs came onto the market in the late 1950s and 1960s, including Doriden (glutethimide), Quaalude (methaqualone), Noludar (methyprylon), and Placidyl (ethchlorvynol).[11] The new drugs were called minor tranquilizers to distinguish them from the discredited barbiturates, which had been called sedatives. (Chlorpromazine and other antipsychotic drugs were called major tranquilizers.)

The distinction between minor tranquilizers and sedatives turned out to be more important for drug promotion than for medical treatment. As experience accumulated with the minor tranquilizers of the 1950s, it became obvious that they were no more effective, just as sedating, just as addictive, and just as toxic as the barbiturates that preceded them.[12]

THE BENZODIAZEPINES

In 1960 and 1962 Roche Laboratories introduced two more minor tranquilizers, Librium (chlordiazepoxide) and Valium (diazepam).[13] These drugs are members of the chemical family called benzodiazepines. Librium and Valium soon captured a large share of the market for anxiolytics, and other companies followed suit with additional drugs of the benzodiazepine family. In the ensuing three decades, thousands of benzodiazepines have been synthesized; over 100 have been tested for medical use, and 8 (listed in the appendix) are approved for anxiety relief in the United States.[14]

By the early 1970s the benzodiazepines had nearly replaced barbiturates and all other contenders as the drug of choice for excessive anxiety. Furthermore, the use of prescription anxiolytics had become more widespread. In 1972 Valium ranked first and Librium third on the list of most-prescribed drugs in the United States.[15] About 85 million prescriptions were written for benzodiazepine anxiolytics in the United States in 1975[16]; 10 to 20 percent of adults in Western Europe and North America took benzodiazepines on a fairly regular basis. As remarked by D. J. Greenblatt and R. I. Shader, two prominent benzodiazepine researchers, there was a benzodiazepine bandwagon (Figure 16–1).[17]

The first report of benzodiazepine addiction appeared in 1963, three years after the introduction of Librium. Additional reports trickled in thereafter.[18] At first the drug companies and medical authorities discounted these reports as cases in which the original addiction had developed as a result of using a nonbenzodiazepine drug like alcohol. Nonetheless, as the use of benzodiazepines continued to grow, unfavorable publicity about addiction to "tranquilizers" appeared more and more frequently in the media.

A wave of concern about benzodiazepine overprescribing swept through the medical community in the mid-1970s.[19] In 1975 the U.S. drug enforcement authorities placed benzodiazepines on the list of controlled substances, as they had earlier placed the barbiturates and other minor tranquilizers.[20] The annual number of benzodiazepine prescriptions began to decline sharply. Then in 1981 the decline reversed to very gradual growth (Figure 16–1). In the late 1980s the annual number of prescriptions for benzodiazepine anxiolytics was about 60 million,[21] down from a peak of about 85 million. In 1989 the two top-selling benzodiazepines (Xanax and Valium) occupied fourth and thirty-third places on the list of most-

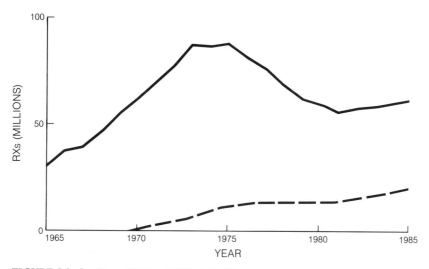

FIGURE 16-1   From 1965 to 1985, 1.5 billion prescriptions were written in the United States for benzodiazepines. The benzodiazepine bandwagon ran from the early 1960s until 1975. Solid line: prescribed as anxiolytics. Dashed line: prescribed as hypnotics. The sum of anxiolytic and hypnotic prescriptions reached about 100 million in 1975. From U.S. Food and Drug Administration. *Drug Utilization in the United States, 1985, 7th Annual Report* (Washington, D.C.: U.S. Department of Health and Human Services, 1986).

prescribed drugs.[22] The decline in use of benzodiazepines has caused some psychiatrists to express concern that excessive fear of addiction is preventing proper medication for patients who could safely benefit from anxiolytics.[23]

The explosion in the use of anxiolytics beginning in the mid-1960s is a social phenomenon whose causes are not fully known. Perhaps, for the first time, people began to believe that maladaptive anxiety is a disorder that should be treated medically rather than overcome by an act of character. Perhaps the sophisticated advertising of Roche Laboratories was a factor.[24] The pitch was that Librium and Valium relieved anxiety with fewer bad side effects and with greater safety than drugs previously available, and apparently most physicians were persuaded. Furthermore, people who took benzodiazepines seemed to be pleased with the results.[25] According to a survey conducted in Europe, people who used benzodiazepines were only one-half to one-third as likely as people who never took these drugs to believe that the drugs "do more harm than good."[26] Women were twice as likely to use benzodiazepines as men, and older people were more likely to use them than young people.[27] Instead of benzodiazepines, the young people of the era were involved with marijuana, LSD, and psilocybin. ᒪᔑ HₙᵤₘS

In one respect, there is universal agreement that the benzodiazepines are an improvement over the barbiturates. They have less potential for use as suicide pills. Some authorities doubt that anyone has ever died as a result of an overdose of benzodiazepine *alone*.[28] Ingesting 50 or 60 times the anxiolytic dose does not arrest respiration, and it is almost always possible to arouse a person from a benzodiazepine stupor. Accordingly, benzodiazepines cannot be used for surgical anesthesia. By contrast, the lethal dose of alcohol, barbiturates, or the nonbenzodiazepine minor tranquilizers is 10 to 20 times the anxiety-relieving dose.[29] People who seek medical help for excessive anxiety are much more likely to have suicidal impulses than are those who do not seek such help.[30] Considering the vast number of people who take benzodiazepines, the rarity of lethal overdose is a remarkable fact that, more than any other, justifies the wide acceptance of benzodiazepines by physicians and patients.

Benzodiazepines, however, can be a contributing cause of death when they are combined with other drugs. A dose of barbiturate, alcohol, opiates, or nonbenzodiazepine anxiolytic that would not be lethal by itself can become lethal when a benzodiazepine is added.[31] As explained below, benzodiazepines suppress nervous activity by a mechanism that is different from that of barbiturates and other drugs. While not lethal by itself, the benzodiazepine action can add to the action of the other drugs, resulting in a lethal combination.

Effectiveness of Benzodiazepines Compared to Barbiturates

Scientific studies leave no doubt that benzodiazepines bring anxiety relief. Anxiolytic efficacy can be demonstrated easily in laboratory animals. Under the influence of the benzodiazepines, rats or monkeys become less fearful of punishment. A standard test, called the Geller test, is to train a hungry rat to press a bar to obtain a bit of food. When this behavior is well learned, the researcher throws a switch so that every time the rat presses the bar, it receives a mild electric shock on the feet (punishment) as well as the food. A drug-free rat slows down or stops pressing the bar soon after the first shock. If, however, the experimenter injects a benzodiazepine before the test, the rat, as if unencumbered by fear, will press and eat, shock notwithstanding (Figure 16–2).

Using the Geller test and similar animal techniques, researchers have been able to screen hundreds of compounds in search of new

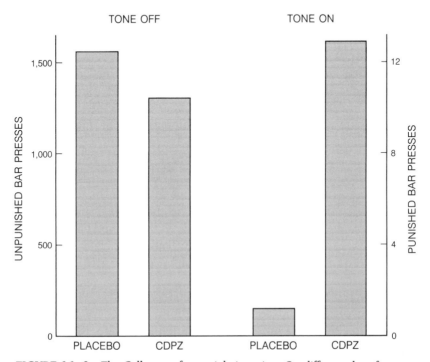

FIGURE 16–2   The Geller test for anxiolytic action. On different days four rats were given either placebo or the benzodiazepine chlordiazepoxide (CDPZ). The rats were then tested for number of bar presses under two conditions. (1) When a tone was on, every bar press was rewarded with a sip of milk and punished with a mild electric shock lasting 0.25 seconds. These are called punished bar presses. Normal rats emit very few punished bar presses. (2) When the tone was off, there was no punishment, and bar presses were sometimes rewarded with a sip of milk. The time between rewarded bar presses varied, with an average of one rewarded bar press every two minutes. These are called unpunished bar presses. Normal rats press the bar rapidly on this schedule of rewards. The tone was off (no punishment) for 15 minutes and then on (punishment) for 3 minutes. This off/on cycle was repeated five times. The graph gives the average number of bar presses made during a 15-minute unpunished period and a 3-minute punished period. Note that the rats emitted many more punished bar presses when given chlordiazepoxide than when given placebo. The chlordiazepoxide did not increase the number of unpunished bar presses. This result is an example in which an anxiolytic drug facilitates a behavior that is inhibited by punishment. Data from I. Geller, J. T. Kulak, and J. Seifter, "The Effects of Chlordiazepoxide and Chlorpromazine on a Punishment Discrimination," *Psychopharmacology* 3(1962):374–85.

anxiolytics that have fewer bad side effects. This is the method by which the anxiolytic efficacy of benzodiazepines was discovered, and it has led recently to new drugs that have fewer side effects than diazepam.[32]

In human anxiety patients the efficacy of benzodiazepines has been demonstrated in experiments in which a benzodiazepine is compared with a placebo or some other active drug. A good example of such an experiment was reported in 1970 by Peter Hesbacher, Karl Rickels, and several of their colleagues at the University of Pennsylvania Medical School. They compared diazepam (Valium) to placebo and to the barbiturate, phenobarbital. The study involved 472 patients, all of whom sought treatment for chronic excessive anxiety. Since the study was published 10 years before the *DSM-III*, we cannot report the diagnosis that these patients would receive today. Many of them would probably satisfy the *DSM-III-R* criteria for GAD or adjustment disorder with anxious mood. In the terminology of the day, the patients were said to be psychoneurotic. Some of the patients were treated in a medical clinic that served patients with low incomes; others were treated by private physicians in general practice, and still others were treated by psychiatrists in private practice.

At the beginning of treatment, each patient filled out a data sheet consisting of about 60 common symptoms of anxiety (headache, diarrhea, feeling tense, and so on). The patients were asked to rate on a scale of one to four how much each symptom had bothered them during the past week. The patients then had an interview with one of the participating physicians, and the physician scored the severity of the anxiety symptoms on a scale of one to seven.

The physician next gave each patient some capsules containing either diazepam, phenobarbital, or placebo. He explained that the capsules contained a new drug that had been supplied free by a drug company and that it would be "good for your nerves." One capsule was to be taken with breakfast, lunch, and dinner, and two more were to be taken at bedtime. The physician further explained about possible side effects, such as drowsiness and difficulty keeping one's balance, and warned about the hazard of driving a car or operating dangerous machinery while taking the drug. The capsules had been coded by the participating pharmacist, but neither the physician nor the patient knew whether the capsules contained placebo, diazepam, or phenobarbital. The drug that a particular patient received was determined at random. Patients receiving an active drug took 10 mg per day of diazepam or 150 mg per day of phenobarbital.

The patients returned for evaluation after two weeks and again after four weeks. During these follow-up visits, physicians evaluated the improvement of symptoms and the occurrence of side effects. The physicians also counted the remaining capsules to determine whether the patients had used the drug as directed.

When the data were analyzed, it was clear that both active drugs were superior to placebo in relieving symptoms, but neither of the active drugs was consistently superior to the other (Figure 16–3). Patients taking diazepam reported fewer side effects than did patients taking phenobarbital. Diazepam was superior to phenobarbital in patient acceptability. More diazepam patients than phenobarbital patients took their capsules as prescribed, and fewer diazepam patients dropped out of the study. Also, there were fewer diazepam dropouts than placebo dropouts. Presumably the phenobarbital dropouts were dissatisfied with bad side effects, while the placebo dropouts were dissatisfied with their lack of improvement.[33]

Numerous studies similar to the one by Hesbacher and colleagues have been reported. In most of these studies the benzodiazepine was more effective than placebo; placebo was never more effective than the benzodiazepine. When a benzodiazepine was compared with a barbiturate, the benzodiazepine was usually equal or superior to the barbiturate in relieving anxiety symptoms. The barbiturates usually produced more side effects than did the benzodiazepines.[34] We may conclude, therefore, that the benzodiazepines are indeed an effective treatment for anxiety symptoms, they are as effective as barbiturates, and they produce fewer complaints about side effects.

Side Effects of Benzodiazepines

The most feared side effect is drug dependence and addiction. The most common side effect is excessive sedation in the form of drowsiness, loss of mental acuity, and motor incoordination. The problem of dependence and addiction is broad and complex, involving much more than just the treatment of anxiety. Accordingly, we have given it an entire chapter of its own (Chapter 18). In this chapter we discuss the common side effect of unwanted sedation and the less common side effect of release of impulsive aggression.

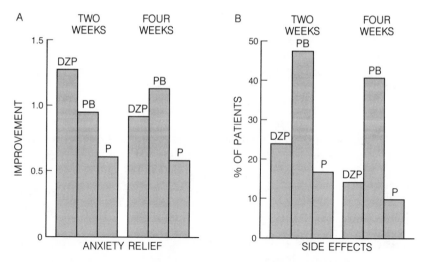

FIGURE 16-3 Anxiolytic efficacy and frequency of side effects in chronic anxiety patients treated with diazepam (DZP), phenobarbital (PB), and placebo (P). Data obtained two weeks and four weeks after beginning of drug treatment. A. Symptomatic improvement rated on scale of 0 to 3, where 0 = no improvement, 3 = very much improvement. B. Percentage of patients experiencing either drowsiness or dizziness during the preceding two weeks of treatment. Note: Phenobarbital and diazepam are not consistently different in relieving symptoms, but diazepam evokes significantly fewer side effects than does phenobarbital. Diazepam and placebo are not significantly different in evoking side effects. Data from P. T. Hesbacher, K. Rickels, P. E. Gordon, B. Gray, R. Meckelnburg, C. C. Weise, and W. J. Vandervort, "Setting, Patient, and Doctor Effects on Drug Response in Neurotic Patients. I. Differential Attrition, Dosage Deviation, and Side Reaction Responses to Treatment," *Psychopharmacologia* 18(1970): 180–208; P. T. Hesbacher, K. Rickels, J. Hutchison, E. Raab, L. Sablosky, E. M. Whalen, and F. P. Phillips, "Setting, Patient, and Doctor Effects on Drug Response in Neurotic Patients. II. Differential Improvement," *Psychopharmacologia* 18(1970): 209–26.

EXCESSIVE SEDATION.   At the beginning of benzodiazepine treatment, patients may experience difficulty remaining alert, learning new verbal material, thinking, making judgments, reading, or carrying on complex discussions. Reflexes and skilled movements are somewhat impaired. Driving a car or flying a plane may be hazardous. The patient may not be aware of the impairment.[35]

In the case of diazepam, cognitive side effects after a single dose are maximal about one hour after taking the drug and have largely subsided by three hours. With other benzodiazepines, the effects may last considerably longer. Differences between drugs are caused by differences in their rate of elimination by the liver and kidney, the degree to which they are stored in different tissues of the body, and the ease with which they penetrate the brain. With multiple daily doses there is buildup of the active drug in the blood, resulting in persistent unwanted sedation.[36] The side effects become more severe and last longer as the dosage is increased. At toxic dosages the syndrome is similar to alcoholic drunkenness and stuporousness.[37]

In most patients, unwanted sedation is diminished by the development of tolerance. That is, the side effects diminish as drug treatment continues. Some patients show less rapid tolerance than others; for most patients, excessive sedation has diminished considerably, though perhaps not totally, after six to eight weeks of treatment. At the University of Pennsylvania, Irwin Lucki and Karl Rickels investigated the question of excessive sedation in a group of patients who had been taking benzodiazepines for many years for generalized anxiety disorder. The patients were tested on cognitive tasks that are very sensitive to the sedative effects of benzodiazepines, barbiturates, and alcohol. Their performance on the cognitive tasks was just as good as the performance of a matched group of anxiety patients who had not been treated with drugs. Thus, in this experiment, tolerance for the sedative side effects appeared to be complete after years of treatment.[38] Tolerance develops less readily in the elderly than in the young, and therefore the elderly must be given lower doses.[39]

In contrast to sedation, little tolerance develops for the desired anxiolytic effect. This point is exemplified in another study by Rickels and colleagues, in which patients with chronic generalized anxiety were given diazepam for 6 to 22 weeks. At arbitrary times between 6 and 22 weeks some of the patients were switched, double blind, to placebo. Those patients who were switched to placebo showed a higher rate of relapse than did those who were not, and those who were maintained on diazepam continued to experience relief from anxiety from the sixth through the twenty-second week. These results indicate that detectable tolerance does not develop for the therapeutic benefit for at least 22 weeks of treatment.[40]

The comparatively new drug alprazolam (Xanax), introduced in 1981,[41] appears to produce somewhat less sedation at anxiolytic dosages than the older benzodiazepines. Aden and Thein compared alprazolam, diazepam, and placebo in nonhospitalized anxiety patients who were randomly assigned, double blind, to placebo, alprazolam, or diazepam groups. Anxiety symptoms and side effects were evaluated by structured interviews and checklists at the beginning of treatment and after one, two, or four weeks of treatment. Alprazolam was equal to diazepam, and both drugs were better than placebo for producing relief of anxiety. As usual, drowsiness was the most frequently mentioned side effect, and there were no severe side effects in any of the groups. Fewest side effects were reported by patients receiving alprazolam, somewhat more by placebo patients, and the most by diazepam patients. These differences in side effects were apparently not statistically significant.[42] In studies like this, side effects are so infrequent, even for diazepam, that it is hard to demonstrate the statistical significance of the differences between groups. Similar trends in favor of alprazolam have been observed in many studies.[43] When patients are asked if they would like to continue with the medication they have experienced during the study, they are more likely to answer yes when the drug has been alprazolam than when it has been diazepam.[44] In an interesting animal study, Soderpalm found that tolerance for the sedative action, but not for the anxiolytic action, develops more rapidly with alprazolam than with diazepam.[45] Thus research suggests that alprazolam causes less unwanted sedation than the previously available benzodiazepines.

DRUG-RELEASED AGGRESSION. It is generally believed that social restraint and judgment are impaired by anxiolytics. The drugs may permit people to take risks or engage in behaviors they normally would suppress for fear of embarrassment.[46] These effects are predictable from the animal studies, showing that anxiolytics increase behaviors that are inhibited by fear of punishment. The relief from social fear is one of the main goals sought by those who take anxiolytics, of course. But this benefit is a two-edged sword. Living harmoniously with others requires a certain amount of social restraint. Drug-induced impulsiveness can be disastrous, as is well known from the association of alcohol with violent crimes and suicide. Less well known are the cases in the psychiatric literature in which prescription anxiolytics appear to have released ill-considered hostility or aggressiveness.

Peter exemplifies a patient who became unusually hostile while taking an antianxiety drug. Peter was about 40 years old and worked as a tree trimmer. In an accident at work he injured his back, and his family doctor prescribed Valium at 20 mg per day to relieve some of the anxiety associated with the pain. After about three days on Valium, Peter began to be unusually argumentative. Arguing with his wife was not normal behavior for him, and he thought the cause was being cooped up at home all day. So he went back to work. However, he immediately got into an argument with a coworker that escalated into a fist fight. Peter had not gotten into a fight since high school. His wife then insisted that he see a psychiatrist.

The psychiatrist thought that Peter had been harboring resentments and that the Valium was decreasing inhibitions and releasing the expression of hostility. Peter's Valium was discontinued, and the argumentativeness went away after a couple of days. The psychiatrist encouraged Peter to see a counselor in his neighborhood mental health clinic so that he could ventilate some of his resentments. Whether the psychotherapy was undertaken or was beneficial was not reported.[47]

A few case histories are not proof, of course, that benzodiazepines can release aggressiveness. The aggressive behavior might have occurred anyway, given the particular personality and the particular situation. In an effort to evaluate rigorously whether benzodiazepines could release aggressiveness, Carl Salzman and several colleagues from the medical schools at Harvard and New York University performed an experiment in which aggressive behaviors were measured in small groups of young men who were subjected to mild frustration.

For a week prior to the critical experimental day, the men in some groups were given a small daily dose of chlordiazepoxide, while the men in other groups received a placebo. On the day of the experiment, the experimenter asked the men in each group to spend 10 minutes making up a story about a picture they were shown. At the end of the discussion, the experimenter created a frustrating situation by telling each group that its story was inadequate and that a new story had to be prepared. At this point, one of the men (who had taken chlordiazepoxide) became furious and walked out of the study, but the remaining men controlled themselves sufficiently to finish a second story. Later, the psychologists scored videotapes of the group discussions to find out whether hostile or assaultive behavior had increased after the men had been told that they had to make up new stories.

On the average, the frustration had caused a greater increase in hostility and assaultiveness in the men who had taken Librium than in those who had taken placebo. This study was double blind — neither the observers nor the subjects knew who had taken chlordiazepoxide and who had taken placebo.[48] Thus it appears that low dosages of benzodiazepine sometimes release social aggressiveness.

EFFECTS OF BENZODIAZEPINES ON ORGANS OF THE BODY. In contrast to alcohol and barbiturates, benzodiazepines have little known action outside the brain and spinal cord. The benzodiazepines do not induce drug-metabolizing enzymes in the liver, so they do not significantly interfere with drug treatment of nonpsychiatric illnesses. The most frequently reported nonneural effect of benzodiazepines is skin rash, and even this is very rare. It is unclear whether rashes are due to the action of the drug on the skin itself or to an action on the central nervous system that secondarily results in a rash. The freedom from threatening nonneuronal side effects gives the benzodiazepines a genuine therapeutic advantage over other drugs available for the treatment of anxiety and justifies the popularity of benzodiazepines with physicians and patients. The use of other drugs, such as meprobamate, barbiturates, glutethimide, and so on, for the treatment of anxiety is now virtually obsolete.[49]

How Benzodiazepines and Barbiturates Act on Neurons

Before 1977 neuropharmacologists knew rather little about how benzodiazepines and barbiturates act on neurons to produce relief from anxiety. Recently, however, there has been a leap forward in this area. As mentioned in Chapter 2, recent research indicates that anxiolytic drugs modulate synaptic transmission that is mediated by the transmitter GABA. GABA is a very common transmitter in the brain. It is especially common in the cerebral hemispheres where the neural mechanisms of anticipatory anxiety are thought to reside.

At GABA synapses, as at all others (see Chapter 2), the transmitter molecules must attach, or bind, to postsynaptic receptor molecules in order to cause a change in the nerve impulse activity of the postsynaptic cell. A postsynaptic receptor is a particular type of protein structure that is imbedded in the membrane of the postsynaptic cell. For each type of transmitter there are corresponding types of postsynaptic receptors that readily bind to the particular transmitter; these receptors do not bind readily to most other chemicals or other transmitters.

When GABA binds to its postsynaptic receptors, it has an inhibitory effect; that is, when the axon terminal of a GABA-secreting nerve cell releases GABA into the synaptic cleft, the postsynaptic nerve cell responds by reducing its output of nerve impulses. This inhibitory effect stops promptly when GABA detaches from its receptors. Because the attachment is not exceedingly tight, GABA does detach fairly readily under normal circumstances. When GABA becomes detached, it may be removed from the synaptic cleft by being taken up into the presynaptic terminal, thus terminating inhibition by removal of the transmitter from the vicinity of the receptor.[50]

The GABA receptor, it turns out, is a complex assembly of several (probably five) protein molecules (Figure 16–4). These GABA receptor molecules associate with one another to form a multimolecular mechanism called the GABA receptor complex. When fully assembled, the GABA receptor complex forms a channel or pore through the membrane that can be either open or closed. When the channel is open, ions can flow through the channel across the postsynaptic membrane, resulting in inhibition of impulses in the postsynaptic neuron. The attachment of GABA to its binding site on the receptor increases the probability that the channel will open, thus causing inhibition. Detachment of GABA restores the probability of opening to its low resting value, which relieves inhibition.

A key observation about the action of benzodiazepines is that they enhance synaptic inhibition at GABA synapses.[51] This point was made as early as 1971 by Stratten and Barnes, working at Indiana University. Measuring the effectiveness of synaptic inhibition in suppressing nerve impulses at a GABA synapse in the cat spinal cord, they found that an injection of diazepam enhanced inhibition.[52] Robert E. Study and Jeffery L. Barker, working at the National Institutes of Health in Bethesda, Maryland, extended this work by observing how GABA and diazepam act on the ion channel. Using neurons isolated from the mouse spinal cord, they found that GABA evokes more openings of the channel in the presence of diazepam than in the absence of diazepam.[53] Diazepam is a GABA helper. Diazepam alone has no effect on the channel.[54]

Meanwhile, investigators in Denmark and Switzerland found that there is a protein in the brain that has a high-affinity binding site for

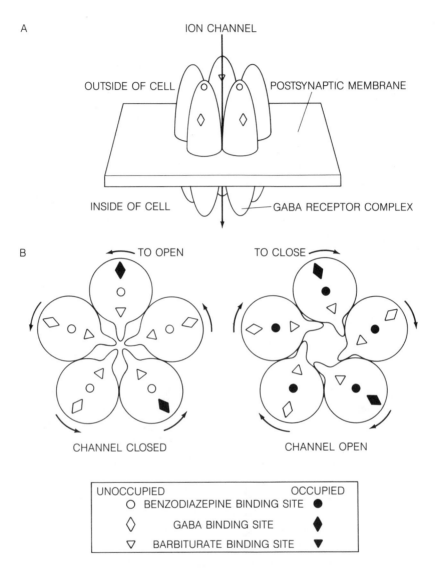

FIGURE 16–4 Diagram of the GABA receptor complex in the postsynaptic membrane. A. Position of the receptor complex in the membrane. It is likely that the receptor complex consists of five elongated protein molecules arranged in the shape of a cylinder that forms an ion channel through the membrane. Each of the proteins probably has binding sites for GABA, benzodiazepines, and barbiturates. Binding of GABA facilitates the passage of ions through the channel. The flow of ions causes inhibition of the postsynaptic neuron. The pathway taken by the ions is shown by the arrow. B. Cross sections of the GABA receptor complex in the plane of the membrane, showing the channel either open or closed. It is hypothesized that opening and closing of the channel may occur by a tilting of the receptor complex that imparts a twisting motion to the receptor proteins. Binding of benzodiazepines

diazepam. This diazepam-binding protein had properties that would be expected of a specific receptor for benzodiazepines. It was especially abundant in parts of the brain containing many GABA synapses and less abundant elsewhere. Furthermore, when a large series of benzodiazepines was tested, a good correlation was found between the affinity of the benzodiazepine for the protein and the anxiolytic potency of the compound. This indicates that the anxiolytic action of benzodiazepines is produced when the drug binds to the identified protein.[55] (It is interesting that a similar type of experiment showed that antipsychotic drugs act at dopamine receptors. See Chapter 7.) Further experiments at Cambridge University in England showed that the benzodiazepine-binding protein is a part of the GABA receptor complex (Figure 16–4).[56]

In summary, this and other evidence indicates that benzodiazepines enhance inhibition at GABA synapses by binding directly to the GABA receptor complex. The sites where benzodiazepines bind are distinct from the sites where GABA binds. When benzodiazepines alone bind to the receptor, there is no inhibition. But when GABA binds, there is greater inhibition if the benzodiazepine sites are also occupied by diazepam than if the benzodiazepine sites are unoccupied.[57]

There are additional binding sites on GABA receptors. These sites have a high affinity for barbiturate drugs and may be called barbiturate binding sites. When barbiturates are bound to the barbiturate sites, the action of GABA is enhanced, much as it is enhanced by benzodiazepines. Barbiturates, however, are more than just GABA helpers. Barbiturates can open the ion channel and evoke inhibition by themselves in the absence of GABA.[58] Scientists also suspect that barbiturates can suppress neural activity in other ways at non-GABA synapses.[59]

Because barbiturates can suppress the activity of neurons in at least two ways while benzodiazepines do so in only one way, one can

---

increases the probability of channel opening when GABA is also bound. Binding of barbiturates will open the channel even in the absence of GABA. The open channel is depicted with two GABA sites occupied (filled symbols) and all five benzodiazepine sites occupied. The depicted shape of the channel wall and positioning of the binding sites are diagrammatic. The actual shape of the channel and position of biding sites are unknown. Based on N. Unwin, "The Structure of Ion Channels in Membranes of Excitable Cells," *Neuron* 3(1989): 665–76; R. W. Olsen and A. J. Tobin, "Molecular Biology of GABA$_A$ Receptors," *FASEB Journal* 4(1990): 1469–80.

expect barbiturates to be more disruptive of normal brain function than the benzodiazepines. This expectation is borne out by the clinical observation that barbiturates produce more numerous side effects than do benzodiazepines. At low dosages barbiturates relieve anxiety, with some unwanted sedation as a side effect. The anxiolytic action at low dosages is thought to be caused predominately by enhancement of GABA inhibition. At higher dosages barbiturates induce a deep coma and arrest respiration. These high-dosage effects are probably caused by both enhancement of GABA inhibition and direct neural suppression produced by the barbiturate alone. One reason why benzodiazepines are not lethal, even in massive overdose, is that they enhance only natural inhibition; they do not suppress neural activity in the absence of naturally secreted GABA. Another reason why benzodiazepines are not as dangerous as barbiturates is that many GABA receptors may lack the high-affinity binding site for benzodiazepines. These inhibitory synapses therefore are not acted upon by benzodiazepines. In contrast, nearly all GABA synapses have binding sites for barbiturate. Barbiturates thus act on more synapses than do benzodiazepines.

Low doses of alcohol also relieve anxiety. Is it possible that these actions of alcohol are due to enhancement of GABA-mediated inhibition? Some recent data indicate that the answer may be yes. Peter Suzdak and collaborators at the National Institutes of Health have applied low concentrations of alcohol to preparations of synaptic membrane from the brain of rats. These membranes contain GABA receptor complexes, and application of GABA to the membranes causes opening of ion channels as it does at intact GABA synapses. Addition of a low concentration of alcohol to the preparation enhances channel opening evoked by GABA. The concentration of alcohol that produces this enhancement is similar to that which causes anxiety relief.[60]

We may hypothesize that anxiety corresponds to a high level of nerve impulse traffic in particular brain circuits serving fear and vigilance. The anxiolytic drugs would then relieve anxiety by enhancing the inhibition of activity in these circuits. Several groups of investigators have marshaled evidence that they think points to specific brain loci where the fear circuits may reside.[62] We will have a bit more to say about these brain loci in our discussion of agoraphobia, panic disorder, and obsessive-compulsive disorder in Chapter 18.

Ever since the discovery that the benzodiazepines modulate synaptic inhibition at GABA synapses, scientists have wondered if there may be a natural compound in the brain that modulates the action of GABA. Such a compound might play the role of a natural anxiolytic by which the brain could regulate its own anxiety level. The benzodiazepines might simply mimic the action of this natural compound. The GABA receptor might even have evolved as a physiological fear regulatory site.[61]

No compound has yet been identified that unequivocally plays the role of a natural anxiolytic. A compound has been extracted from the brain, however, that binds to the benzodiazepine site on the GABA receptor complex. The discoverers of the compound, Erminio Costa and colleagues at the National Institutes of Health, call it DBI, which is short for diazepam binding inhibitor. When DBI is present, it occupies the benzodiazepine site and prevents the binding of diazepam. When injected into test animals, DBI causes them to display signs of excessive fear and vigilance. DBI enhances the power of very mild electric shock to interrupt a rat's bar pressing for food or water. Thus DBI is not an anxiolytic agent like diazepam, but an "anxiogenic" one.[63] Costa and his colleagues cite a variety of indications that, to their minds, suggest that DBI or its by-products are released by neurons to suppress GABA inhibition and enhance fear.[64] Many investigators, however, are not yet convinced.

Other anxiogenic compounds that bind to the benzodiazepine site are known. Although these compounds are not present in the brain, they do suppress inhibition by GABA.[65] These compounds, like DBI, arouse anxiety in animals[66] and people.[67] Their anxiogenic efficacy is blocked by anxiolytic benzodiazepines.

BUSPIRONE, AN ANXIOLYTIC WITH A DIFFERENT MECHANISM

In psychology, psychiatry, and neuroscience the most common mistake is oversimplification. This point is brought home by the fact that there are several drugs with anxiolytic action that have no direct effect on the GABA receptor complex.

One of the most interesting of these drugs is buspirone, an anxiolytic introduced in 1986 by the Meade Johnson pharmaceutical firm under the trade name of BuSpar. Buspirone is not a member of the benzodiazepine family,[68] and it does not bind to the GABA receptor complex.[69] In double-blind, random assignment studies, buspirone has been found equal to diazepam for relieving anxiety in patients with GAD and other forms of excessive anxiety.[70] Thus, there is more than one way to relieve anxiety, and not all the ways involve direct modulation of the GABA receptor.

A difference between buspirone and benzodiazepines is that buspirone has a long delay of benefit. Anxiety relief occurs only after several weeks of use. In contrast, benzodiazepines are effective within an hour of drug taking. This means that buspirone is inappropriate for treating brief episodes of anxiety. Patients cannot be instructed to take the pill as needed to control their current state.[71] Another drawback is that patients given buspirone may be inclined to quit taking the drug when it fails to produce immediate relief. Indeed, there is considerable evidence that patients drop out of buspirone treatment more frequently than they drop out of benzodiazepine treatment.[72]

The side effects evoked by buspirone are markedly different from those evoked by diazepam. In a review of side-effect data from a number of double-blind studies comparing buspirone with benzodiazepines for treatment of GAD, Newton and coworkers identified eight side effects that were mentioned by the buspirone patients significantly more frequently than by the placebo patients. These were dizziness (9 percent of patients), headache (7 percent), nervousness (4 percent), light-headedness (4 percent), tingling feeling (2 percent), diarrhea (3 percent), excitement (2 percent), and sweating (1 percent). By contrast, benzodiazepine patients experienced drowsiness, weakness, and fatigue significantly more often than buspirone patients.[73] Interestingly, the buspirone side effects are similar to anxiety symptoms and could represent a partial failure of anxiety relief.

Buspirone produces less cognitive and motor impairment than do other anxiolytics. Cognitive and motor skill can be tested in many different ways. In studies of buspirone and diazepam, cognitive and motor tests have included measurements of the ability to stand upright without body sway and the ability to make quick stops and skillful turns on driving simulators that work like video games. A divided-attention test used in a study by Herbert Moscowitz and Alison Smiley required subjects to press a button whenever the digit 2 appeared in numbers that periodically flashed on four different video screens. While watching for 2's the subjects also used a joy-stick to control the position of a moving visual target on a fifth video screen. In tests like these, buspirone at an anxiolytic dosage does not impair and sometimes improves performance in normal subjects. Benzodiazepines uniformly impair performance on these tasks. A very interesting finding is that buspirone in combination with alcohol produces no greater impairment than does alcohol alone.[74]

Normal experimental subjects who are given an anxiolytic dose of diazepam often report that they do not feel sedated and do not believe their cognitive ability and motor performance are impaired. In contrast, subjects who are given buspirone often complain of feeling tranquilized and intellectually impaired. When these complaining subjects are tested objectively, however, they perform as well as placebo subjects. Subjects who are blindly given either buspirone or diazepam are more likely to say the drug feels like a tranquilizer when the drug is buspirone than when it is diazepam. Thus it appears that benzodiazepines (like alcohol) can cause mental impairment without the drug user's awareness. With buspirone the problem seems to be an awareness of impairment when little impairment objectively exists.[75]

The actions of buspirone suggest the possibility that anxiety relief may be achievable in the absence of sedation. In the past, many theorists believed that anxiety relief and sedation are inextricably intertwined. They reasoned that relief from anxiety is the same as relief from vigilance, and relief from vigilance is, almost by definition, sedation. This could be wrong, of course. Anxiety and vigilance may be governed by distinct but interconnected brain circuits, and these circuits could be modulated independently. Perhaps there is a fearless vigilance and a fearful vigilance: Fearless vigilance is exhibited by a person who is listening closely for the next wisecrack from a stand-up comic; fearful vigilance is exhibited by a soldier who stands guard at night against surprise by a well-armed enemy.

There are several classes of neurons in the brain whose activity is involved with the emotions of arousal, vigilance, fear, and depression. We have mentioned these neurons already in several parts of the book. They are the norepinephrine-secreting neurons, the dopamine-secreting neurons, and the serotonin-secreting neurons. On the basis of a great deal of animal and human data, activity in these neurons is known to be involved in the regulation of sleep, arousal, vigilance, and pain.[76]

Brain recordings from animals show that buspirone and benzodiazepines influence the activity of these cells in different ways. For the dopamine- and norepinephrine-secreting neurons, buspirone causes an increase in activity, whereas benzodiazepines cause a decrease. Buspirone and benzodiazepines both cause a decrease in activity of the serotonin-secreting neurons.

The clinical difference between buspirone and the benzodiazepines may be due to the different effects that the two types of drugs have on the norepinephrine and dopamine neurons. The benzodiazepines, by suppressing activity in the norepinephrine and dopamine cells, may cause sedation and loss of mental alertness. Buspirone, by activating these same cells, may preserve alertness and mental acuity. Both classes of drugs may relieve anxiety by suppressing the activity of the serotonin cells. According to this line of thinking, buspirone may bring about an alert, vigilant nonanxious state, whereas the benzodiazepines may bring about a sedate, relaxed nonanxious state.[77]

The cellular mechanisms that explain buspirone action on neural activity are not fully understood. Buspirone interacts with dopamine receptors at concentrations that are achieved with anxiolytic doses. It displaces antipsychotic drugs from dopamine-binding sites in preparations of synaptic membranes. In tests of drug action on animal behavior, buspirone mimics the actions of drugs that are known to act at dopamine receptors.[78] Buspirone is not an effective antipsychotic, however, nor does it produce the motor side effects that are common with antipsychotic drugs (see Chapter 8). It is unknown whether binding to the dopamine receptor is necessary or sufficient for producing anxiety relief. Buspirone also interacts with serotonin receptors,[79] and it may have actions at other sites as well. Much more research is needed on the mechanism of action of buspirone.

In the century-long search for an anxiolytic that is free of sedation, buspirone may be the closest approach to success. Many psychiatrists are advising that the benzodiazepines be abandoned in favor of buspirone for the treatment of chronic anxiety as in GAD.[80] Dull wits and accident-proneness are high prices to pay for anxiety relief if an alternative is available that does not exact these penalties. Buspirone, however, has its disadvantages in comparison to the benzodiazepines. One is that buspirone has a significant delay of benefit. This means that it is not effective for immediate relief of intermittent anxiety on an as-needed basis. It also has some unpleasant side effects, such as dizziness and headache. These unpleasant side effects and perhaps the lack of drug-induced relaxation and sleep make buspirone less desirable than benzodiazepines to many patients.

17

ALCOHOL, ANXIOLYTIC DRUGS, AND ADDICTION

—

A ddiction and dependence are the most feared negative consequences of anxiolytic drugs. Authors of popular books and magazine articles have lavished attention on this problem. The danger has been proclaimed under headlines like "Danger! Prescription Drug Abuse" and titles like *The Tranquilizing of America*.[1] In 1979 social concern found an outlet in the United States Congress. The Senate Subcommittee on Health and Scientific Research held what was known as the Valium Hearing to consider the "growing and very serious public health problem" of benzodiazepine abuse. At this hearing, Senator Edward Kennedy said, "If you require a daily dose of Valium to get through each day, you are hooked and you should seek help."[2] Drug scares, of course, have been a staple of popular culture since long before the invention of minor tranquilizers. On some occasions the media and the government have been profoundly misleading. In the late 1930s, for instance, numerous popular magazine articles, prepared with the help of the U.S. Federal Bureau of Narcotics, played an important role in convincing the American public that marijuana is an addictive killer drug. Marijuana, while not praiseworthy, is not an addictive killer drug.[3]

In this chapter we evaluate the risk and seriousness of addiction to anxiolytic drugs. Our focus is on the benzodiazepines, which are the most commonly prescribed anxiolytics today. We compare the benzodiazepines with alcohol, which is the most used anxiolytic, with the barbiturates, which are the older prescription anxiolytics, and with buspirone, the newest prescription anxiolytic. We try to identify some of the inducements that lead people to overuse drugs. Then we ask to what extent these inducements are associated with the various kinds of anxiolytic drugs. This approach has the advantage of focusing attention on some of the presumed causes of addictive behavior and provides a basis for judgment about how potentially addictive drugs can be used with minimal risk. In the final part of the chapter we offer recommendations for minimizing the risks of addiction during treatment for excessive anxiety.

WHAT WE MEAN BY ADDICTION

There is a continuum of drug-taking habits ranging from proper medical use through overuse to addiction. No clear lines separate medical use from overuse, and overuse from addiction. Nonetheless, we find it useful to define addiction by three criteria. First, a person with an addiction uses the drug much more frequently and in larger quantities than is medically justified by illness (excessive use). Second, the excessive use causes social, psychological, and/or physiological impairment that is not justified by the benefits (harmful use). Third, the addict is unwilling to quit taking the drug; the prospect of running out of the drug arouses anxiety and strenuous efforts to obtain an adequate and continuous supply (compulsive use). Thus, addiction involves (1) excessive use, (2) harmful use, and (3) compulsive use. According to this definition addiction is an illness in the sense that it is distressing, disabling, and difficult to stop. This definition of addiction is similar, though not identical, to the definition given in the *DSM-III-R* for the disorder called psychoactive substance dependence.[4]

Note that our definition does not equate addiction with mere "physiological dependence." We use the term "physiological dependence" to stand for the physiological state in which the sudden withdrawal of a drug results in a particular collection of symptoms. The entire collection of symptoms is called a withdrawal syndrome. Many people with physiological dependence are in no sense drug addicts. A person who is physiologically dependent on morphine as a consequence of treatment for intractable pain is not correctly called an addict. When the source of pain is removed, such a patient can gradually withdraw from morphine without incident, and the morphine will have been a benefit, not a harm. Moreover, it is possible to be addicted without being physiologically dependent. For example some users of marijuana and LSD are addicts even though the sudden withdrawal of these drugs does not usually result in a distressing withdrawal syndrome.[5]

An addiction is much harder to combat than physiological dependence. If addiction were nothing more than physiological dependence, the addict would simply check into a hospital, undergo a medically supervised gradual drug withdrawal, and then walk out cured. Anyone who has had experience with Alcoholics Anonymous, or any other addiction treatment program, will tell you that surmounting the withdrawal illness is only the first of many hurdles encountered by the recovering addict.

It is easy to avoid harmful, compulsive overuse of some drugs because the drugs fail to produce a pleasant experience and because there are few inducements for drug taking. Addiction to quinine, for instance, will never be a problem since it tastes terrible and produces no pleasant experience. The anxiolytics are dangerous because their effects and the social patterns of their use may encourage people to increase their drug consumption even when good health would require that consumption be reduced or terminated.

PREVALENCE OF ANXIOLYTIC ADDICTION

Alcohol, the most popular anxiolytic, accounts for most cases of anxiolytic addiction. When used in small amounts, at the proper time and place, it can relieve anxiety and help people enjoy themselves. But some people use excessive amounts without regard for the impropriety and harmfulness of their intoxication.

Alcohol is often used as a self-medication for phobic disorders such as agoraphobia, social phobia, and panic disorder.[6] This kind of self-medication contributes significantly to the harm done by alcohol. If these self-medication patients could be switched to less harmful drugs or taught how to cope with anxiety without drugs, great human benefit would be realized.[7]

About 18 million Americans suffer serious consequences of alcohol addiction. Alcoholism is the most prevalent of all psychiatric disorders. It promotes accidents, disease, occupational failure, wife beating, child abuse, divorce, violent crime, and suicide. The monetary cost of alcohol problems in the United States was estimated to have totaled about $117 billion in 1983. No dollar figure can be attached to the human suffering involved. There is some hope that these problems will diminish in the future as the per capita consumption of alcohol has declined somewhat since 1981. There has also been a recent downward trend in the number of alcohol-related car accidents.[8]

Abuse of prescription anxiolytics also occurs. A favorite subject in popular journalism is the pill addiction of celebrities like Elvis Presley, Betty Ford, and Kitty Dukakis.[9] The famous cases tell us little, however, about the numerical prevalence of pill addiction in the general population. They also fail to make clear whether pill addictions are the result of medically supervised treatment of anxiety or of misjudgment brought on by the excessive use of alcohol. People who abuse pills usually overuse alcohol as well, but they may be more embarrassed to admit their alcoholism than to admit their abuse of drugs "the doctor ordered." Betty Ford and Kitty Dukakis openly acknowledged that their problems involved both alcohol and prescription drugs.[10]

Some data illustrating the prevalence of multiple drug use among anxiolytic abusers were published by Christer Allgulander of the Department of Clinical Alcohol and Drug Research of the Karolinska Institute in Stockholm, Sweden. Allgulander studied patients admitted to the institute's Department of Psychiatry during a two-year period for treatment of addiction to anxiolytic drugs. These patients constituted about one-third of the psychiatric admissions for all causes. Sixty-eight percent of them had been overusing alcohol and no other drug. Another 23 percent had been using alcohol in combination with prescription drugs. Only 9 percent were addicted to prescription drugs alone. Of these prescription addicts, who numbered 55, about one-half had used 10 or more different prescription sedatives; only four patients had used fewer than four different prescription drugs. Allgulander's data indicated that, under the conditions existing in Stockholm, alcohol is the only sedative-hypnotic that leads to addiction when taken alone. Among the prescription drugs, it was impossible to conclude which had the greatest addiction liability since these drugs were always used in combination.[11]

ADDICTION LIABILITY OF VARIOUS TYPES OF ANXIOLYTICS

Ideally we would like to know how probable it is that a person would become addicted if he or she were to use a particular drug to control a single episode of anxiety. For many reasons, such knowledge does not exist. The variables that influence the development of addiction are so numerous that simple answers are not meaningful. For example, the likelihood of becoming addicted may depend on the sex, age, health, and ethnic status of the user, the type of drug, the amount and duration of use, the illness for which the drug is prescribed, and the concomitant use of other drugs, among other variables.

In the following text, we compare the addiction liability of alcohol, barbiturates, benzodiazepines, and buspirone by asking whether each of the drugs has properties that encourage excessive, harmful, and compulsive use. The drugs of reference are the benzodiazepines as they are the most widely prescribed anxiolytics.

There are seven properties of drugs that we think are relevant to addiction liability:

1. Euphoria: The drug produces a subjective high or other desirable feelings.
2. Rapid action: The drug takes effect rapidly after it is taken.
3. Unsupervised use: The drug can be used at will without medical supervision of dose and dosage schedule.
4. Social encouragement: Settings are frequently encountered in which use of the drug is socially encouraged as a means of obtaining pleasure, amusement, friendship, or conformity to group standards.

5. Tolerance: The dose required for the desired effect increases with repeated use.
6. Physiological dependence: discontinuing the drug causes an unpleasant or even life-threatening withdrawal syndrome.
7. Cross-tolerance and cross-dependence: In the production of tolerance and dependence the drug can substitute for other addictive drugs.

Property 1: Euphoria

As a euphoriant, buspirone is probably the least effective of the anxiolytics. Benzodiazepines appear to have some euphoriant action, and barbiturates and alcohol appear to be the most euphoriant. This opinion is based on two kinds of studies. First, there are studies in which animals are given an opportunity to work for injections of various drugs at various doses. Second, there are studies of volunteer human subjects who take various drugs and report on the subjective experience that the drug produces.

In a typical animal study, a monkey is trained to administer drugs to itself through a tube that is inserted into a vein or the stomach. By pressing a lever, the monkey activates the injection of either a small dose of a drug or an equal amount of saline solution (placebo). Cocaine, amphetamines, or opiates are strong euphoriants; monkeys press the bar much more vigorously and reliably when they self-inject these drugs than when they self-inject saline solution.[12] With benzodiazepines the results are less clear. Under some conditions, monkeys or baboons will press the lever more frequently for diazepam than for saline, but the reward value of diazepam is weak. Self-injection is maintained only under fairly restricted conditions of dose and pacing of injection.[13] Self-injection of barbiturates or methaqualone is much more robust.[14] With these compounds animals will regularly and voluntarily anesthetize themselves.[15] Using buspirone, it is difficult to get animals to self-inject above the placebo rate. In fact, at higher doses buspirone sometimes suppresses bar pressing below the placebo rate, which indicates that buspirone is unpleasant.[16]

Experiments with humans suggest the same conclusions. One such experiment compared the desirability of placebo, amphetamine, and diazepam. The participants, healthy college students, reported to the laboratory in the morning, three times per week for three weeks. On the first four laboratory visits, the students took the various drugs to experience their effects. Each drug was presented in a different colored capsule so that the participant could associate the effects of the drug with the appearance of the capsule. On the remaining five visits, the participants were shown two colored capsules and asked to choose the one they preferred to take. Thus, on each of five drug comparison trials, the participants judged the preferability of two drugs or drug dosages, identifying them by color. Neither the experimenter nor the participants knew which drug was in which colored capsule. The participants showed no preference between 2 mg (a very small dose) of diazepam and placebo. They preferred placebo, however, to either 5 or 10 mg of diazepam, and they preferred amphetamine to placebo. Apparently, these normal, presumably anxiety-free, non-drug-abusing college students positively disliked diazepam.[17]

Drug-choice experiments have also been done with human drug abusers, a population who, by definition, are susceptible to addiction. John D. Griffith and colleagues gave single doses of placebo, diazepam, or buspirone in a double-blind fashion to a group of men who were in the hospital recovering from long-standing alcoholism. At several intervals following each drug ingestion, the men filled out questionnaires that recorded how the drug made them feel. In the questionnaire the men responded with agreement or disagreement to statements like "Things around me seem more pleasing than usual" or "My head feels as it does during a hangover." Diazepam in doses of 10 or 20 mg produced more euphoria than did buspirone at doses of 10, 20, or 40 mg. Buspirone did not produce more euphoria than did placebo, and at the high dose buspirone produced subjective unpleasantness.[18]

Similar results were obtained by Cole and coworkers when they compared buspirone, diazepam, and methaqualone using nonaddicted college students as subjects. Methaqualone is a 1960s model nonbenzodiazepine minor tranquilizer that is no longer on the market. Methaqualone was most euphoric; diazepam was next, and buspirone was either not different from placebo or dysphoric at high doses.[19]

The overall impression from these studies is that buspirone is ineffective as a euphoriant. As the dosage is increased, the drug becomes unpleasant. Thus, it appears unlikely that patients would be tempted to use buspirone to excess. Small doses of benzodiazepines are usually more pleasant than placebos, and their pleasantness appears to increase with the dose. Barbiturates and the nonbenzodiazepine minor tranquilizers are more strongly euphoriant than benzodiazepines. They present a significant incentive for recreational use, which is reflected by their position in the illicit drug market. Where alcohol fits into this continuum is not clear. Our guess is that alcohol's effectiveness as a euphoriant is comparable to the barbiturates and nonbenzodiazepine minor tranquilizers.

Property 2: Rapid Action

When a pleasant feeling follows immediately after drug taking, the user will like the drug more than if the pleasant feeling is long delayed. If the delay is long enough, the user will decide the drug is worthless. Also, if a drug is absorbed slowly, the onset of action will be gradual, and the user will have difficulty appreciating the effect; there will be no sudden "rush." Slow onset of action also reduces a drug's suitability for use in recreational settings. Recreational users do not want to take the drug hours or days before the planned time for the drug experience. For most addicting drugs, the delay between ingestion and effect is much less than 30 minutes.

Alcohol can be effective within minutes of drinking.[20] Rapidly acting benzodiazepines, begin to take effect about 30 minutes after pill taking and reach their peak effectiveness at about one hour. Some benzodiazepines are slower. This fairly long delay is due to the slow absorption of benzodiazepines from the stomach and intestine.[21] Some barbiturates and nonbenzodiazepine minor tranquilizers take effect more rapidly than benzodiazepines.[22] The delay can be shortened to seconds by injecting the drug into a vein, a procedure that enhances the addiction liability of benzodiazepines, barbiturates, and any other drug with addiction potential.

Buspirone has an extremely long delay of benefit. In double-blind studies comparing benzodiazepines with buspirone for the relief of anxiety in patients with GAD, benzodiazepines appear to bring anxiety relief within about an hour of taking the first pill, whereas buspirone brings relief only after a delay of two to three weeks.[23] Thus the delay of benefit for buspirone appears similar to that of the antidepressants for relief of depressive symptoms. As we mentioned in Chapter 11, such long delays may cause the patient to become discouraged and quit taking the drug before it has a chance to work. The delay of benefit for buspirone is not due to delayed absorption from the stomach and intestine, as shown by the fact that side effects commence within one hour of pill taking.[24] Thus we would not predict that the addiction liability of buspirone would be increased by injecting the drug intravenously.

Property 3: Unsupervised Use

The use of a potentially addictive drug without medical supervision is more risky than the medically supervised use of the same drug. The requirement for a physician's prescription is a significant barrier to addiction.

There is no prescription barrier, of course, for alcohol. With anxiolytic pills, the barrier can be circumvented by determined drug users. Many people can obtain a small amount of benzodiazepine by going to the medicine cabinet and taking pills that are left over from a previous illness. A supply for sustained overuse, however, requires additional measures, such as going to several different physicians and getting a separate prescription from each of them. Nonbenzodiazepine minor tranquilizers and barbiturates are less available through multiple prescriptions simply because doctors do not routinely prescribe them. They are rather commonly available on the illicit market, but the necessity of dealing with the criminal element of society deters many from this route of drug access. Buspirone is probably not available on the illicit market.

Precise figures on the extent of illicit use of prescription drugs are hard to obtain. Questionnaire surveys indicate that about 15 percent of high school students and young adults have used a benzodiazepine nonmedically at least once. About 17 percent have used barbiturates or the nonbenzodiazepine minor tranquilizers. About 94 percent have used alcohol. The surveys also show that the nonmedical use of benzodiazepines and barbiturates has been declining in recent years.[25]

In summary, alcohol is the anxiolytic with the greatest potential for unsupervised use. Barbiturates, benzodiazepines, and nonbenzodiazepine minor tranquilizers are next. Buspirone is least available. On the dimension of unsupervised use, buspirone again presents the least abuse potential of presently available anxiolytics.

Property 4: Social Encouragement

There is a greater temptation for overuse when a drug is taken among friends as an aid to conformity, companionship, and pleasure than when a drug is taken for medical purposes only. By custom, alcohol is the anxiolytic most used socially for pleasure. It is ideally suited to this purpose. There are enjoyable customs surrounding drinking; the same drug taken blind in a hospital setting during a pharmacology experiment would have considerably less euphoric impact. Alcohol is also well suited for use as a party drug by virtue of its rapid absorption and metabolism. The alcohol high begins within a few minutes of drinking, and the drug promptly disappears from the blood after the party is over. Many barbiturates and the nonbenzodiazepine minor tranquilizers can also be used illicitly for pleasure in social settings. These drugs are good euphoriants, and they are rapidly absorbed and metabolized.

The benzodiazepines are less desirable as party drugs. They are unwieldy because of their slow onset of action, and they are metabolized more slowly than alcohol and the recreationally used barbiturates.[26] The slow metabolism is especially troublesome, since many days may be required to clear benzodiazepines from the blood. During this time there may be impaired intellectual and motor function. Buspirone is more rapidly metabolized than benzodiazepines. Its two-week delay of benefit, however, would seem to preclude its use by people seeking a brief period of anxiety relief during a party or social gathering. Chronic treatment of GAD with buspirone, of course, might appreciably enhance the patient's ability to enjoy a good party, and such would be a legitimate use of the drug.

Property 5: Tolerance

Many drugs, including many of the anxiolytics, produce tolerance, which means that the effect of the drug decreases if the drug is continuously present in the blood for a long time. Tolerance is caused by several factors. The prolonged presence of the drug may stimulate an increase in the capacity of the liver and kidney to metabolize and eliminate the drug. Also, the presence of the drug may stimulate brain cells to biochemically compensate for the drug's effects. As tolerance develops for a desired drug effect, a person must escalate the dosage to continue experiencing the effect. The longer the drug is used and the higher the dosage, the greater the tolerance that develops. Tolerance for the desired effect increases addiction liability.

Most people have had personal experience with the development of tolerance. When one inhales cigarette smoke for the first time, the nicotine typically evokes a precipitous drop in blood pressure. One may experience a visual blackout and even faint. With a little experience smoking, though, blood pressure becomes so resistant to the effects of nicotine that inhaling cigarette smoke no longer even evokes dizziness. The process is similar with alcohol tolerance. If you are naive to alcohol, you may stagger and sway after drinking a single beer on an empty stomach. If you are a heavy drinker, a single beer will have almost no effects.

Tolerance may develop more rapidly and more completely for some drug effects than for others. We have already pointed out examples of this variation in previous chapters. For example, tolerance develops for the sedative effects of phenothiazines and tricyclic antidepressants but not for the antipsychotic and antidepressant effects.

With alcohol, barbiturates, and the nonbenzodiazepine minor tranquilizers, tolerance develops for the sedative and anxiolytic actions but not for the lethal dose. Therefore, people suffering from severe alcoholism or barbiturate addiction are caught between a severe withdrawal illness if they cut down their intake and a life-threatening intoxication if they increase it ever so slightly. They get no anxiety relief because tolerance has developed for the anxiolytic effect.[27] A drug with potential for tolerance can be used only for a brief course of treatment.

A question of prime importance is whether tolerance develops for the anxiolytic effect of benzodiazepines and buspirone.

Tolerance for the anxiolytic action of benzodiazepines develops less rapidly than does tolerance for the sedative action. David Margules and Larry Stein of Wyeth Laboratories clearly demonstrated this point in animals. They trained rats to press a bar to obtain milk as a reward. After this behavior was well learned, the researchers introduced a tone stimulus, and while the tone was on, the rats got a mild electric shock to the feet every time the bar was pressed. Milk continued to be delivered as well. Placebo-treated rats rapidly learned to stop pressing when the tone was on. A dose of benzodiazepine, however, caused rats to be less impressed with the electric shock, and they continued pressing the bar even when the tone was on. As mentioned in Chapter 17, this release from the suppressive effect of punishment is considered to be analogous to the antianxiety effect of benzodiazepines in humans.

When the dose of benzodiazepine was increased, the sedative effect became prominent. The rats slowed down their bar pressing even when the tone was off. They acted tired and lethargic. This is analogous to the sedative effect of the benzodiazepines in humans. When Margules and Stein gave the rats high doses of benzodiazepine for several days, tolerance developed for the sedative effect but not for the antianxiety effect; that is, after several days of high doses, the rats resumed pressing the bar at the normal or supernormal rate when the tone was off (tolerance for the sedative effect) and continued right on pressing when the tone was on (no tolerance for the antianxiety effect) (Figure 17-1).[28]

Understandably, experiments with such clear-cut results have not been performed with humans, but the accumulated clinical opinion is that tolerance for the sedative effect of benzodiazepines develops after a few days or at most a few weeks, while tolerance for the antianxiety effect develops much more slowly.[29] Of course, if the dose were sufficiently low and use sufficiently intermittent, significant tolerance would not develop at all for either the sedative or the antianxiety effect. Conversely, if the dose were excessively high, tolerance could probably be demonstrated even for the antianxiety effect.

In the 1960s there was little professional concern about the possibility of tolerance for the antianxiety effects of benzodiazepines. In the discussion of benzodiazepines in the 1970 edition of Goodman and Gilman's *The Pharmacological Basis of Therapeutics*, the standard textbook of medical pharmacology, the problem of tolerance was not even mentioned.[30] In the late 1970s, during the height of negative publicity about addiction to "tranquilizers," conflicting opinions began to appear in the medical literature. In his book *Chemotherapy in Psychiatry*, published in 1977, Ross J. Baldessarini of the Harvard Medical School stated, "The benzodiazepines, like all of the sedative-tranquilizing agents, are limited by the development of tolerance to their main or desired antianxiety effect as well as to the degree of sedation they produce. This aspect of their actions limits the length of time they are clinically useful and contributes to their abuse."[31] Baldessarini did not give any estimation of the dose and duration of use that he thought might lead to tolerance for the anxiolytic effect in humans.

One of the first empirical studies of tolerance in humans was published in 1981 by Leo E. Hollister and three colleagues of the Stanford Medical School. They selected a group of 106 hospital

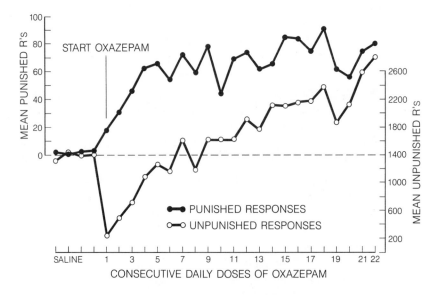

FIGURE 17-1 Effect of daily injections of oxazepam, a benzodiazepine, on punished and unpunished bar pressing in rats. Y axis shows mean number of bar presses given during each daily session in a group of five rats (solid line, punished responses; dotted line, unpunished responses). X axis shows consecutive daily testing sessions. Prior to the experiment the rats learned to press the bar for milk and, when a tone was on, to avoid shock (punishment) by ceasing to press. On the first four days shown, the rats were given an injection of saline solution (placebo) prior to the bar-pressing session. In this placebo condition, the mean number of punished bar presses was zero or one per day, and the mean number of unpunished bar presses was about 1,400 per day. On the fifth day and for 21 days thereafter, the rats were given an injection of oxazepam before the session. Note: On the first day of benzodiazepine there was an increase in the number of punished bar presses, and there were additional increases on subsequent days (anxiolytic effect). Tolerance for the anxiolytic effect did not occur. The benzodiazepine caused an initial decrease in the number of unpunished bar presses (sedative effect), but pressing recovered to normal after about five daily doses (tolerance for the sedative effect) and even accelerated to a supernormal rate as days passed. It is thought that the supernormal rate of unpunished bar pressing is due to the continuing development of the anxiolytic effect, which allows the rats to press with increasing abandon, uninhibited by the fear of punishment in the same surroundings when the tone is on. From D. Margules and L. Stein, "Increase of 'Antianxiety' Activity and Tolerance of Behavioral Depression During Chronic Administration of Oxazepam," *Psychopharmacology* 13(1968): 74–80.

patients who had been taking diazepam to relieve anxiety and tension associated with back pain. The patients had been taking diazepam for 1 month to 16 years; half the patients had been using diazepam longer than 5 years. Dr. Hollister and his colleagues tried to find out if these patients tended to escalate their dose above the recommended range, thus indicating tolerance.

The daily doses the patients claimed to be taking were within the normally prescribed range and did not reflect a tendency for dose escalation. People who overuse drugs, however, often try to conceal this fact. Thus, more critical data came from measurements of diazepam in the blood. The blood levels were not excessively high. Dosage escalation apparently had not occurred. Eighty-seven percent of the patients thought the diazepam was beneficial, suggesting that they were not tolerant to the anxiolytic effects of the drug. In summarizing their results, Hollister and colleagues wrote, "Even with long-term use, diazepam seemed to retain its efficacy and did not lead to any clear-cut abuse." [32]

A recent and more definitive study of tolerance for the anxiolytic action of benzodiazepines has been carried out by Karl Rickels and his associates. One hundred eighty outpatients with GAD or atypical anxiety disorder (*DSM-III*) participated in the study. For the first six weeks they were given diazepam at the conventional therapeutic dose. At the end of the sixth week some of the patients were switched, double blind, to placebo. Another group of patients was switched to placebo at the end of 16 weeks. The third group of patients was switched to placebo at the end of 22 weeks. The intensity of the anxiety symptoms was measured at monthly intervals using the Hamilton Anxiety Scale and other measures. During the eight weeks following the switch to placebo it was possible to compare those patients who were switched with those who were being maintained on medication. The question was whether the patients who were maintained on diazepam would show a reappearance of their anxiety symptoms (tolerance) at the same rate as those who were switched to placebo.

The results were clear. During the first few weeks the patients improved markedly while taking diazepam, and they experienced no reappearance of symptoms during the entire 22 weeks of treatment. During this time they did not escalate their dosage. In contrast, about 50 percent of the placebo patients experienced renewed anxiety during the first eight weeks on placebo. The investigators were careful to distinguish between drug withdrawal reactions and re-newed anxiety symptoms. Rickels and colleagues concluded that tolerance did not develop for the anxiolytic effect of diazepam for 22 weeks in this patient population.[33]

An interesting feature of Rickels's data is that about half the patients who were switched to placebo did *not* experience renewed anxiety following drug termination. This indicates that up to half the patients in the 22-week diazepam group were taking a drug they did not need to maintain their relatively nonanxious state. Accordingly, it appears that long-term treatment with diazepam is undesirable in patients with GAD or atypical anxiety disorder. It would be better to give a short course of drug treatment, withdraw the drug, and then restart it again as necessary to control a renewed outbreak of anxiety.

Some patients, however, take benzodiazepines continuously for years. Does tolerance develop in these very long-term patients? The data available on this question are ambiguous. As we saw in the study by Hollister and colleagues, long-term patients often say that their drug continues to be effective. This observation has been repli-cated.[34] Some investigators, however, have uncovered a population of long-term patients who say that they experience a return of their old symptoms while still taking benzodiazepines.[35] Haskel and col-leagues found that long-term benzodiazepine users scored as high in symptoms of anxiety as did patients who are just entering treatment for GAD or panic disorder with agoraphobia. These same patients, however, said they believed their benzodiazepine was beneficial.[36] In summary, the jury is still out on the question of whether tolerance develops for the anxiolytic benefit of benzodiazepines after years of use. What we know is that significant tolerance does not occur with continuous use for as long as 22 weeks.

What about the side effects of sedation and cognitive impair-ment? Does tolerance develop for these in humans? There is general agreement that patients complain the most about drowsiness and cognitive impairment during the first few weeks of benzodiazepine treatment.[37] Tolerance is probably not complete, however. Hoehn-Saric and McLeod assessed cognitive skill and subjective feelings of drowsiness in normal volunteer subjects who had received a modest daily dose benzodiazepine for six weeks. Subjects receiving benzo-diazepine reported more feelings of drowsiness than did subjects receiving placebo. The drug group also had impaired performance on the digit-symbol substitution test, a popular test of mental acuity, in which subjects must scratch out, as quickly as they can, all occurrences of a particular letter, for example, *o*, on a sheet of text and replace it with a particular digit, say, *3*; their score is the number of correct substitutions.[38]

Lucki and coworkers administered tests of cognitive skill to a group of normal placebo subjects and to a group patients with GAD who had been taking therapeutic doses of benzodiazepines for an average of over five years. The drug group had high levels of benzodiazepine in the blood at all times, but the highest blood level occurred every day about one hour after taking their daily medication. When they were tested before taking their daily dose, there were no differences between the drug group and the drug-free group on most measures of cognitive performance. When the tests were run one hour after the daily dose, however, the drug group was impaired with respect to the control group on the digit symbol substitution test and a test of ability to memorize a list of nouns. This experiment probably indicates that tolerance is nearly complete with respect to the drug that is present between doses while the drug content of the blood is declining. Tolerance is not complete with respect to the drug that is present during the time of rising blood level just after pill taking.[39] Cognitive difficulty just after pill taking can be minimized by taking the drug at bedtime.

An advance in the pharmacotherapy of anxiety could be achieved by finding a new drug that shows even slower development of tolerance to the anxiolytic benefit while showing more rapid tolerance for the side effects. Bo Soderpalm of the University of Goteborg, Sweden, has made tests in animals indicating that the new benzodiazepine, alprazolam, may be such a drug. In rats, Soderpalm assessed tolerance for the anxiolytic effect and the sedative effect using diazepam and alprazolam. The test for the anxiolytic effect was whether the drug suppressed the action of punishment on drinking, and the test of the sedative effect was whether the rats could maintain their balance while standing on a rotating rod. Soderpalm found that tolerance for the sedative effect was greater for alprazolam than for diazepam, but tolerance for the anxiolytic effect was less for alprazolam than for diazepam.[40] These data reinforce the opinion stated previously, that alprazolam can relieve anxiety, with fewer side effects, than can other benzodiazepine drugs.

Tolerance for the effects of buspirone has not been studied as extensively as for the effects of benzodiazepines. Buspirone is a very new drug, and knowledge has not had time to accumulate. An early report by John Feighner, however, suggests that tolerance does not limit buspirone's efficacy in the long-term treatment of GAD. Feighner's study involved 700 patients from several hospital clinics who were given buspirone daily for one year. Anxiety symptoms, measured by the Hamilton Anxiety Scale and other measures, steadily improved for the first six months of the study and then held steady for the remainder of the year. Feighner states that few increases in dose were required to maintain the low anxiety state for one year, but the data are not explicit on this point.[41]

Property 6: Physiological Dependence

A drug produces physiological dependence if a withdrawal syndrome occurs when a habitual user suddenly stops taking the drug, provided, of course, that the illness is not simply a reappearance of an illness that was controlled by the drug. Withdrawal symptoms are different for different drugs. The symptoms of opiate withdrawal, for instance, are different from the symptoms of alcohol withdrawal. In addition, the higher the dosage of the drug and the longer the drug has been continuously present in the blood, the greater the likelihood of physiological dependence and the more severe the withdrawal illness. The illness is also more severe when the drug is withdrawn suddenly—when the patient goes cold turkey—than when drug taking is diminished little by little over a long period. In some cases the illness can be circumvented entirely by gradual drug withdrawal. There are many psychoactive drugs that do not produce significant physiological dependence; marijuana, LSD, lithium, and phenothiazines are examples.

Alcohol, barbiturates, meprobamate, and the benzodiazepines, to varying degrees, all present a risk of physiological dependence. The withdrawal symptoms are similar for all of these drugs, and the withdrawal syndrome, called the sedative-hypnotic withdrawal illness, can be dramatic. Its most intense and life-threatening expression can be seen following sudden alcohol withdrawal in a patient who is severely dependent. The following is a typical case.

Henry had been drinking more than 600 ml of whiskey a day for eight years. Whenever he tried to stop drinking, or even when he just tried to cut down, he got sick within a few hours. His illness always disappeared, however, shortly after he took another drink. Henry found he could also prevent his withdrawal illness by taking barbiturates or benzodiazepines, which he had done on several occasions when trying to convince his family that he was cutting down on his drinking.

When Henry was forced to stop drinking, cold turkey, his withdrawal illness unfolded inexorably.[42] A few hours after his final drink, Henry started to get anxious, shaky, and sweaty. He felt weak and sick to his stomach. Knowing well the cause of his problem, he started to search for alcohol. He begged and pleaded with family and friends, but they refused him. Had he been permitted to do so, he would have begged on the street for a drink or for money to buy it. Not obtaining a drink, Henry started to have cramps, and he had an episode of vomiting. His heart began pounding. Desperate and panicky, he looked for Valium, Librium, barbiturates, or Miltown, but he found neither drugs nor sympathizers. Henry's hands started shaking. It was so bad he could not lift a glass to his lips without spilling half the water. His reflexes became supersensitive; he jumped uncontrollably at unexpected sounds or other stimuli. He felt a tingling sensation in his skin. When he closed his eyes, he could see things. He hallucinated fire burning out of control. At this time, a little more than a day after his last drink, Henry knew his visions were not real and that they were caused by his need for alcohol. He was not yet disoriented: He knew where he was, who he was, and what was happening to him. It was at about this time that Henry had his first grand mal seizure. He lost consciousness, and the muscles throughout his body rhythmically and uncontrollably flexed and writhed; if a recording machine had been attached to Henry's scalp, abnormal brain waves similar to those seen in patients who have epilepsy would probably have been recorded. Had Henry been seen by a physician at this stage, his condition would have been diagnosed as *acute alcoholic halluncinosis.*

If Henry had been lucky, his withdrawal illness would have started to get better at this stage. But Henry was not lucky, and his illness got worse. He started to drift in and out of consciousness. When he was conscious, he was confused, disoriented, and weak. He did not know who he was or where he was. He lost the insight that he was ill and began to believe that his terrible hallucinations of persecution were real. He believed he was being tormented by the most unimaginably evil persecutors, that he was burning in the fires of hell. He was terrified. It was then the third day after his last drink, and a physician would have said that Henry had *delirium tremens*. At this stage, even a large dose of alcohol or some other sedative-hypnotic would probably not have suppressed the withdrawal symptoms as it would have earlier.

During delirium tremens, Henry had a high fever, and he was exhausted. His life was in danger: His heart was racing and could have failed at any time. But now Henry was lucky: His heart did not fail; instead, he began to improve. Six days after his last drink, Henry was fine. He had never felt better. With an alcohol-free brain, he could think and speak more clearly than he had been able to in years. Henry could remember the horrible visions he had had while in delirium tremens. They were so vivid he almost believed they had been real.

Fortunately, people seldom have to suffer the worst symptoms. A nonalcoholic sedative-hypnotic can be prescribed to relieve the withdrawal symptoms if the illness has not progressed to delirium tremens. Later, the dosage of the prescribed drug is diminished slightly each day in steps so small that they do not evoke threatening symptoms. Finally, no drug at all is needed, and the patient is no longer physiologically dependent. Loss of physiological dependence, however, does not mean that the addictive behavior is cured. A relapse into drug overuse is possible at any time. In the language of Alcoholics Anonymous, Henry will always be called a recovering alcoholic.

One of the few differences between the withdrawal illness for alcohol and the withdrawal illness for barbiturates and other sedative-hypnotics is that with prescription drugs, seizures are more likely during the stage of acute hallucinosis. Other differences relate to the rate at which the particular drug disappears from the brain after the last dose. The more rapidly the drug disappears, the more severe is the withdrawal illness. Alcohol disappears from the brain more rapidly than do most prescription sedative-hypnotics. In consequence, the illness following alcohol withdrawal develops more rapidly, is more severe at its peak, and is shorter in duration than the withdrawal illness of many prescription sedative-hypnotics.

With benzodiazepines, the liver and kidney can remove from the blood about half of the active drug in a day and a half. Up to two weeks may be required to eliminate the drug completely. Withdrawal symptoms typically do not appear until about a day and half after the last benzodiazepine pill, and the peak of the illness may not occur until the sixth or seventh day. At its peak, the illness may reach an intensity similar to acute alcoholic hallucinosis, but full delirium tremens or death is very unlikely. At least two weeks are required for full recovery, and in some cases months may be required.[43] Despite intense interest and speculation, the biochemical mechanisms for the development of the sedative-hypnotic withdrawal illness are poorly understood.

Although it has long been known that prolonged use of high doses of benzodiazepine give rise to physiological dependence,[44] it has been unclear whether significant dependence develops when benzodiazepines are used at the low dosages prescribed for anxiety relief. When withdrawal symptoms are mild, it is difficult to prove that they are actually withdrawal symptoms and not a return of the anxiety for which the drug was originally prescribed. It is now clear, however, that low-dosage dependence sometimes occurs. One of the first convincing accounts of it was published in 1981 by a group of psychiatrists headed by Andrew Winokur at the University of Pennsylvania.[45] The report describes a young man of 26 who lived in Chicago. We shall call him Eric.

Eric was referred to Winokur by a neurologist who had examined Eric to find out if a neurological problem might be responsible for the severe shaking and dizziness that he had been experiencing. These symptoms had begun at approximately the same time that he had discontinued the Valium he had been taking—15 mg per day for six years. Eric's internist had originally prescribed the Valium to help Eric with his "nervous upset stomach." The nervous stomach responded well, and Eric had been taking the medicine as prescribed ever since, never increasing or decreasing the dose. On one occasion, he stopped taking the Valium, and his nervous stomach seemed to come back. Accordingly, his doctor advised him to continue with the Valium. Finally, Eric got tired of taking the medicine and resolved to quit. This act of assertiveness was followed by a flare-up of his nervous stomach, dizziness, ringing in the ears, blurred vision, and generalized shakiness. Alarmed, Eric went to the neurologist, thinking that he might have some menacing neurological disease that Valium had been controlling.

The neurologist found no neurological problem and, recognizing the possibility of a Valium withdrawal illness, referred Eric to Winokur's group. Winokur suggested that Eric participate in a rigorous experiment to find out if he did indeed suffer from Valium dependence or whether Valium was controlling a more ominous underlying problem. Eric agreed and entered the hospital. Winokur's plan was to terminate the Valium for several days, then restore it, and then terminate it again while Eric was in the hospital and under professional observation. Every day a psychiatrist talked with Eric and recorded any apparent symptoms of anxiety, the sedative-hypnotic withdrawal illness, or any other psychiatric disturbance. The nurses on the ward, who were trained in behavioral observation, also kept detailed notes on Eric's behavior. Twice a day, at 8:00 A.M. and 8:00 P.M., a nurse took a blood sample that was analyzed for its benzodiazepine content. The entire procedure was carried out double blind; only the hospital pharmacist knew whether the pills Eric took four times a day contained diazepam or an inert substance. In fact, Eric was kept on diazepam for 4 days, then switched to placebo for 4 days, then put back on Valium for 4 days, and finally put back on placebo for 21 days.

The results were clear. On the first day in the hospital Eric was a bit nervous, as might be expected of one who has just been incarcerated in a strange place, but he was relaxed on the second, third, and fourth days. On the fifth day, the first day of placebo, Eric continued to have no problems. By the middle of the sixth day, however, Eric began to complain of anxiety, dizziness, blurred vision, ringing in the ears, constipation, and heart pounding; an increase in anxious behavior was also apparent to the nurses and the psychiatrists. The symptoms got worse on the third and fourth day of drug withdrawal. Eric became extremely anxious and irritable. He began to sweat. His hands began shaking. Soon the shakiness spread to his arms and body. He got a severe headache and could not sleep. Then he became so agitated that he could not verbalize his thoughts coherently. Eric became supersensitive; he could not tolerate the sound of a clock ticking or the smell of an orange peel. At one point, he became so sensitive to touch that even the feeling of his clothes against his body was intolerable. Diazepam was restored on the ninth day. Thirty minutes after the first pill, Eric announced, "I feel remarkably better, never felt better." He remained normal for the next three days while taking Valium.

The second placebo period began on the thirteenth day in the hospital. Exactly as before, Eric felt fine on the first placebo day, but in the middle of the second, began to complain of anxiety. Again, the symptoms got worse, and on the fourth placebo day Eric became uncooperative and wanted to quit the experiment. The symptoms continued to be severe for 11 more days. During this time in addition to all the symptoms he had previously had, Eric became disoriented. He could not tell where he was or what time it was. He could not find his way to the nursing station, and his hands and body shook so uncontrollably that he could not take his pills (now placebos) without help. On the sixteenth placebo day, he finally felt healthy again, with a normal level of anxiety. He was discharged from the hospital.

The blood tests showed that Eric began to have withdrawal symptoms when the blood level of diazepam fell to about half the value that had prevailed while Eric was taking the drug. This blood level was reached in about the middle of the second placebo day. By the sixteenth placebo day, when Eric's symptoms began to improve, no detectable diazepam remained in his blood.

How common is it for patients to take benzodiazepines for more than a few months, and when they do so, how commonly do they become physiologically dependent? Glen D. Mellinger and co-workers surveyed a representative sample of adults in the United States to determine the prevalence of benzodiazepine use, the illnesses for which benzodiazepines were prescribed, and the duration for which they were used. The survey involved interviews with, 3,161 people and was conducted in 1979, a year in which the annual number of benzodiazepine prescriptions was about the same as it is today but was much lower than during the peak year of 1975. The data indicated that 11 percent of Americans between the age of 28 and 79 took benzodiazepines at least once during the year. Fifteen percent of these (about 4 million people) had been using benzodiazepines daily for one year or more. Many of the chronic users were taking the drugs to relieve anxiety associated with long-term illnesses such as arthritis and cardiovascular disease.[46] (The long-term use of benzodiazepines is greater in Europe than in the United States.[47])

What proportion of these long-term users would we expect to be physiologically dependent? This is not an easy question. The proper experiment would be to find a representative sample of long-term benzodiazepine users who would volunteer as subjects. They would be divided into two groups, a drug withdrawal group and sham withdrawal group. The drug withdrawal group would have a placebo substituted for their daily medication, while the sham withdrawal group would continue their medication, and we would observe the number of patients in each group who experienced symptoms following drug withdrawal or sham withdrawal. We would expect symptoms to be more numerous and more severe in the drug withdrawal group than in the continuation group.

Withdrawal symptoms would have to be distinguished from a resurgence of the original anxiety symptoms. Three criteria that can help make this distinction are (1) the time course, (2) the intensity, and (3) the quality of the symptoms. A withdrawal symptom is expected to occur between 5 and 10 days following drug withdrawal and recede thereafter, while an original anxiety symptom could arise at earlier or later times and last much longer. A symptom that reappears after drug withdrawal at an intensity greater than it had had prior to drug use may be counted as a withdrawal symptom. A symptom that appears following withdrawal that was not present prior to benzodiazepine use can also be classified as a withdrawal symptom. For example, a patient might feel a tingling sensation in the skin following drug withdrawal while never having experienced tingling as a part of the anxiety illness.

Peter Tyrer, Robert Owen, and Shiela Dawling have carried out a study of this type in a group of benzodiazepine patients who were judged ready to be taken off drugs. They had been taking benzodiazepines for an average of over two years. Some of the patients were switched to placebo beginning at the second week of the study, and some were switched at the eighth week. The switch was gradual; that is, the drug dose was first cut in half for two weeks, then cut to one-quarter for two more weeks before being cut to zero for the remainder of the study. At two-week intervals, blood samples were taken to monitor the amount and rate of change of benzodiazepine in the blood. Forty-four percent of the patients showed withdrawal symptoms, as distinguished from resurgent anxiety symptoms. The symptoms were not very severe, however; they consisted of insomnia, apparent sadness, reduced appetite, worrying over trifles, and perceptual anomalies, such as feeling that things were not real or that one was outside one's body.[48]

A recent study by Karl Rickels and colleagues appears to use very sensitive criteria for identifying withdrawal reactions after abrupt discontinuation of diazepam. In this study patients with the diagnosis of GAD or panic disorder were treated with diazepam for six months, then switched to placebo. Twenty-seven percent of the patients showed withdrawal symptoms that included insomnia, nervousness, sweating, loss of appetite, and "feeling strange."[49] Previous studies by Rickels indicated that benzodiazepine treatment for four to six months can lead to withdrawal symptoms in about 10 percent of patients.[50]

The overall picture based on currently available evidence is that taking benzodiazepines continuously for a month or two presents an acceptably low risk of physiological dependence. The withdrawal symptom that is most likely following brief exposures to benzodiazepines appears to be insomnia. If treatment is extended beyond about three months, the number of patients that have withdrawal trouble rises above 10 percent. If use stretches on into years, about half the patients experience withdrawal symptoms. In some very long-term users these symptoms may be severe, as in Eric's case, but they usually do not include the delirium or seizures observed during withdrawal from alcohol or barbiturates.[51]

Finally, we must consider the risk of physiological dependence with buspirone, the new nonbenzodiazepine anxiolytic. Rickels and colleagues, in the study cited above, directly compared the dependence liability of buspirone with clorazepate, a slowly eliminated benzodiazepine. Being slowly eliminated, clorazepate probably is less likely than most benzodiazepines to evoke withdrawal symptoms. Patients with GAD or panic disorder were treated for 24 weeks with either clorazepate or buspirone, double blind. This treatment brought about substantial improvement in anxiety symptoms as indicated by changed scores on the Hamilton Anxiety Scale and other measures. The patients were then switched to placebo and observed for an additional four weeks. During the first two drug-free weeks anxiety and other withdrawal symptoms appeared in the clorazepate group but not in the buspirone group. The difference between the two groups was statistically significant. The symptoms in the clorazepate group diminished markedly during the third and fourth placebo weeks. Thus, withdrawal of buspirone failed to evoke any withdrawal symptoms, and in this respect it is meaningfully superior to a benzodiazepine (Figure 17–2).[52]

Property 7: Cross-Tolerance and Cross-Dependence

Development of tolerance or dependence for a sedative, hypnotic, or anxiolytic drug usually results in at least some degree of tolerance or dependence for other drugs that have similar actions. For example, a heavy drinker who has developed tolerance for the anxiolytic effect

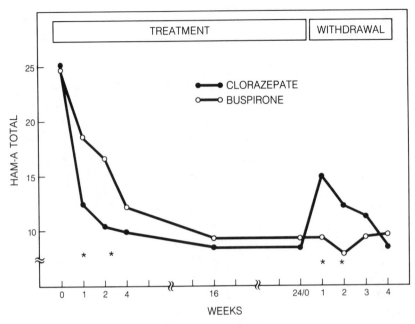

FIGURE 17-2 Effect of clorazepate, a benzodiazepine, and buspirone on anxiety symptoms during drug treatment and drug withdrawal in anxiety patients. Y axis shows mean score on Hamilton Anxiety Scale; a high score indicates numerous and severe anxiety symptoms. X axis shows weeks of treatment or weeks of withdrawal. At outset all patients had diagnosis of GAD or panic disorder. Patients received drug treatment for 24 weeks with either clorazepate (40 patients) or buspirone (21 patients). Patients were switched to placebo for four weeks of withdrawal at the end of treatment. Asterisks are time points at which a difference between the two groups is statistically significant. Notes: (1) Buspirone has a longer delay of benefit than does the benzodiazepine. (2) In withdrawal there is a rebound of anxiety in the benzodiazepine group but not in the buspirone group. The fact that the withdrawal anxiety occurred only in the clorazepate group shows that the withdrawal symptoms are evoked by benzodiazepine termination and are not a return of the original illness. From K. Rickels, E. Schweizer, Edward, I. Csanalosi et al.,[4] "Long-Term Treatment of Anxiety and Risk of Withdrawal," *Archives of General Psychiatry* 45(1988): 444–50.

of alcohol will be tolerant also for the anxiolytic effect of a barbiturate the first time he or she takes it. Accordingly, we say that barbiturates and alcohol show cross-tolerance. The fact that alcohol withdrawal symptoms can be relieved by taking a barbiturate indicates that alcohol and barbiturates show cross-dependence.[53]

The existence of cross-tolerance among the sedative-hypnotic drugs increases addiction liability for two reasons. First, taking one drug can increase the person's motivation for taking another. Second, by taking two cross-tolerant drugs at the same time, tolerance can be established more quickly than would be expected from one of the drugs alone. Two cross-tolerant drugs have the same effect on the development of tolerance as taking a higher dose of a single drug. Alcohol and benzodiazepines are frequently used together, thus enhancing the risk of tolerance and an increase in alcohol consumption when benzodiazepine treatment ceases.

Cross-dependence contributes to addiction because it provides a standby method for remaining addicted. When drug abuse becomes obvious and embarrassing or when the preferred drug becomes unavailable, the user can switch to a cross-dependent drug to avoid the withdrawal illness. A woman who wants to conceal her drinking from the family might substitute some diazepam for her morning eye opener. A methaqualone addict whose illicit supplier has landed in jail might satisfy his need by switching to alcohol.

Among the currently available anxiolytics, buspirone is unique in that it produces little sedation and hypnosis (Chapter 17). It does not give rise to symptoms of the sedative-hypnotic withdrawal illness, nor is it presently known to evoke other withdrawal symptoms. A most interesting observation is that buspirone does not potentiate the effects of alcohol intoxication.[54] These facts suggest that buspirone may not show cross-dependence with sedative-hypnotics.

Leslie A. Riblet and coworkers found that buspirone will not substitute for barbiturates or benzodiazepines for relief of sedative-hypnotic withdrawal symptoms in mice.[55] Schweizer and Rickels have shown, additionally, that buspirone does not relieve the benzodiazepine withdrawal illness in human patients.[56] They made the especially interesting observation that anxiety caused by benzodiazepine withdrawal was not relieved by buspirone. This observation was replicated by Lader and Olajide.[57] As buspirone does relieve the anxiety symptoms of GAD, it appears that the withdrawal anxiety is physiologically and pharmacologically distinct from the symptoms of GAD.

Although more research is needed on buspirone, the current data suggest that this new anxiolytic, which neither causes sedation nor hypnosis, does not increase one's motivation for using sedative-hypnotics.

SUMMARY OF ADDICTION RISKS

Considering all seven of the factors contributing to addiction liability, it seems clear that buspirone is the least addictive drug. The benzodiazepines are second, and the barbiturates and the nonbenzodiazepine minor tranquilizers are third. Alcohol is the most addictive.

Table 17–1 summarizes the reasoning behind this ranking. The factors contributing to addiction are the rows in the table. The four types of anxiolytic drugs are the columns. Each drug type is given a zero or one to four plus signs. A zero means that the drug has no value on the particular factor; for example, buspirone gets a zero for euphoria, since there is no evidence for a euphoric action of buspirone. The plus signs indicate addiction liability; the more pluses, the greater the liability in comparison to drugs with fewer pluses. For example, alcohol is most distinct from the other agents in the rapidity of its action, freedom from supervision, and social setting. One might disagree with the exact number of pluses we have placed in each cell of the table, but even if the assignments were adjusted somewhat, the relative standing among the four drug categories would likely remain as shown.

Since buspirone apparently does not produce cognitive impairment and has low risk of dependence and since cognitive impairment and dependence are the main problems with benzodiazepines, it might seem appropriate to recommend that buspirone replace the benzodiazepines as the workhorse anxiolytic in the physician's ar-

TABLE 17-1 Addiction Liability of Anxiolytic Drugs

	ALCOHOL	NONBENZODIAZEPINE PILLS	BENZODIAZEPINES	BUSPIRONE
Euphoria	++	+++	+	0
Rapid action	+++	++	+	0
Unsupervised use	++++	++	++	0
Social encouragement	++++	++	+	0
Tolerance	++	++	+	0
Physiological dependence	++++	+++	++	0
Cross-tolerance and cross-dependence	+++	+++	+++	0
Total	22	17	11	0

mamentarium. Indeed, this recommendation has been made by at least one research psychiatrist, John Feighner, who points out that a switch to buspirone would result in a significant reduction in the annual number of deaths due to automobile crashes.[58]

It is too soon, however, to launch a buspirone bandwagon. Buspirone is a very new drug, and unforeseen problems may come to light as time goes on. Also, buspirone has some known drawbacks. Unlike benzodiazepines, the long delay of benefit makes buspirone nearly worthless for immediate short-term relief of anxiety. Furthermore, patients reject treatment with buspirone more frequently than they reject benzodiazepines. Those who have had experience with benzodiazepines are especially intolerant of buspirone. This lack of patient acceptability may be due to buspirone's greater delay of benefit, to its occasional dysphoric side effects, or to its lack of euphoric effects in comparison with benzodiazepines. It may also be due to buspirone's ineffectiveness in relieving withdrawal anxiety that follows termination of drinking or long-term benzodiazepine therapy. Patient satisfaction with buspirone might be improved by supportive psychotherapy and proper education about the delay of benefit, low addiction risk, and lack of cognitive impairment. Further research and clinical experience will determine buspirone's role during the decade of the 1990s.[59]

PROPER USE OF ANXIOLYTICS

There is no easily applied test that tells whether drugs or nonpharmacologic measures are best for the relief of maladaptive anxiety. The effectiveness of nonpharmacologic methods must be considered, and the risks and benefits of the drugs must be weighed. If the drug route is indicated, how does one design a treatment for anxiety that secures the drug benefits while avoiding the harms? The following are some guidelines for this decision-making process.

Do not think of anxiolytics as cures. These drugs are optimally used to give temporary relief until the cause of the anxiety can be removed.

Do not think of anxiolytics as the main treatment. Think of them instead as a supporting treatment. Get appropriate medical, psychological, or pastoral help.

Do not take anxiolytics without first having a psychiatric examination to make sure that the anxiety is not being caused by a mental health condition like depression, bipolar disorder, or alcoholism. Those disorders can be treated directly.

Never use alcohol or barbiturates for the relief of anxiety. These drugs have been superceded by benzodiazepines and buspirone.

Do not take benzodiazepines continuously for more than two months without a drug holiday lasting several weeks. Use psychotherapy and other methods to survive the drug holidays. Buspirone is probably safer than benzodiazepines for long-term treatment. Benzodiazepines are good for immediate short-term relief.

Do not use benzodiazepines if you are a heavy drinker or have suffered from any form of sedative-hypnotic addiction. Buspirone, by contrast, may be a safe anxiolytic for those who have overused sedative-hypnotics.

Do not use benzodiazepines for insomnia for more than four nights in a row.

Do not increase the dose of a benzodiazepine without consulting a physician. Do not get your benzodiazepine prescription refilled without revisiting the physician.

Do not drive under the influence of sedative-hypnotics. Whatever you do, do not drive under the combined influence of benzodiazepines and alcohol.

The decision to use a risky treatment depends on the severity of the patient's suffering, the likelihood that the treatment will work, and the negative consequences of treatment, If, by risking dependence on a benzodiazepine, one could avoid certain addiction to alcohol, the costs would be worth the benefit. Indeed, some authorities believe there are patients with generalized anxiety for whom benzodiazepine dependence is a justifiable price to pay for the peace of mind that can be obtained in no other way. These authorities point out that benzodiazepine dependence is not threatening to health and can often be terminated by tapered withdrawal. Furthermore, they feel that many patients are suffering unnecessarily because they irrationally fear addiction, which is much worse than simple dependence.[60] Although long-term benzodiazepine use may have a high risk of dependence, the risk of addiction may be fairly low. This line of argument calls attention to the fact that a decision to obtain a medical treatment is a value judgment that each individual must make for him- or herself after receiving advice from a physician and carefully evaluating the options.

18

TREATMENT OF PANIC DISORDER AND OBSESSIVE COMPULSIVE DISORDER

—

I n the two preceding chapters drugs were conceived as agents for controlling anxiety symptoms that could arise from a variety of circumstances, such as pain in the back, anticipation of surgery, GAD, or situational stress. In this chapter the targets of drug treatment are two particular anxiety disorders defined in the *DSM-III-R*: panic disorder and OCD.

In the following text, we discuss the efficacy of drug treatments, the efficacy of psychotherapy, and biological hypotheses about panic disorder and OCD. Our discussion of psychotherapy is intended as a supplement to the pharmacological and biological information. A more thorough treatment of psychotherapy for these disorders can be found in *Fears, Phobias and Rituals* by Isaac M. Marks.[1] As with other mental illnesses, good therapy for panic disorder and OCD involves personal advice and support for the patient. Drugs alone are not the optimal treatment.

PANIC DISORDER AND AGORAPHOBIA

A seminal observation about panic disorder was made by Donald F. Kline in 1964. By careful study of symptoms and drug treatments dispensed for mental patients in the Hillside Hospital, Glen Oaks, Long Island, Klein noticed a group of patients that had an unusual response to drugs. These patients suffered from what we now call panic disorder with agoraphobia. They were stricken with panic attacks at unexpected times and for no apparent reason. Fearful that they would be rendered helpless by one of these attacks, they were excessively dependent on others for reassurance and support. Prior to hospitalization, the patients had been afraid to travel alone away from home, and they had never been anxiety free, even while at home. The psychiatrists of the day judged that these patients needed tranquilizers, and they prescribed phenothiazines or sedatives along with psychotherapy. These treatments, however, were either ineffective or problematic. Klein decided to try other drugs that at the time were not known to relieve anxiety. When he tried imipramine, he and his patients were rewarded.

Imipramine relieved the panic attacks within 3 to 14 days. The drug did not, Klein believed, relieve the emotional dependence and fearful avoidance behavior that the patients expressed between the panic attacks; that is, the drugs did not relieve the agoraphobia. Klein noted, however, that the phobic symptoms could be relieved to some extent by intense persuasion and therapeutic support after the panic attacks had been stopped with imipramine. Indeed, in this early work, and in all later work by Klein and his colleagues, the panic/agoraphobia patients have received psychotherapy of one kind or another along with drug treatment.

Klein went on to do a small drug efficacy study in which seven panic patients were given imipramine and six controls were given placebo. As measured by several rating scales after five weeks of treatment, the imipramine patients improved markedly in comparison to the placebo patients. The patients tended to relapse when the drug was discontinued.[2]

In second- and third-generation studies Klein's initial observations have been largely confirmed. In particular, there is now widespread agreement that imipramine (a tricyclic antidepressant), phenelzine (a MAOI), and alprazolam (a benzodiazepine) can all reduce the frequency of panic attacks.[3] Of these drugs, phenelzine may be the single most effective agent, although this point is not proved beyond doubt. Benzodiazepines other than alprazolam are not effective for the relief of panic attacks.[4]

A study by David V. Sheehan, James Ballenger, and Gary Jacobsen of the Harvard Medical School represents the newer work nicely. In this study, patients suffering from panic disorder with agoraphobia were treated with imipramine, phenelzine, or placebo. The drug treatments were double blind, and the patients were randomly assigned to a placebo, imipramine, or phenelzine group; there were about 20 patients in each group. The presence and intensity of panic attacks, phobias, and anxiety were assessed by several rating scales before drug treatment, after 6 weeks of treatment, and after 12 weeks of treatment, when the study ended. The patients participated in supportive group psychotherapy at two-week intervals during the treatment. There was no effort to see how long the patients stayed well after treatment ended.

All three groups improved significantly by the end of the twelfth week (Figure 18–1). The improvement was greatest in the phenelzine group and least in the placebo group. The differences between the drug-treated groups and the placebo group were statistically significant on nearly all rating scales, but the difference favoring phenelzine over imipramine failed to reach statistical significance on most scales. The drug groups were significantly improved by the sixth week and had improved even more by the twelfth week. The placebo group failed to show significant improvement until the twelfth week. The improvement occurred in both the symptoms of agoraphobia and in the frequency of panic attacks.

The patients in this study were severely ill prior to treatment. On the average they had suffered from panic attacks for about 12 years and were seriously disabled in their work and family life. Ninety-eight percent of the patients had received prior treatment with benzodiazepines or other minor tranquilizers. Ninety-five percent had previously seen a psychiatrist, and together they had accumulated 215 years of weekly psychotherapy of various types. These prior treatments had been unsuccessful.[5]

Studies like this one by Sheehan and his colleagues do not show that imipramine or phenelzine are cures for panic disorder with agoraphobia. Although patients typically get better than they would have been without treatment, they often fail to become normal. They may retain a propensity for excessive fearfulness and dependence.[6]

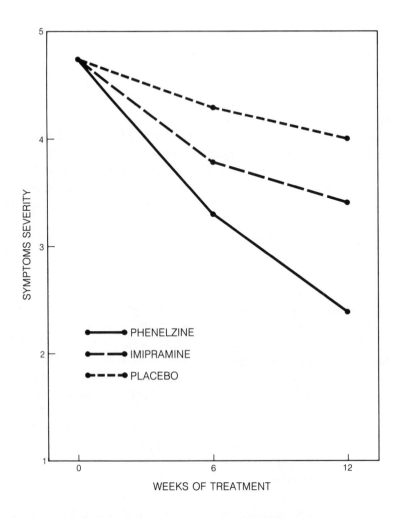

FIGURE 18-1   Efficacy of phenelzine, imipramine, and placebo for treatment of panic disorder with agoraphobia. Severity of symptoms rated on scale in which 1 = no fear felt when confronted with threatening situation, 2 = mild symptoms that do not interfere with confrontation of threatening situation, 3 = less mild symptoms that interfere in minor ways, 4 = marked interference, and 5 = panic when confronted with threatening situation. Threatening situation is defined specifically for each patient. Graph gives mean scores for the three groups. Significant differences between the groups: Phenelzine is superior to placebo at 6 and 12 weeks, imipramine is superior to placebo only at 12 weeks, and phenelzine is superior to imipramine at 12 weeks. Data from D. V. Sheehan, J. Ballenger, and G. Jacobsen, "Treatment of Endogenous Anxiety with Phobic, Hysterical, and Hypochrondriacal Symptoms," *Archives of General Psychiatry* 37(1980): 51–59.

There is also a tendency for patients to relapse when the drug treatment is discontinued. The addition of psychotherapy, however, may give some protection against relapse.[7] The study by Sheehan and colleagues did not report on how long the patients remained panic free following drug treatment. More information is needed about the frequency of relapse and how it is best prevented.

Klein has proposed that in most patients who suffer from panic disorder with agoraphobia the unprovoked panic attacks are the primary problem, and the agoraphobia is secondary. The fearful dependence and the refusal to leave home, he thinks, are brought about by the patient's fear of having an unprovoked attack in an unprotected environment. Further, Klein has proposed that imipramine and the other effective drugs primarily relieve the panic attacks while having little direct impact on the agoraphobia. In the absence of the panic attacks, however, the agoraphobia can be unlearned (extinguished, habituated) with the aid of psychotherapy.[8] This view of the relationship between panic disorder and agoraphobia is consistent with the results of many studies of drug treatment of panic disorder with agoraphobia. In these studies psychotherapy is given concurrently with drug or placebo. The relief of the agoraphobia that occurs may be a benefit of psychotherapy acting in a context that is free of panic, thanks to the drug action.

Klein's views, however, are not consistent with all the data. First of all, there are some patients who have agoraphobia without panic attacks.[9] Thus agoraphobia is not always caused by fear of panic attacks. Whether imipramine, phenelzine, or alprazolam would relieve the agoraphobia in such patients is unknown. Second, a recent double-blind study has shown that imipramine can relieve both the panic and the agoraphobic symptoms under conditions that involve no psychotherapy whatsoever.[10] In this study the investigators purposely withheld psychotherapy so that the drug action could be measured without being confounded with the effects of psychotherapy. The drug improved both the panic symptoms and the agoraphobic symptoms more than did placebo. Thus imipramine appears to be efficacious for agoraphobia for reasons that go beyond simply facilitating psychotherapy.

It is equally clear that psychotherapy in the absence of drugs can lead to improvement of agoraphobia in many patients.[11] Effective psychotherapy for agoraphobia and other phobias employs the principles of exposure and habituation. The fearful patient must be exposed to the situation that evokes his or her fear, and the patient must remain in the situation long enough to learn that nothing bad will happen. Thus, in the case of snake phobia, exposure and habituation require the patient to bring him- or herself into the close proximity of a snake and to stay near the snake until feelings of anxiety begin to subside or habituate. This exercise is repeated until the initial anxiety evoked by a snake, or by the mere possibility of seeing a snake, no longer occurs or is no longer debilitating. The role of the psychotherapist is to help the patient have enough courage to endure the initial exposure.

In the case of agoraphobia, the therapist coaches patients to plan how they are going to venture out of the house and into the feared public place. Like a cheerleader, the therapist congratulates and rewards patients for their successful courageous behavior. Studies by Isaac M. Marks, of the Maudsley Hospital in London, indicate that psychotherapy leads to more permanent improvement than does treatment with drugs alone. Agoraphobia patients may remain symptom free for many years following termination of successful exposure therapy, but in the absence of exposure therapy, the symptoms may reappear soon after drug treatment is stopped.[12]

Marks found that exposure therapy in the absence of drugs brings about improvement in both agoraphobia and panic attacks in patients who suffer from both. This appears to conflict with Klein's opinion that psychotherapy is ineffective for panic disorder. The root of this particular controversy may be that Marks and Klein have not used the same diagnostic criteria for defining panic disorder. Klein has used a definition similar to that in the DSM-III-R, which requires that at least some of the panic attacks occur without provocation by a feared stimulus and that there be four attacks within a period of four weeks. Marks, in contrast, has not regarded panic disorder as a condition that is separate from agoraphobia; rather, he has conceived a single illness, agoraphobia, that includes panic attacks as one symptom. When Marks has given his patients exposure therapy, he has found that panic attacks are reduced in frequency along with other anxiety symptoms.[13] It could be that the panic attacks experienced by at least some of Marks's patients occurred rather infrequently and never spontaneously. In these patients, who do not strictly satisfy Klein's criteria for panic disorder, drug treatment may not be essential. Obviously, more research is required to determine the relative importance of drugs and psychotherapy for the relief of panic and agoraphobic symptoms. All agree, though, that the best clinical results are obtained when drugs and exposure therapy are combined for the treatment of panic disorder with agoraphobia.

Biological Basis of Panic Disorder

Animal research, supported by neurological observations in human patients, has allowed neuroscientists to identify several regions of the brain that are heavily involved in the expression of intense emotions like anger and fear. These brain centers are located in the upper portion of the brain stem (locus ceruleus), along the floor of the frontal lobes (orbital frontal cortex), and deep in the forward portion of the temporal lobe (amygdala) (Figure 18–2). A reasonable hypothesis, therefore, is that patients who suffer from panic disorder might have a malfunction in one or more of these brain regions.[14]

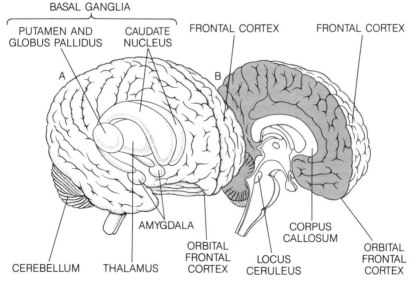

FIGURE 18–2 Views of the brain showing structures likely to be involved in panic disorder and OCD. A. Three-dimensional view of the right side of the brain. The basal ganglia and amygdala lie beneath the surface and are shown as they would look if the overlying cerebral cortex were transparent. B. The brain has been cut down the midline into a right and left half-brain. The cut surface of the left half-brain is shown. The locus ceruleus lies below the surface at the indicated position.

Whatever the malfunction might be, however, we know it does not involve a large anatomical abnormality in the brain that is easily seen by simple inspection. The problem is more subtle, perhaps arising from some abnormality in the way neurons are interconnected or in the way they release or respond to synaptic transmitters. Recently, evidence has begun to accumulate in support of this view.

The phenomenon of lactate susceptibility is one indication that panic disorder patients are biochemically different than nonpanic patients. As originally discovered by F. N. Pitts and J. N. McClure, at Washington University in St. Louis, injection of excessive lactate, a natural product of metabolism, will trigger panic attacks in many patients who suffer panic disorder. In Pitts and McClure's original study, a group of 14 panic disorder patients and 10 normal controls, were given injections of a solution containing lactate or of a control solution containing glucose. In response to lactate, 13 of the 14 panic disorder patients experienced symptoms that were subjectively similar or identical to the symptoms they experienced when they had one of their spontaneous panic attacks. Only 2 of the 10 healthy control subjects experienced severe nervousness or panic, and the rest of the control subjects experienced only very mild symptoms. The glucose injection had no anxiety-provoking effect in either the controls or the patients. Pitts and McClure's finding has been replicated in many subsequent studies. These studies show that about two-thirds of panic disorder patients are susceptible to lactate, while other types of psychiatric patients and normal controls are much less likely to be susceptible.[15]

Lactate is produced in the body as a metabolic by-product during periods of intense muscular exercise. Pitts and McClure suggested that spontaneous attacks in panic disorder patients may be caused by an abnormal sensitivity to lactate that is released during exercise or muscle tension due to stress. Recent research lends only vague support to this hypothesis. Several agents other than lactate have been found to provoke attacks in panic disorder patients. Elevation of carbon dioxide in the blood, for example, can trigger panic attacks. High blood carbon dioxide occurs naturally as a result of intense exercise or deprivation of fresh air. Other agents that can provoke attacks include caffeine, yohimbine, and norepinephrine, which are known to act on neurons in the locus coeruleus that are a part of the brain circuitry that is active during natural fear. Activity of these neurons would result in secretion of the hormones of stress and secretion of neurotransmitters that are normally released during times of natural fear, vigilance, or panic.[16]

We speculate that panic attacks may be caused by the inappropriate triggering of brain circuitry that orchestrates the instinctive panic response that appropriately occurs only when there is a shortage of air, the immediate prospect of death, or some other calamity. It is as if this calamity response is set on hair trigger. Agents like elevated blood lactate or carbon dioxide, which conceivably could signify a shortage of air, might trip the hair-trigger of the panic response. An important research strategy would be to figure out what synaptic transmitters are involved in triggering panic responses and then try to develop a drug treatment that would reduce the activity of the transmitter. Animal research has already shown that the transmitter norepinephrine is involved in the expression of fear and vigilance.[17] We also know that the tricyclic antidepressants and MAOIs reduce the sensitivity of postsynaptic nerve cells to norepinephrine. Perhaps this reduction in sensitivity to norepinephrine is a part of the explanation for why tricyclic antidepressants and MAOIs are effective treatments for panic disorder.

The possibility of provoking panic attacks on demand by giving lactate or carbon dioxide has provided an opportunity to study the physiology of panic attacks experimentally in the laboratory. In volunteer subjects, measurements of respiration, blood circulation, muscle activity, secretory activity, and brain activity can be made prior to a panic attack and then during the lactate-evoked attack. Instances when lactate provokes an attack can be compared with instances when lactate fails to provoke an attack. Normal volunteers or volunteers with various psychiatric diagnoses can be compared with patients who have panic disorder.

In a recent interesting experiment of this type, Reiman and colleagues, at Washington University in St. Louis, assessed neural activity in various brain regions before and during lactate injection. The measurements of neural activity were made using the new radiological technique of positron emission tomography (PET), explained in Chapter 5. The subjects were a group of patients who had panic disorder without agoraphobia and a group of controls who had no psychiatric illness. As expected, some of the panic disorder patients experienced a panic attack during the lactate injection and others did not. None of the normal patients had panic attacks in response to lactate.

Even before lactate injection, lactate-sensitive patients had a higher level of neural activity throughout a large portion of the brain than did the control subjects or the panic disorder patients in whom lactate did not evoke panic. During the lactate injection, those who responded with panic showed a further increase of neural activity on both sides in the temporal lobe near the amygdala, in the brain stem near the locus coeruleus, and in a few other locations. These brain locations are known to be important parts of the brain circuitry for vigilance, fear, and anger. No lactate-induced changes occurred in the normal subjects or in panic disorder patients who were not sensitive to lactate.[18]

The PET methods for localizing the changes in neural activity are new, and they require calculations that rely on assumptions that may be questioned by experts. Therefore there is some uncertainty about the size of the changes and their precise locations in the brain. Further refinements and replications will be required to support the findings of the Reiman group. At present, these experiments make the point that panic disorder, like other mental disorders, can be understood as a biological entity that involves unusual activity in the brain. The portions of the brain involved are those that, through animal research, are known to be a part of the circuitry for intense emotions like fear, anger, and rage.

Some important questions for future research are whether treatments that are effective for panic disorder normalize the activity near the amygdala and locus coeruleus, and whether these abnormalities occur only in patients with panic disorder or also in patients with other closely related psychiatric disorders, such as agoraphobia without panic attacks.

OBSESSIVE COMPULSIVE DISORDER

As shown in Chapter 15, OCD is a chronic debilitating illness that, prior to 1980, had the reputation of being unresponsive to treatment. Insight psychotherapy, anxiolytic drugs, and antipsychotic drugs had a poor record of success. The psychoanalytic hypothesis that obsessions and compulsions are caused by unconscious conflict also had not been helpful in relieving symptoms of the disorder.

Clomipramine Therapy

Recently, obsessive compulsive disorder has attracted considerable attention due to the discovery that the tricyclic antidepressant clomipramine (Anafranil) can bring significant relief for many patients. As early as 1967 uncontrolled observations indicated that clomipramine might have efficacy in OCD. Properly designed, objective studies, however, were not available until 1980, when two papers were published from research teams headed by Peter Thoren of Stockholm, Sweden,[19] and Isaac M. Marks of London, England.[20]

In the 1980 study by Thoren and colleagues, clomipramine was compared with placebo and with another tricyclic antidepressant, nortriptyline. There were only 24 subjects, 8 each in a clomipramine group, a placebo group, and a nortriptyline group. Although the study predates the *DSM-III*, all the patients satisfied the criteria for OCD in the Research Diagnostic Criteria, which are similar to the *DSM-III* criteria. As is typical in OCD, many of the patients also had symptoms of depression, but depression was considered secondary to the OCD. All the subjects were severely debilitated. They were all hospitalized; they had suffered from OCD for an average of over 10 years, and they had failed to respond to at least one other form of treatment. These other treatments had included psychoanalysis, behavior therapy, electroconvulsive shock, and other drug therapies.

The number and severity of OCD symptoms were assessed at the beginning of the study and at weekly intervals using rating scales that were filled out by the hospital personnel and by the patients themselves. For the first week all patients received placebo to allow time for washout of any drugs they had been taking prior to the study. At the beginning of the second week, patients in the two drug groups were started on either clomipramine or nortriptyline, and they remained on the drug for five weeks. Then the patients were given the option of continuing treatment, nonblind, using clomipramine in combination with exposure therapy. During the initial six weeks there was no formal psychotherapy, but patients were encouraged to resist their obsessions and compulsions.

Five replicable features of clomipramine therapy were revealed in the 1980 study by Thoren and colleagues. The principal result was that the group of patients receiving clomipramine experienced an improvement of obsessive compulsive symptoms after five weeks of drug treatment (Figure 18–3). Their average score on the OCD

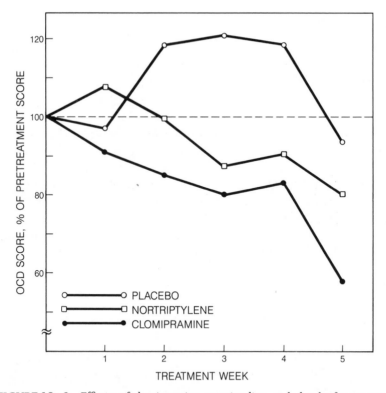

FIGURE 18-3   Efficacy of clomipramine, nortriptyline, and placebo for treatment of OCD. Plotted points give mean score on a scale of OCD symptom severity presented as a percent of pretreatment score. Scores of less than 100 percent indicate improvement; those greater than 100 percent indicate worsening. The score for clomipramine at five weeks is significantly different from that for placebo. Data from P. Thoren, M. Asberg, B. Cronholm, L. Jornestedt, and L. Traskman, "Clomipramine Treatment of Obsessive-Compulsive Disorder," *Archives of General Psychiatry* 37(1980): 1281–85.

symptom rating scales declined by about 50 percent, while the average score in the placebo group did not decline at all. This difference between the clomipramine patients and the placebo patients was statistically significant.

The second point is that clomipramine is more beneficial than other tricyclic antidepressants for relief of OCD. Thoren's patients treated with nortriptyline improved somewhat, but the improvement was less than that of the patients treated with clomipramine. Fur-

thermore, the difference between the placebo group and the nortriptyline group was not statistically significant.

The third important observation was that the benefit of clomipramine occurs only after a long delay. The improvement of the
clomipramine patients in comparison to the placebo patients did not
become large enough to be statistically significant until the fifth week
of drug treatment. This is meaningfully longer than the two- to
three-week delay that is typical of tricyclics when used for the
treatment of depression. In studies in which drug treatment has
lasted longer than five weeks, the benefit of clomipramine continues
to increase as time goes on. The full drug benefit probably requires
about 10 weeks of treatment.[21] In Thoren's study there was further
improvement during the nonblind voluntary extension beyond the
fifth week of clomipramine treatment. During the extension, however, Thoren's patients received both clomipramine and exposure
therapy, so we do not know whether the additional improvement
was due to an extension of the clomipramine, the addition of exposure therapy, or a placebo effect.

The fourth observation of Thoren and colleagues is that the
efficacy of clomipramine in relieving OCD does not depend on the
coexistence of depressive symptoms. As we have said, many obsessive compulsive patients also meet the *DSM-III-R* criteria for major
depression. Clomipramine is just as likely to help OCD patients who
are not depressed as it is those who are depressed. Thus, clomipramine does not appear to be simply acting as an antidepressant when
it brings relief to obsessive compulsive patients.[22]

The fifth observation by Thoren and colleagues is the bad news:
Clomipramine is only partially effective. Only about half the clomipramine patients showed clear improvement after five weeks. In
other studies the maximum percentage of patients reported to benefit is about 75 percent.[23] All workers agree that complete recovery
does not occur. While on drug treatment, patients usually continue
to be aware of their problems, but the obsessions and compulsions
become less intrusive and less damaging to everyday life. A patient in
a study by Flament and colleagues said, "The thoughts are still there,
but they don't bother me any more.[24]"

Thus, though the benefits are neither immediate nor complete,
clomipramine can relieve the suffering of OCD. This benefit is in
addition to the drug's benefit in the relief of major depression. As we
explain below, psychotherapeutic techniques that are effective for

OCD have also been developed. Indeed, for many patients psychotherapy may be superior to clomipramine. For other patients clomipramine may be superior to psychotherapy, and for many patients the best treatment may be clomipramine and psychotherapy combined.

Psychotherapy for Compulsive Rituals

In psychotherapy for OCD the therapist encourages patients to expose themselves to situations that arouse the performance of rituals. While exposed to the arousing stimulus, the patient must forego performing the rituals for long enough to allow the resulting anxiety and tension to habituate. The willful suppression of the ritual is called response prevention. At first, the patient is made very anxious and uncomfortable by exposure and response prevention. After many trials, though, most patients learn not to be so discomforted and can avoid performing rituals to relieve the discomfort.

For example, a person with a hand-washing compulsion would be assisted in the confrontation and toleration of dirt. In a case described by Marks, the therapist took a compulsive patient to the hospital dust bin, reached into the dust bin, got his hands thoroughly covered with dirt, and rubbed the dirt on his face and hair. The therapist then asked the patient to do the same. If the patient could not do it, the therapist tried a less challenging (less dirty) task. Several sessions of demonstration and encouragement were required before the patient could tolerate direct contact with the dust bin; but no pain, no gain. Although patients may have to approach the threatening situation by small degrees, eventually they must endure the anxiety long enough to allow it to subside in the presence of the provoking stimulus without succumbing to the urge to perform the ritual. In many cases the patient can manage the treatment as a series of homework assignments. The therapist gives coaching and encouragement at weekly or biweekly sessions.[25] The patient may have to practice several hours per day. Properly supervised exposure therapy, though not easy, can be very effective. Up to 80 percent of patients who practice conscientiously receive lasting relief, without drugs, from rituals.[26]

Important questions are whether exposure therapy is more effective than drug therapy and whether the combination of exposure and drug therapy is better than either alone. Two studies from the group headed by Marks have attempted to get at these issues. In a 1980 study, patients were treated with either clomipramine or placebo. The drug group and the placebo group were further subdivided such that half the patients in each group also got relaxation psychotherapy, while the other half got exposure therapy. All the patients had overt rituals at the outset; there were no purely obsessive patients. After 10 weeks of treatment, the greatest improvement had occurred in the patients who received clomipramine combined with exposure therapy. Exposure therapy plus placebo and clomipramine plus relaxation therapy were both better than placebo plus relaxation. These results suggest that both exposure therapy and clomipramine can be effective stand-alone treatments for compulsions and that the combination of exposure plus clomipramine is superior to either alone.[27]

In a 1988 study by Marks and colleagues, groups of ritualizing patients received (1) clomipramine with exposure, (2) placebo with exposure, or (3) clomipramine with "antiexposure." Antiexposure consisted of instructing the patients to avoid any contact with the situations that made them anxious or made them feel the urge to perform rituals. The antiexposure patients were also instructed that whenever they felt the urge to perform rituals, they were to indulge themselves in ritualizing until the need had been fully satisfied. The exposure treatments were carried out as homework assignments. (In a small part of this complex study, the effect of adding a live therapist to assist with exposure was evaluated; the live therapist brought little benefit). The treatment lasted 27 weeks, and there were follow-up assessments of the patients' symptoms at intervals throughout 25 additional weeks. None of the patients had previously received exposure treatment, and none of them had obsessions without rituals. From a standpoint of experimental design and methods, this study by the Marks group is an example of excellence in clinical research.

The outcome of the 1988 Marks study suggests strongly that exposure therapy is more potent than clomipramine, with clomipramine adding a small additional benefit. All groups receiving exposure therapy improved significantly. Clomipramine combined with antiexposure was significantly worse than placebo combined with exposure. Clomipramine combined with exposure was significantly better than placebo combined with exposure. The advantage of clomipramine plus exposure over placebo plus exposure, however, was not overwhelming. Clomipramine was better than placebo only during the first 8 weeks of treatment. As the treatment continued to

17 weeks and beyond, the placebo plus exposure group caught up with the clomipramine plus exposure group. The improvement of all patients who received exposure was sustained without decline at the fifty-second week follow-up evaluation. Thus, in this well-designed study, the benefit of clomipramine was to accelerate the relief of symptoms, but not to increase the enduring long-term benefit.[28]

If we were to follow the implications of this study, the best treatment for ritualizing OCD patients would be a combination of clomipramine and exposure therapy for at least eight weeks, with withdrawal of the clomipramine no later than the seventeenth week. Clomipramine is not a benign drug that one can take at no cost: It is a tricyclic antidepressant and evokes all the side effects that are characteristic of this class of drugs (see Chapter 13). The side effect that patients most often complain about is dry mouth; other side effects include constipation, weight gain, blurred vision, orthostatic hypotension, urinary retention, and delayed or absent orgasm.

Patients who have obsessive thoughts without overt rituals are more difficult to treat with exposure therapy than are overt ritualizers. It is harder for a therapist to help a patient resist a compulsive thought than to resist hand washing or checking door locks. Also, obsessions may not be brought on by specific situations (e.g., dirt, leaving home), and therefore it may be impossible for patients to expose themselves to the circumstances that evoke obsessional thoughts. Sometimes patients who have both obsessions and rituals say that their obsessions persist even after their rituals have been brought under control with exposure therapy.[29] It is our impression that while exposure therapy is quite effective for a specific ritual, it is less impressive in bringing broad relief from the many emotional and subjective aspects of OCD.

Obsessive compulsive patients who have additional psychological problems are less likely to respond favorably to exposure therapy than are patients who, aside from OCD, are psychologically healthy. These additional complicating problems include depression, anxiety, and poor adjustment at school, at work, or socially.[30] Unfortunately, depression, anxiety, and poor adjustment often coexist with obsessive compulsive symptoms.

An important advantage of exposure therapy over clomipramine is that exposure provides more long-lasting relief. When clomipramine is discontinued, patients typically relapse within a few weeks.[31]

Improvement in response to exposure therapy, however, may persist several years after the end of the active treatment.[32]

We might hope that the benefits of exposure therapy, once acquired, become a permanent resource for the patient, a lesson well learned. The evidence cited above suggests that this may be true. It is tempting to think that psychotherapy generally works like the processes of training and education; people can remember learned skills and knowledge for a lifetime. (Drugs, by contrast, start disappearing from the brain as soon as they are introduced.) As reasonable as this idea seems, however, only studies of the long-term benefits of psychotherapy will tell us if it is generally correct.

Choosing Between Exposure and Clomipramine

It seems clear that when the main problem is compulsive rituals with few emotional complications, patients respond more reliably to exposure therapy than to drug therapy alone. For these patients, then, exposure with response prevention is the treatment of choice. Drugs are desirable for patients who are not helped enough by exposure therapy. Among these are people who are troubled by severe obsessions and who have intense coexisting depression and anxiety. For these people the soundest advice would be to seek combined exposure and clomipramine therapy. Clomipramine could relieve the broad spectrum of symptoms including obsessions and the secondary depression. In the presence of this relief, further gains might then be made with exposure therapy.

A possibility is that clomipramine weakens the impulse to rehearse the rituals and obsessions, and as a result patients can successfully engage in response prevention. In most studies using clomipramine, the patients are encouraged to resist their obsessions and compulsions, thus giving themselves exposure therapy. Indeed, obsessions and compulsions are subjectively obnoxious, and patients don't have to be instructed to resist them. Flament and coworkers, for example, report that their clomipramine patients say that the drug helps them resist their compulsions without experiencing so much anxiety.[33] Goodman and colleagues have noted the same opinion among their clomipramine-treated patients.[34] Thus, clomipramine treatment may be a case in which a drug allows patients to engage in psychotherapy more productively.

Serotonin and OCD

One way to learn about the biological mechanisms of OCD is to ask what physiological or biochemical responses clomipramine evokes in brain cells. Clomipramine has several different actions on brain cells. Like other tricyclic antidepressants, the drug and its active metabolites prevent the uptake of serotonin and norepinephrine and interfere with transmission at acetylcholine synapses. There are probably additional cellular actions that are unknown. The question is, which of these actions are essential for relieving OCD, and which are unrelated to OCD?

A key observation is that clomipramine is superior to several other antidepressants for relieving obsessive compulsive symptoms. Thoren and colleagues found that clomipramine, but not nortriptyline, relieved obsessive compulsive symptoms.[35] Other workers have found that clomipramine is superior to amitriptyline, imipramine, desipramine,[36] and the antidepressant MAOI, clorgyline.[37]

Clomipramine's capacity for relieving OCD correlates with its capacity to block reuptake of serotonin and not with other known actions. Of all the tricyclic antidepressants, clomipramine is the most potent serotonin reuptake blocker. Desipramine, by contrast, is a weak serotonin reuptake blocker, and desipramine is significantly worse than clomipramine for relief of obsessive compulsive symptoms.[38] Since desipramine is a good norepinephrine reuptake blocker, it is unlikely that the efficacy of clomipramine for OCD is based on norepinephrine reuptake blockade. Other actions that are shared by clomipramine, desipramine, and other tricyclics (e.g., blockade of acetylcholine synapses) are also unlikely causes of OCD relief. We cannot rule out, however, that some unknown action of clomipramine, and not serotonin uptake blockade, is actually the critical event.

Clomipramine is not superior to other antidepressants for the treatment of major depressive disorder. This difference between depression and OCD in response to clomipramine indicates that the two illnesses are somewhat distinct physiologically. We may draw this conclusion despite the fact that many OCD patients also have depression and many depressed patients also have obsessions. Clomipramine's efficacy against depression, like that of other tricyclic antidepressants, is presumably due to its blockade of both sertonin and norepinephrine reuptake.

If clomipramine's anti-OCD action is based on its serotonin uptake blockade, we would predict that all drugs blocking serotonin reuptake should also relieve obsessive compulsive symptoms. Fluoxetin (Prozac), fluvoxamine, and zimelidine are three recently developed drugs that are known to block serotonin uptake. These drugs are not tricyclic antidepressants; they do not block acetylcholine synapses or norepinephrine reuptake, and they presumably have a different spectrum of unknown effects than tricyclics. In double-blind controlled studies of fluvoxamine and zimelidine, both have been shown to relieve OCD.[39] In one study with zimelidine, the drug failed to have a significant effect[40]; this study involved only a small number of patients, however, and a positive drug effect may have been missed. The efficacy of fluoxetine has yet to be demonstrated in controlled studies, but informal observations indicate that fluoxetine treatment also is associated with improvement of OCD.[41]

Another strategy for testing the hypothesis that clomipramine works at serotonin synapses is to see if there are correlations between the response to treatment and changes in serotonin metabolism in the brain. The reasoning is that changes in serotonin transmission will cause changes in serotonin release. This, in turn, will cause changes in the amount of serotonin broken down and changes in the amount of serotonin synthesized to replace that which is broken down. Although it is not possible to measure the rate of serotonin synthesis in the human brain, it is possible to measure the products of serotonin breakdown. The main breakdown product is 5-hydroxy-indole acetic acid (5-HIAA). The amount of 5-HIAA can be measured in samples of the cerebrospinal fluid taken from psychiatric patients and volunteer control patients.

Thoren and associates measured the amount of 5-HIAA in the cerebrospinal fluid of OCD patients before treatment and after three weeks of treatment with clomipramine. They found that patients whose OCD symptoms improved markedly tended to show a correlated decrease in the amount of 5-HIAA in the brain. Also, patients who had the highest level of 5-HIAA prior to treatment were most likely to respond well to treatment.[42] This suggests that a decrease in the release of serotonin may be related to the therapeutic response to clomipramine. Recently results similar to Thoren's have been obtained by Flament and associates.[43]

Another strategy for revealing a possible link between serotonin and OCD has been applied by Joseph Zohar and his colleagues at the

NIMH. They asked whether drugs that are known to interact with postsynaptic serotonin receptors cause changes in the intensity of obsessive compulsive symptoms. Unlike clomipramine, these drugs do not prevent serotonin uptake, but act directly on serotonin receptors either to mimic or block the action of serotonin. As a serotonin mimic, Zohar and colleagues gave the drug mCPP; as a serotonin blocker they gave metergoline. Some of the subjects were obsessive compulsive patients, and some were controls who had no psychiatric illness. Zohar and colleagues found that mCPP, the serotonin mimic, evoked a worsening of symptoms in the obsessive compulsive patients but had no tendency to evoke obsessions or compulsions in the control subjects. Metergoline, in contrast, failed to worsen obsessive compulsive symptoms.[44] Eric Hollander and his colleagues have also observed worsening of OCD symptoms in response to mCPP.[45] A group led by Dennis Charney, however, failed to replicate the obsession-provoking effect of mCPP.[46]

Zohar and colleagues have suggested that patients with OCD may be abnormally sensitive to serotonin. In these patients serotonin may evoke obsessions and compulsions when it is secreted at synapses. The therapeutic benefit of clomipramine may be based on the drug's ability to evoke desensitization of serotonin receptors. In support of this suggestion, Zohar and colleagues conducted a study in which mCPP was given to OCD patients before and after treatment with clomipramine. The OCD patients were much less sensitive to the symptom-provoking effects of mCPP after three and one-half months of clomipramine treatment than they were before treatment. The data are consistent with the hypothesis that clomipramine brings about subsensitivity of serotonin receptors or in some other way makes the brain less sensitive to serotonin.[47]

It is easy to overinterpret Zohar and Insel's work with mCPP, however. The situation in the brain is exceedingly complex and all experiments are not in agreement. A recent study, for example, indicates that metergoline (a serotonin blocker) can worsen obsessional symptoms in OCD patients who are under treatment with clomipramine.[48] How are we to explain the fact that metergoline, a serotonin blocker, and mCPP, a serotonin mimic, both cause obsessional worsening? Despite problems like this, the experiments with mCPP and metergoline raise the level of sophistication about the sertonin hypothesis of OCD.

In summary, at the present state of the art, a good hypothesis is that physiological changes at serotonin synapses can play a role in relieving obsessive compulsive symptoms. Experiments that might have ruled out this hypothesis have failed to do so. The hypothesis is not without difficulty, however. Benefit in addition to that obtained from clomipramine can be achieved with psychotherapy. Therefore we know for certain that mechanisms in addition to serotonin uptake blockade are involved.

The Orbital Cortex, the Basal Ganglia, and OCD

The basal ganglia consist of several large clusters of neurons located beneath the surface of the frontal lobes (Figure 18–2). One of the most prominent of these clusters is the caudate nucleus. The functions of the basal ganglia are not well understood, but a wealth of circumstantial evidence indicates that they play an important role in the voluntary initiation and cessation of movements. Evidence for this view comes from knowledge about Huntington's disease and Parkinson's disease. In both of these diseases, synapses degenerate in the basal ganglia, resulting in loss of voluntary control over muscular activity. In Parkinson's disease, patients become unable to initiate movements voluntarily. In Huntington's disease, patients are unable to prevent themselves from making large, purposeless, jerky movements of the arms and face. Much animal research also indicates that problems in the basal ganglia lead to impairment of the appropriate initiation and cessation of movement. Surgical damage to the caudate nucleus on one side of the brain, for example, will cause an animal to circle endlessly and compulsively in the direction away from the side of the damage.

OCD involves a loss of voluntary control of behavioral and mental routines. Patients are unable to prevent themselves from performing routines such as hand washing or checking the stove. They are unable to prevent themselves from thinking useless thoughts over and over again. In some cases the patient becomes stuck and cannot perform a simple voluntary act like crossing the street due to an inability to stop checking for oncoming cars. These losses of voluntary control make it reasonable to speculate that the basal ganglia could be involved in OCD as they are in Parkinson's disease and Huntington's disease. The research question is, then, do the symptoms of OCD ever occur in association with known pathology of the basal ganglia in humans? Judith L. Rapoport and others have looked into this question by reviewing the medical and scientific literature. They find that, indeed, obsessive compulsive symptoms are often associated with basal ganglia pathology and with other illnesses that are known to involve basal ganglia dysfunction.[49]

One of the most interesting examples is the movement disorder known as Sydenham's chorea. This illness occurs as a complication of rheumatic fever in children. As an aftermath of rheumatic fever a mixup can occur in the body's immune system resulting in the production of antibodies against a protein that occurs exclusively in neuron cell bodies of the caudate nucleus. This antibody binds to the caudate nucleus neurons and impairs their function. The behavioral result is that the patient involuntarily emits jerky movements similar to those of Huntington's disease. For our purposes, however, the more interesting fact is that these patients also experience obsessive compulsive symptoms. They ruminate on obsessive thoughts and irresistibly perform compulsive rituals.[50] These obsessive-compulsive symptoms are probably caused by the antibodies that attack the neurons of the caudate nucleus.

Tic disorders are also often accompanied by symptoms of OCD. This is true of the syndrome known as Gilles de la Tourette disorder. In this disorder, the patient makes involuntary utterances that may consist of nonsense noises, barks, grunts, words, and especially swear words. The patient may also make grimacing movements of the face and jerky movements of the hands. In these patients, the uncontrolled swearing is by far the most socially debilitating symptom. Tourette's patients also often meet the criteria for OCD by performing involuntary repetitive rituals and experiencing worthless and repetitive thoughts. The association of OCD with involuntary verbal and motor tics suggests again the involvement of the basal ganglia.[51]

Confirming these speculations and correlations, evidence is beginning to come in from brain-imaging laboratories that OCD patients may have abnormalities in the basal ganglia and in closely related parts of the frontal and temporal lobe. PET studies of OCD patients carried out at UCLA[52] indicate that there is more metabolic activity in the cerebral hemispheres of OCD patients than in normal healthy subjects or in subjects with primary major depression. This abnormally high level of activity is especially prominent in the head of the caudate nucleus and in the orbital cortex. The orbital cortex is a part of the frontal lobe that lies on the floor of the brain just above the eyes (Figure 18–2). The orbital cortex is richly connected with the basal ganglia. Extra-high metabolic activity in the orbital cortex and related structures was also found by a group of investigators at the NIMH.[53]

Evidence relating the basal ganglia to OCD is also available from studies using the CT technique. Luxenberg and colleagues used CT to measure the size of the caudate nucleus in the brains of 10 obsessive compulsive patients and 10 healthy control subjects. The caudate nucleus of the OCD patients was, on the average, about 25 percent smaller than the caudate nucleus of the normal subjects. The data from this study are especially convincing in that caudate size in 9 of the 10 OCD patients was below the mean of the normal group. Some of the normal subjects, however, had smaller caudate nuclei than some of the OCD patients. Normal subjects and OCD patients were not significantly different in other brain dimensions, such as size of the whole brain and size of structures other than the caudate nucleus. This study falls short in that it has no control group other than healthy volunteers. Thus, an important unanswered question is whether the caudate nucleus differs in size between obsessive compulsive patients and patients with other types of psychiatric illness.

OCD has attracted a great deal of research attention in the past decade, and the research has been gratifying. New drug treatments and new psychotherapies have been developed. A large group of patients who only 10 years ago had no hope of normal life have been freed of their bondage. Indeed, we would nominate the treatment of OCD as the mental health research success of the 1980s. It is to be hoped that during the 1990s progress will be as great and that it will lead to the successful treatment of nearly all OCD patients rather than just the subgroups that respond to current treatments.

This chapter and the preceding two chapters raise the conceptual issue of whether anxiety is best conceived as a symptom of illness, the illness itself, or a painful response to a threatening situation. In Chapters 16 and 17 we discussed the benzodiazepines as if they are drugs that merely relieve symptoms. In this chapter we have discussed drugs as if they relieve underlying illnesses as defined by the *DSM-III-R*. A similar ambiguity exists with respect to depression. Is depression a symptom, an illness, or a response to depressive conditions?

Another conceptual issue concerns the distinction between anxiety disorders and mood disorders. As we have seen, drugs known previously as treatments for depression, a mood disorder, are now known to be effective also for panic disorder and OCD, which are anxiety disorders. Where, we may ask, is the boundary that separates anxiety disorders from mood disorders?

Categorical distinctions are difficult in psychiatry and psychology. Indeed, no one knows exactly where the boundary is between mood disorders and anxiety disorders or between symptoms and illnesses. There may be no such boundaries. Fortunately, all puzzles do not have to be solved in order to make progress in the relief of suffering. A practical clinical strategy is to ask whether a drug or psychotherapy can be used beneficially in a particular, well-defined situation. This simple approach allows us to seek clinical benefits without paralyzing ourselves with doubt concerning the ultimate causes and the proper categorization of suffering. As time goes on, both treatment strategies and classification schemes will be improved in light of the new knowledge.

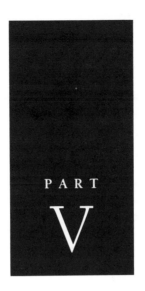

PART

V

GENERAL ISSUES

THE MEDICAL MODEL OF MENTAL ILLNESS

—

I n explaining the use of drugs for mental illness we have emphasized their benefits, risks, mechanisms of action and conditions for their proper use. Three take-home lessons are (1) psychiatric drugs are remarkably effective in relieving the suffering of several significant mental illnesses, (2) their side effects are manageable under the conditions prevailing for most patients, and (3) they work by modifying the strength of synaptic transmission between brain cells.

These lessons support the medical model of mental illness, which states that psychiatric illnesses are similar in important respects to illnesses treated in general medicine. Both types of illness are thought to result from physiological malfunction that leads to the patient's distress and disability. Both types of illness can be observed and studied through scientific research. The goals of the mental health profession are the same as the goals of the general health profession: to relieve suffering, to promote good health, to prolong life, and to learn more about the causes and treatment of illnesses so that superior benefits will be available in the future.

According to the medical model, the major distinction between mental illness and bodily illness is that mental illness arises from the brain rather than from other organs. The symptoms of mental illness appear as psychological and behavioral problems rather than as problems in respiration, metabolism, fertility, and so forth. There are, of course, many diseases of the brain that are not usually called mental illnesses. These include brain tumors, epilepsy, Parkinson's disease, and other disorders of movement and consciousness. Why these brain disorders are not called mental illnesses is not entirely clear, but by custom, the term mental illness usually refers to brain illnesses whose main expression is impairment of the *rational control* of behavior, thought, perception, and emotion. Rational control is preeminently a function of the brain, especially of the frontal and temporal lobes of the cerebral cortex.

As we pointed out in Chapter 1, the expansion of drug treatment and the increasing influence of the medical model of mental illness have met stiff resistance from people holding opposing beliefs. Four of these beliefs were also mentioned in the first chapter: (1) Drugs and other organic treatments are not appropriate in psychiatry because biological treatments cannot correct psychological problems; (2) since psychotherapy is the appropriate treatment, drugs replace the best treatment with a second-rate one; (3) the drug side effects are worse than the illnesses; and (4) psychiatric drugs are not treatments for illness, but agents used by authorities to control troublemakers. In the following sections of this chapter, we further describe these opposition beliefs and attempt to rebut them. We believe that the medical model is a valid and humanitarian conception of mental illness and its treatment.

MENTAL ILLNESS: BIOLOGICAL OR PSYCHOLOGICAL?

It is common to talk about the mind as if it were different from the body. When a person complains of a headache, for instance, someone may ask, "Do you think it's real or just psychological?" Or someone may say, "She's not really sick; she just wants attention." Conventional wisdom suggests that pills should be given if the person is "really" sick, but if the symptom is "just" psychological, medication is inappropriate. Thus, the propriety of using pills to treat depression, mania, and schizophrenia is called into question.

This resistance to drug treatment springs from denial of the central axiom of the medical model. This axiom asserts that mental illnesses are the behavioral and psychological expression of conditions in the brain. Most people today believe this axiom to be true when they stop to think about it. However, the 1,000-year-old English language codifies the ancient belief that the mind and body are separate. In contrast, the biological conception of humanity, which unifies mind and brain, is only 150 years old, dating approximately from the publication of Darwin's *Origin of Species*.

According to the biological conception, if the mind exerts rational control over behavior, then it is the nerve cells, in their ceaseless synaptic interactions, that are exerting rational control. If the mind experiences depression, then the nerve cells have fallen into a particular physiological state. If the mind hears voices, real or imagined, it is the nerve cells, in a particular pattern of secretion, that perform the task of hearing. These notions imply that agents that change the state of activity in nerve cells will change the psychological state of the mind. The converse is also true. Agents that change the state of the mind will change the state of corresponding brain cells.

We say that the unity of mind and brain is an axiom rather than a scientific fact because there is no fully rigorous scientific proof that *all* the experiences occurring in the human mind are *nothing but* conscious expressions of corresponding neural activity. Such proof would amount to a complete explanation of *how* the brain can generate *all* the conscious states that humans experience. Neuroscientists cannot provide such a complete explanation at present. No one can yet say exactly which nerve cells cause depression or how the cells interact with each other during a hallucination. Nature compels contemporary scientists to be satisfied with small incursions into the ordered tangle of the brain. Rigorous conclusions must be modest, for example, "Increasing the amount of transmitter or decreasing receptor sensitivity at norepinephrine and serotonin synapses is frequently correlated with relief from depression." This statement is considerably less than a valid proof that all aspects of depression can be explained by the details of synaptic transmission.

Nevertheless, there is ample evidence for the general proposition that changes in the state of the mind directly correspond to changes in the amount and the pattern of neural activity in the brain. Relationships between psychological functions and brain mechanisms, in fact, can easily be the subject for a sequence of six or seven college courses. Indeed, tens of thousands of scientists are currently working full time trying to obtain more knowledge about mind–brain relationships, and they are progressing rapidly.

The effectiveness of drugs for the treatment of mental illness is one of the best pieces of evidence for the unity of brain and the mind. As we have illustrated in this book, psychological entities such as mood (depression, mania, anxiety), perception (hallucinations), and thought (delusions, incoherent speech, obsessions) can be significantly influenced by molecules that change the efficacy of synaptic transmission.

Other evidence also exists. Gross physical damage to the brain caused by head injury, brain tumor, or stroke, modifies thought, mood, and perception. Specific types of brain damage can cause a person to become blind, angry, peaceful, hungry, irresponsible, or forgetful. Surgical disconnection of one cerebral hemisphere from the other leads to a condition that might be described as "two brains–two minds." The two hemispheres engage in separate and independent trains of thought; one half of the brain may have no knowledge of what the other half is thinking. Again, electrical stimulation of the living brain, as performed by surgeons during some operations for epilepsy, can evoke conscious sensations and the recollection of memories, and electroconvulsive shock treatment reliably relieves depression. A person's genetic inheritance influences his susceptibility to schizophrenia, bipolar disorder, and anxiety disorders. We could continue mentioning such facts, but elaboration is unnecessary to make the point that evidence for the unity of mind and brain is voluminous.

By contrast, there is little evidence for the dualist proposition that the mind is independent of the brain. The potential for separation of the mind from the body is an ancient belief, still present in many cultures. In the West, dualism's most intellectually impressive proponent has been René Descartes, the seventeenth-century philosopher and mathematician. His arguments in support of dualism were entirely philosophical. In Descartes's time no scientific methods for exploring the relationship between mind and brain existed, and so philosophical speculation was the only method of investigation available. However, even in the realm of pure philosophy, the doctrine that mind and body are separate led Descartes into irreconcilable contradictions.

Descartes saw that the body, including the brain, is made of physical matter. He inferred, therefore, that the body must obey the laws of physics as do rocks and other physical objects. All matter occupies space and has weight, as does the body. This implies that the movements of the body are actually the movements of a complex machine. The parts of a machine move and function because they push and tug on each other with physical force. In contrast, Descartes continued, the mind does not act like a machine. The mind doesn't work with moving wheels and levers, but with ideas. These ideas come and go under the influence of reason and will. Reason, will, and ideas have no weight and occupy no space. Therefore, the mind is not a material thing. Reason and will cannot cause movement; they cannot pull on a rope or turn a wheel.

Descartes's theory sounds plausible until one considers how the mind controls the machinery of the body. According to dualism, the body, being a machine, does not respond to reason or will; only the mind can do that. The mind, in its sphere, cannot move a machine. Hence, the mind may see beautiful images, think logical thoughts, and elaborate the most intense will, but it will not be able to move the body. The body will continue to behave like a nonthinking robot, completely outside the influence of ideas. Thus, for example, the mind cannot control the machinery of speech. Reason and will cannot govern the prayers one raises, the promises one makes, or the lover one takes. The mind cannot control the body of an athlete, the hands of a painter or a musician.

Dualism clearly fails because it gives rise to absurd conclusions. Defenders of the medical model assert simply that dualism is wrong. The brain is, beyond doubt, the machinery of the mind, and the brain can cause movement of the body.

All this, you may say, is common sense. Yes, it is now. It is interesting, nonetheless, to observe how much common beliefs can change with the passage of 300 years. The English language and other cultural practices have not yet forgotten dualism.

PSYCHOTHERAPY OR DRUG THERAPY?

Major resistance to drug treatment has come from the supporters of the long tradition of talk therapy in psychology and psychiatry. From the time of Freud, 90 years ago, until the late 1950s, various schools of psychotherapy dominated thinking about mental health in the United States. Freud's theories of psychoanalysis held sway in U.S. medical schools, and numerous non-Freudian psychotherapies were spawned in university graduate schools of clinical psychology. The general public acquired the expectation that psychiatrists and psychologists would provide only psychotherapy. There was scarcely an inkling that mental illness could be treatable with any other technique. In an environment of such undaunted beliefs, it is not surprising that drug treatments initially inspired some objections.

One often-heard objection was that drug treatments could bring about only superficial relief of symptoms, not genuine cures. A second objection was that the sedative action of the drugs would dull the patient's mind so much that he or she would be unable to participate in psychotherapy or other activity requiring significant effort. Third, drugs were just a cheap and easy way to paper over problems without really solving them. Really solving them, people believed, would take psychotherapy and hard work.

In the following sections, we defend drug therapy against these criticisms and discuss our beliefs about the proper role of psychotherapy in the treatment of mental illness.

Drugs: A Superficial Relief of Symptoms?

Biologically oriented psychiatrists and psychologists are the first to point out that the drugs now available do not bring about cures, but only symptomatic relief of mental disorders. In fact, the drugs often do not even relieve all the symptoms. For example, phenothiazines fail to alleviate the symptom of flat or inappropriate affect, and they often do not relieve hallucinations; the patient may only develop sufficient insight to know that the voices are not real. Of all the drug treatments, lithium for bipolar disorder is probably the most successful in restoring a state of normality to patients who are markedly incapacitated without treatment. But current drugs never cure a mental illness in the sense that drug treatment can be discontinued without risk of relapse.

In support of the medical model, we emphasize that the relief of symptoms is a genuine benefit that must not be dismissed as trivial. The objective of using medicine is to relieve suffering, encourage good health, and prolong life. Sometimes diseases, such as bacterial pneumonia and syphilis, are cured as these goals are reached. More often there is no cure, only relief of symptoms. Illnesses such as cancer, rheumatoid arthritis, diabetes, heart attacks, and the flu can be relieved but not often cured. However, relief is a good thing.

The treatment of choice is the one that gives the essential benefit with the fewest side effects, even when the treatment is not a cure. Morphine cannot cure anything, yet it is an appropriate treatment for intolerable chronic pain. A person with a withered leg is thankful for a brace even though it is an awful nuisance and fails to restore normal function. For patients with schizophrenia or mania, drug treatments are unquestionably the best available alternative. Psychotherapy provides no measurable benefit, not even superficial relief, for these disorders (see Chapters 6 and 14). For patients suffering from depression and anxiety disorders, both drugs and psychotherapy are effective. The treatment of choice for these patients depends, therefore, on how one evaluates the benefits, risks, and costs of the two forms of treatment.

Does Sedation Impair Psychotherapy?

Some people oppose drug treatments on the grounds that the sedative action of the drugs impairs the patient's ability to engage in psychotherapy or other pursuits requiring attention and mental effort. In other words, one of the side effects of psychiatric drugs is unacceptable. We ask, "Unacceptable in comparison to what?" In medicine, you must always compare the undesirability of drug side effects with the undesirability of the symptoms that the drug relieves. You then choose the lesser of two evils. If the symptoms are as debilitating as incoherence, hallucinations, manic rages, or suicide attempts, some degree of sedation is a small price to pay for relief.

In addition, the sedation may not be as debilitating as the opponents of drug treatment claim. First, sedation declines considerably over the first few weeks of treatment through the development of tolerance. If excessive sedation persists longer, there is a good chance that the drug dosage is too high. Second, during the initial stages of treatment for mania, schizophrenia, or agitated depression, the sedative effects are desirable because the objective of treatment at this stage is to calm excessive agitation.

Criticism of excessive sedation is probably most valid when directed toward drug practices in public mental hospitals, veterans hospitals, and nursing homes. Most of the patients in these institutions are chronically ill with schizophrenia, Alzheimer's disease, or other types of dementia. In the absence of drugs, many of them are belligerent or assaultive. Underfunding and understaffing make it impossible for the institutional staff to give patients individual attention and to adjust the drug dosage for optimal balance between desired and undesired effects. As a result, some patients are probably overdosed most of the time, accounting for their "zombie-like" appearance. One must remember, however, that the flat affect of schizophrenia itself can produce "zombie-like" behavior, and this symptom often does not respond well to drug treatment.

Drugs: An Ineffectual Substitute for Psychotherapy?

Our defense against the criticism that drugs deflect patients from psychotherapeutic solutions, varies according to the illness. For schizophrenia and bipolar disorder, our rebuttal is simply that known methods of psychotherapy are not effective for relieving the acute episodes of illness. Therefore, drugs do not displace a psychotherapeutic solution. However, psychotherapy in these illnesses can be helpful. Psychotherapy can teach the patients cognitive and social skills to help them cope with the problems of living. This therapy often prevents relapses. But most patients are not able to reap the benefits of psychotherapy until drugs have reduced irrational behavior and thinking.

Both psychotherapy and drug therapy are effective for depression, and it is legitimate to ask which form of treatment is better. At present, there is no compelling evidence favoring one over the other. As we have previously pointed out, the two forms of the treatment should not be conceived as competing with one another. The best treatment for depression is probably a combination of psychotherapy and drug therapy.

For the treatment of anxiety disorders, drugs should never be the only form of therapy (see Chapter 16). Talking with a professional therapist to design solutions for life's problems is indisputably helpful. Exposure therapy is effective for phobias and compulsions. Clomipramine is beneficial in OCD; phenelzine and imipramine are helpful in panic disorder. Because of the addiction risk and accident proneness associated with benzodiazepines and alcohol, there is a definite danger associated with these drugs. The danger has been reduced considerably, however, by the advent of buspirone, which may replace benzodiazepines for long term drug treatment of excessive anxiety. Perhaps the best strategy for anxiety disorders is to use drugs to control brief, intense episodes of anxiety and to use nondrug methods on a long-term basis to lower the average anxiety level and lengthen the time between intense episodes.

Roles for Psychotherapy

There is always a role for psychotherapy. For some diagnoses, psychotherapy is the primary or perhaps the only form of treatment. For other diagnoses it may play a supporting role. In this book we have focused on disorders for which drugs play an important role, and we have not discussed disorders in which drugs are seldom used. Even when drugs are the main treatment, supportive psychotherapy is important to help patients conform to an optimal treatment plan. Training and advice on how to manage problems of living significantly reduce the stress that bears on mental health patients. Personal attention and emotional support are important in all forms of medical care, especially mental health care. Visitors, unstressful purposeful activities, and aesthetically pleasant surroundings are also helpful. A psychiatrist who hands out prescriptions and dismisses patients without further personal consideration will log few therapeutic successes.

The medical model requires that the efficacy and safety of all therapeutic techniques, both drug and psychotherapeutic, be adequately tested before being released for general clinical use. As we mentioned in preceding chapters, many psychotherapeutic techniques have been tested and have been found to be effective. Proposed drug treatments are often found to be ineffective. If two treatments are equally safe, the more expensive one should be used only if it is more effective. It is unethical for a therapist or physician to administer a treatment that has no known prospects for success; this practice is called quackery, whether it is drug therapy or psychotherapy.

FDA regulates drug use, but laws protecting the public from ineffective psychotherapies are much less rigorous. Anyone who desires can obtain primal screaming therapy, reasoning therapy, realism cure, decision cure, orgasm cure, rest cure, feeling therapy, nude therapy, marathon therapy, nude marathon therapy, and many others. Most of these therapies have never been tested in properly controlled studies. In some cases, the therapy is conducted by people who have not had rigorous training, and the odor of a confidence racket permeates the procedure. The American Group Psychotherapy Association, a highly reputable organization, has taken the stand that many of these untested therapies may actually do more harm than good.[1] About the only protection for the prospective patient is choosing a psychotherapist who is well established and highly regarded in the mental health care community.[2]

People who favor psychotherapy are frequently opposed to biological treatments, yet psychotherapy can be properly thought of as a biological technique that fits neatly into the medical model of mental illness. Psychotherapy produces biological effects just as a drug or electroconvulsive shock does. Through talking and personal interactions, psychotherapy changes the state of the brain. Under the direction of the psychotherapist, the biological mechanisms of learning alter the strength of transmission at some synapses and alter the pattern of activity in some neural circuits. Although the details are not known, psychotherapy is likely to change the amount of transmitter secreted or change the sensitivity of postsynaptic receptors. Whatever the details, effective psychotherapy has to be considered a method of changing synaptic transmission.

SIDE EFFECTS: ARE THE RISKS WORTH THE BENEFITS?

We have already explored in detail the problem of drug side effects and how they can be managed. An important additional point is that the problem of side effects is no different in psychiatry than in other branches of medicine. No medical treatment is free of risk. In selecting a treatment, the magnitude of the expected harms and the probability of their occurrence must always be weighed against the magnitude and probability of the desired benefits. For example, the surgical treatment of appendicitis carries several risks. First, general anesthesia deeply suppresses the activity of the nervous system; occasionally, the patient stops breathing. Second, the abdominal incision can cause uncontrolled bleeding, infection, or damage to vital organs. Nonetheless, because the risk of death due to the treatment is less than the risk of death due to the untreated disease, the surgical treatment is accepted as a humanitarian practice. By contrast, no one would suggest that general anesthesia and surgery be used to relieve stomach gas, though such a procedure might be successful. Treatments for stomach gas are available that have risks commensurate with their expected benefits.

Analogously, the risks of tardive dyskinesia and other side effects are often justified when antipsychotic drugs are used to treat schizophrenia. But such grave risks are not justified in the treatment of anxiety associated with depression, somatic illness, or marital stress even though the drugs might successfully relieve these types of anxiety. Thus, we rebut the charge that psychotherapeutic drugs ordinarily cause harms that are worse than the illnesses they cure. Some psychotherapeutic drugs may have side effects that are more harmful than some mental illnesses, but for schizophrenia, bipolar disorder, major depression, and many types of excessive anxiety, drug treatments can be matched to the illness so that the likelihood of overall benefit far exceeds the likelihood of overall harm. Continued research may bring forth new treatments that have more favorable ratios of benefits to harms than the treatments now available.

PATIENTS' RIGHTS

The Radical Psychiatry Movement

The fourth form of resistance to drug treatment takes the form of a civil rights movement. The aim of the movement is to liberate mental patients from unjust coercive control by psychiatrists and their allies in the sociopolitical establishment. We call this the radical psychiatry movement to emphasize its antiestablishment outlook.[3] Intellectual leaders in this movement have been Thomas Szasz in the United States, R. D. Laing and David Cooper in England, and Franco Basaglia in Italy. The radical psychiatry movement grew and flourished during the 1960s, a time of great dissatisfaction with authoritarian structures in society. A flagship publication of the radical psychiatrists is Thomas Szasz's *The Myth of Mental Illness*, published in 1961.

The radical psychiatrists believe neither that mental patients are ill nor that psychiatrists are healing the sick. Instead, they claim, the unpatients, or clients, are either having trouble solving problems of living or are simply nonconformists. According to this view, schizophrenia and other disorders are just patterns of behavior expressed by particular individuals in response to the conditions of the world. Behavior patterns are not considered to be illnesses. Therefore, psychiatrists are unjustified in their attempts to terminate behavior patterns by giving drugs on the pretense that they are healing the sick. More accurately, claim the radicals, the psychiatrists and psychologists are punishing troublemakers and coercing deviant individuals to behave in conventional ways. Drug treatment of mental disorders does not benefit the patient; it benefits only the established order.[4]

In his role as enforcer, the conventional psychiatrist exercises the police power of society. He plays the roles of the judge, jury, and jailer. The alleged patient is the accused. The radical psychiatrists further claim that conventional psychiatrists call themselves physicians not because they deal with medical problems or make use of medical science, but because they wish to use the prestige and authority of the medical profession as a disguise. In this way, the psychiatrists can intimidate their alleged patients and mislead everyone about their police function. In this system of thought, the accused do not need drugs, just a fair trial. Szasz points out that if John Hinkley had been given a criminal trial as a normal person, he would be out of jail by now. But since he was declared a psychiatric patient, he still languishes in custody with no realistic hope of release. This shows that psychiatric patients have fewer rights than criminals.[5]

If mental illness is a convenient fiction, the radical psychiatrists have a point. The Eighth Amendment of the U.S. Constitution says that the state shall not require excessive bail, excessive fines, or cruel and unusual punishment. Courts have ruled that forcible hospitalization without criminal charge is a form of cruel and unusual punishment and is therefore prohibited, unless there is some unusual circumstance. The Fourteenth Amendment requires that citizens shall not be deprived of life, liberty, or property without due process of law and that all persons shall have equal protection under the laws. The hospitalization of a competent person against his or her will without the benefit of a trial or other legal proceedings is a patent violation of the Fourteenth Amendment.[6]

A central disagreement between the radical psychiatrists and the proponents of the medical model is the definition of illness. Conventional psychiatrists interpret the behaviors of schizophrenia, for example, as evidence of illness that deprives patients of their ability to think rationally. The radical psychiatrists interpret the symptoms of schizophrenia as simple nonconformity or as sane responses to an insane world. Szasz argued that an illness, by definition, is a condition that is caused by an anatomical defect or lesion of the body. This definition, he claimed, is one of the great discoveries of modern medical science. Therefore, schizophrenia is not an illness because there is no known anatomical lesion or physiological defect underlying it.[7]

There are two rebuttals to Szasz's argument that we think are persuasive. First, Szasz's definition of illness is eccentric and not in accord with the understanding of illness shared by the vast majority of medical professionals, legal experts, and the public. Migraine headaches and epileptic seizures are indisputably illnesses; yet many cases of these diseases are not caused by known anatomical lesions. Most people call headaches and seizures illnesses because there is clear suffering and disability. It is not necessary to identify the anatomical, physiological, or biochemical causes to realize that illness exists.[8]

The second rebuttal is that the present state of ignorance about the causes of schizophrenia and other mental disorders is almost certainly temporary. In earlier chapters we described research suggesting that schizophrenic behavior is related to the transmitter dopamine and abnormal activity in the frontal and temporal lobes. Further, risk factors for schizophrenia can be inherited. These facts are a great advance beyond the biological knowledge that prevailed only 25 years ago, when the first edition of The Myth of Mental Illness was published. We believe that research will eventually uncover the precise causes of schizophrenia. Dr. Seymour Kety has pointed out that the biological causes of general paresis (the psychiatric manifestations of syphilis) and pellagrous psychosis (a mental illness caused by a deficiency of the B vitamin niacin) were not known in the nineteenth century. However, these illnesses were probably the most common reasons for psychiatric hospitalizations at that time. Could it be true, Kety asked, that pellagrous psychosis and general paresis were myths before their causes were understood and that they became illnesses only when medical science reached a particular stage of development?[9]

Although we vigorously disagree with the radical claim that mental illness is a myth, we agree fully with the radicals that psychiatry must not be used as a form of police power. Psychiatrists and psychologists who adhere to the medical model want to be healers; they do not want to be judges, lawyers, police, or jailers.

The Case of General Grigorenko

To illustrate what can happen when psychiatry is abused, we can look at a situation that existed in the Soviet Union between about 1960 and 1987. The case of General Pyotr Grigorievich Grigorenko is an example. General Grigorenko rose to the top of the Soviet military in World War II and was highly placed in the Kremlin at the time of Stalin's death. For many years, he had been quietly dissatisfied with the undemocratic nature of the Soviet government. In 1961, during the liberalization of the regime that followed Stalin's death, General Grigorenko made some of his views public in a speech at a party meeting. He advocated democratization of the government. He criticized the exorbitant salaries and special privileges enjoyed by government officials, and he called for rotation of party leaders in office.

General Grigorenko's speech was apparently too extreme, for he was stripped of his duties in Moscow and sent to a minor post in East Asia. There, however, he continued his open dissent by organizing a group that distributed pamphlets urging a return to the principles of Leninism. After three months of this activity, in February 1964, the KGB arrested him on a charge of anti-Soviet agitation, a criminal offense, and sent him to prison to await trial. During this internment, the prosecutor ordered a psychiatric examination. The government psychiatrists, who were supervised by the KGB, pronounced that Grigorenko suffered from a "psychological illness" that was manifested by symptoms of "reformist ideas, in particular for the reorganization of the state apparatus; and this was linked with ideas of over-estimation of his own personality that reached messianic proportions. He felt his experiences with emotional intensity and was unshakably convinced of the rightness of his actions."[10] Further, they said that Grigorenko was not legally responsible, was incompetent to defend himself in court, and was in need of compulsory treatment.

A Soviet court accepted the opinion of the government psychiatrists without dispute. In a proceeding that neither Grigorenko nor any of his relatives was allowed to attend, the court ordered Grigorenko into a special "hospital" that, again, was administered by the national police bureaucracy. At no point during the proceeding was he allowed to consult with a lawyer, participate in the investigation, or confront his accusers.

Grigorenko was discharged from the hospital nine months later, but in 1969, following another episode of dissident activity, he was rehospitalized. Again there was no public hearing or opportunity for appeal. The second incarceration lasted more than five years. When he finally left the hospital, he was 67 years old and in poor health. In 1978 Grigorenko secured a visa to come to the United States to obtain medical treatment and visit his son. While he was in the United States, his Soviet citizenship was revoked, banishing him from his homeland.[11]

Grigorenko had never believed he was mentally ill and was keenly interested in setting the record straight. Accordingly, he approached Walter Reich, a psychiatrist at the Harvard Medical School, and requested a psychiatric evaluation. Reich assembled a team of psychiatrists and experts in psychiatric and neurological diagnosis, including Alan Stone, professor of law and psychiatry at Harvard University, Norman Geschwind, professor of neurology, Harvard Medical School, and Lawrence Kolb, director of New York State Psychiatric Institute. This team exhaustively examined General Grigorenko in December 1978. They found him to be lucid, rational, conscientious, idealistic, nonrigid, nongrandiose, intelligent, and persuadable by reason. According to diagnostic criteria that were broadly accepted in the United States, he had no diagnosable mental illness. Approximately 50 psychiatrists from the United Kingdom, West Germany, and the United States had the opportunity to examine Grigorenko's Soviet case reports. In their opinion, there was no evidence of mental illness.[12]

The case of General Grigorenko is exactly the kind of oppression that the radical psychiatrists warn against. A person with a long-established record of public service was falsely diagnosed as mentally ill and involuntarily confined because he expressed ideas that were not approved by authorities. The inconvenience of a public trial, at which the accused might have embarrassed his accusers, was avoided. Deprived of the right to counsel, the accused had no chance to dispute the charges. The authorities covered their trail by calling Grigorenko a medical patient rather than a political dissident.

Several hundred Soviet cases similar to General Grigorenko's came to the attention of psychiatrists in the West. In response, Western psychiatric organizations, especially those in Britain and the

United States, publicly criticized Soviet abuses of psychiatry. At its international convention in 1977 the World Psychiatric Association condemned the Soviet practice of hospitalizing political dissidents. In 1983 the World Psychiatric Association was on the verge of expelling the Soviet psychiatric association over the issue. The Soviets, however, preemptively resigned from the organization before the expulsion vote could be taken.[13]

Mikhail Gorbachev came to power in 1985, and after a few years his reforms of glasnost and peristroika began to influence the relationship between the KGB and psychiatry. In 1986 articles began to appear in the Soviet press that were critical on the political abuse of psychiatry. In 1987 more than 100 psychiatric prisoners were released. New laws were passed that dissolved the connection between the KGB and the state psychiatric services. Procedures were spelled out giving patients and their families the right to appeal and a right to a public hearing.[14]

Whether these new procedures have been implemented fully is unclear, but considerable reform has occurred. A group of U.S. psychiatrists visited several mental hospitals that had formerly been used to house political dissidents. They interviewed 25 patients and former patients who had been identified as political detainees. The U.S. psychiatrists found little evidence that psychiatric abuse was continuing in the Soviet Union. In the fall of 1989, after the Soviets publicly admitted past errors, the delegates to the Congress of the World Psychiatric Association voted to readmit the Soviet psychiatric association to membership in the worldwide professional association of psychiatrists. It is hoped that the reforms will be permanent.[15]

We should not self-righteously suppose that abuse of psychiatry does not happen in the United States or other Western countries. There are many situations here at home in which mental health professionals are strongly tempted, and even required, to act on behalf of authority rather than on behalf of patients. In many states there are laws requiring mental health workers to protect potential victims of their patients when the mental health worker detects that a patient is about to commit a dangerous act. Thus a therapist may feel it necessary to commit a patient to the hospital in order to protect potential victims and to ensure against malpractice suits.[16] In underfinanced state mental hospitals, the overworked staff has a strong incentive to maintain order in the hospital by giving drugs, even though some patients may be oversedated. A military psychiatrist may have to preserve military discipline rather than restore the soldier's mental health. One of us knew a young psychiatrist who served in Vietnam. Assigned the job of treating shell-shocked troops, he felt he was being asked to rehabilitate the men just enough to get them back into battle. Finally, of course, the general public is fearful of mental patients who behave in bizarre ways. Public authorities are under pressure to keep nonconforming individuals out of shopping malls, off the streets, and generally out of sight.[17] Thus there are incentives to use mental hospitals, as Szasz says, to punish and control deviance.

Civil Commitment in the United States

Prior to 1969 there were few legal restraints on the power of U.S. psychiatrists to send patients to the hospital against their will. The only justification required was the psychiatrists' opinion that the patients needed treatment. In the predrug era, hospital personnel ordered bleeding, purging, cold baths, or whirling chair therapy for patients' own good, without patients' consent.

Since 1969 new laws have forced mental health workers to pay serious respect to patients' wishes. Patients have been awarded the legal right to refuse treatment. The legal changes have focused on the plight of those who are committed to mental hospitals against their will. These are the patients who, like General Grigorenko, are most likely to be victims of unjust coercive control.[18]

In U.S. law, the authority to detain a person who has not been charged with a crime derives from the state's power of *parens patriae*, the ability of the state to act as a substitute parent. According to this doctrine, the state can intervene to take care of people who cannot care for themselves or to protect society and the people themselves from dangerous acts they might commit. Civil commitment, the procedure that legally authorizes the forcible detention of a person under the powers of *parens patriae*, involves a hearing before a judge at which the patient can protest commitment. The judge decides whether the person should be hospitalized.[19]

In cases of civil commitment there is an inherent conflict between the values of individual autonomy and the benevolence of the state. Since 1969 the courts have increasingly resolved this conflict in favor of autonomy. Civil commitment has been largely restricted to those cases in which patients appear to be a danger to society, a danger to themselves, or gravely disabled. Gravely disabled means that the disorder is so severe that the patients' lives are threatened by their inability to keep themselves fed, clothed, and housed. To a large extent, the courts have freed patients to have their mental illness if they want it, as long as they do not become dangerous.[20]

U.S. judges have applied a narrow definition of "dangerous". A dangerous patient is currently construed as one who is imminently likely to become so violent that he or she will do bodily harm to him- or herself or others. A patient who is merely troublesome or embarrassing is not considered dangerous. Property damage, disturbing the peace, and destroying family life do not qualify. Furthermore, judges are requiring that dangerousness be proven "beyond reasonable doubt." This standard of proof is very rigorous, requiring an almost 90 percent certainty that the patient will commit a violent act. Since psychiatrists and psychologists cannot predict beyond reasonable doubt whether a patient is going to become violent several days or weeks into the future, the dangerousness criterion can be satisfied only by those who are already violent, have made a suicide attempt, or have made credible violent or suicidal threats.[21]

This libertarian development has, no doubt, been gratifying to Thomas Szasz. It has also moved legal practice toward the standard set by John Stuart Mill in his famous essay "On Liberty":

> The only purpose for which power can be rightfully exercised over any member of a civilized community, against his will, is to prevent harm to others. His own good, either physical or moral, is not a sufficient warrant. He cannot rightfully be compelled to do or forbear because it will be better for him to do so, because it will make him happier, because, in the opinion of others, to do so would be wise, or even right. These are reasons for remonstrating with him, or reasoning with him, or persuading him, or entreating him, but not for compelling him, or visiting him with any evil in case he do otherwise.[22]

Once committed to the hospital, involuntary patients soon encounter authority figures who want them to take drugs. Thus, another power struggle may ensue. Until recently it was customary for psychiatrists to give drugs forcibly by injection to involuntary patients who would not take them willingly. This practice changed in 1975, when a group of patients at the Boston State Hospital asked the courts to prevent hospital personnel from injecting them with drugs that they didn't want to take. Federal District Judge Joseph L. Tauro immediately issued a restraining order prohibiting psychiatrists at the hospital from giving mental patients drugs against their will, except in emergencies. A final decision in the case was not reached until 1979. A similar case was decided in 1978 by Federal District Judge Stanley S. Brotman in New Jersey.[23]

Judge Tauro and Judge Brotman both ruled in favor of the patients. Except in emergencies, they said, involuntary patients have the right to refuse medication, even though they have been committed for the purpose of treatment and even though the treatment may be in the patients' best interest.

In his written decision Judge Tauro quoted from an opinion written in 1914 by Justice Benjamin N. Cardozo: "Every human being of adult years and sound mind has a right to determine what shall be done with his own body." [24] This doctrine, that a person has the right to control his body, has long been accepted as a part of an individual's common law right to privacy. In general medicine it is accepted that a competent person can refuse medical treatment even if such refusal will certainly lead to his or her death.[25]

When a person seeks the advice of a doctor, it is understood that a contract is formed between physician and patient. A valid contract for treatment can be formed only with the "informed consent" of the patient. Judge Tauro ruled that this kind of contract also exists between involuntarily hospitalized mental patients and their psychiatrists.[26] This doctrine, of course, requires the patients to have mental capacity sufficient to enter into a contractual agreement, a requirement they often do not meet. Patients with schizophrenia who pay attention only to their delusions and cannot speak coherently are not able to form and carry out contractual agreements with other people.[27]

Judge Tauro also found support for his decision in the First Amendment's guarantee of the right of free speech. Since psychiatric drugs have the power to influence the process of thinking, they must also influence speech. Judge Tauro wrote:

> Whatever powers the Constitution has granted our government, involuntary mind control is not one of them, absent extraordinary circumstances. The fact that mind control

takes place in a mental institution in the form of medically sound treatment for mental disease is not, in itself, an extraordinary circumstance warranting an unsanctioned intrusion on the integrity of a human being.[28]

Psychiatrists express consternation at this aspect of Judge Tauro's opinion because, according to their values, the antipsychotic drugs do not control the mind but liberate it. They liberate it from the bonds of delusions, hallucinations, and incoherence.[29]

Both judges stated that drugs could be given against patients' will in emergencies. Emergencies were defined as situations in which there was imminent danger of violent behavior leading to bodily harm to the patients themselves, to other patients, or to the hospital staff. This definition was considerably narrower than state psychiatrists wanted. During the Boston State trial, the psychiatrists proposed that a psychiatric emergency should consist of suicidal gestures even when not seriously meant, property destruction, assaultiveness, extreme anxiety or panic, bizarre behavior, emotional disturbance having potential to interfere with the patient's ability to maintain daily functions, and the prospect of rapid deterioration in the patient's psychological condition. According to the court, the prevention of these nonviolent behaviors was not a sufficient justification to override a patient's desire to remain drug free.

There are several sources of dissatisfaction with the almost exclusive reliance on dangerousness as a justification for civil commitment and involuntary treatment. There is no effective psychiatric treatment for some types of mental disorder in which the person expresses violent and antisocial impulses. In such cases hospitalization of a person to prevent future violence is similar to putting a person in jail before the crime has been committed. Such preventive detention is clearly forbidden in the criminal justice system. Potentially, therefore, psychiatric commitment may be brought in to do some dirty work that is hard to accomplish under the criminal statutes.[30]

Another problem is that dangerousness criteria make the state hospital into an institution that specializes in the care of dangerous patients. Nonviolent voluntary patients tend to go to private hospitals to avoid the violent patients. State hospitals tend to serve young men with paranoid schizophrenia, mania, or antisocial personality disorder. Women with depression and old patients, who are typically less violent, are not committed. It is unsatisfactory, that many of these nondangerous, treatment-refusing patients end up roaming the streets. For these reasons, sole reliance on dangerousness criteria is less than fully satisfactory.[31]

We think a compromise between benevolence and liberty is needed. Mill acknowledged that there are exceptions to the principle that the state ought not coerce individuals for their own good. One exception is when individuals are incapable of thinking for themselves or incapable of rationally deciding on their own course of action. This exception would apply, for instance, to young children who are being abused by their parents or to adults who are mentally retarded or in a coma. It might also apply to mental patients who have illnesses that involve a serious thought disorder. Thus, whether patients are delusional or incoherent should probably be a key issue in judging whether they may be legally treated against their will.[32]

A severely depressed patient, for example, might refuse to go into the hospital because he believes he is so worthless that he does not deserve to recover. A patient with schizophrenia may believe that the doctors are spies from a foreign government who are conspiring to thwart her plans. With these patients, it may be impossible to follow Mill's advice to remonstrate with them, reason with them, persuade them, or implore them to enter the hospital. Their refusal of treatment is not a rational choice, but a product of their illness. Allowing them to exercise their right to refuse may be granting liberty to illness rather than liberty to thought. When their mind is restored through treatment, such patients may have much more freedom of thought and individual autonomy than they ever would have had while ill. Viewed in this light, coerced treatment is a temporary restriction of liberty that results in a larger and longer-lasting increase in liberty.[33]

Courts have generally recognized that when medical patients, because of illness, are not competent to decide for themselves, others must decide on their behalf.[34] Judges Tauro and Brotman both ruled that patients could be given drugs against their will if they had been found incompetent to refuse drugs. The incompetence has to be established in a legal proceeding in which the patient is represented by a lawyer, advocate, or some other outside person who is not employed by the hospital. The function of the patient advocate is to argue that patient's case with a view toward safeguarding the patient's interest and constitutional rights. Legal procedures in this area are still evolving, and the details vary from state to state.[35]

As argued eloquently by Loren Roth, director of the Program in Law and Psychiatry at the University of Pittsburgh, the purpose of civil commitment is to restore competence. The commitment need be only temporary, in no case longer than about three months. If treatment has not restored competence by that time, then the treatment is not going to be effective, and the justification for commitment evaporates. In cases where treatment is not effective and the patient continues to incompetently refuse maintenance care, a special proceeding is needed in which the person is afforded all the protections he or she would have in a criminal trial.[36]

How should incompetence be determined? At present, there is no single test that is universally accepted by all jurisdictions. Words often used in an effort to define competent thinking are "rational," "responsible," "knowingly," "understandingly," and "capable." These words signify the capacity to decide an issue by applying the normal thought process. It is very difficult, however, to evaluate objectively whether the thought process of a mental patient is sufficiently normal to make a particular decision.

Roth and Alan A. Stone, of Harvard, have suggested that judges apply the following three tests to determine whether a patient is competent to refuse treatment. First, the judge should ask the patient questions to determine whether he or she understands what is likely to happen as a result of treatment or in the absence of treatment. For instance, if a patient who has been diagnosed as having schizophrenia says, "I don't want to go to the hospital because the doctors are going to transplant my brain into an android," the patient does not understand what is going to happen. If the patient understands that the treatment will help her keep her job and that without treatment she will lose her job, then she does understand. Second, the judge finds out if the patient understands why a particular form of treatment is being advised. If, after being instructed about the purpose of treatment, the patient thinks the doctors are trying to poison him, then he does not understand; if he can give no explanation, he does not understand; if he thinks the doctors are trying to relieve his delusions, he does understand. Third, can the patient express a choice, yes or no? A patient who cannot decide one way or the other is not competent.[37]

Stone and Roth have suggested that four criteria in addition to incompetence should also be satisfied if a patient is to be forcibly treated. First, the patient must have a reliable diagnosis. Reliable means that numerous psychiatrists agree on the patient's category of illness. If psychiatrists cannot agree on the diagnosis, neither the patient nor the public can be confident that the patient is actually ill. Incarcerating people without a reliable diagnosis would soon lead to the incarceration of inconvenient nonconformists.

Second, the untreated illness promises severe distress and disability for the patient. The distress might be extreme anxiety, panic, depression, or lack of self-care. The rationale for this requirement is that depriving a patient of liberty under the power of *parens patriae* should be allowed only when there is a psychiatric crisis in which the potential exists for significant harm to the patient or others. If little harm is being caused by the illness, or if the illness is likely to get better in a day or two, there is no need for state intervention. When commitment is restricted to cases of great severity, diagnostic reliability is improved, and the chances are further reduced that the objecting patient will be incarcerated for some nonmedical reason.

Third, the state should be required to show that while the patient is committed, the treatment provided is likely to relieve suffering from the illness. Obviously, the state cannot legitimately exercise its power to coerce treatment if there is no treatment that is beneficial.

The fourth and final test is designed to determine whether a reasonable person, given the circumstances of the particular patient, would reject the hospitalization. To make this decision, the judge must weigh all the benefits and harms of coerced treatment with all the benefits and harms of denying involuntary commitment. The judge should reject commitment if the hospital environment is such a snake pit that it is worse to be in the hospital than to be schizophrenic on the street. Unfortunately, the conditions inside many state hospitals are such that this criterion might be difficult to meet. State legislatures and the voters are characteristically reluctant to provide money for quality treatment of mental patients. A recent concept is that the judge should commit the patient to treatment in an environment that is "the least restrictive alternative."[38]

General Grigorenko, whose worst symptom was reformist ideas, would not have been judged incompetent, nor would he have satisfied any of the additional four criteria. Studies have been done in which the Stone–Roth criteria have been compared to the dangerousness criteria that are currently in force in most states. These studies find that the Stone–Roth criteria would result in forcible treatment for the same number of (or perhaps fewer) psychiatric emergency patients as would the existing dangerousness criteria. The patient mix would be slightly different, however. The Stone–Roth criteria would commit those who could benefit from treatment, while the dangerousness criteria commit those who are prone to violence.[39]

The presence of homeless mentally ill people on the streets of our cities has impressed nearly everyone that the mentally ill need care as well as liberty.[40] How do you provide care with the least possible restriction of liberty?

One procedure that has been tried in a handful of states is called outpatient commitment. In outpatient commitment, the court requires the unwilling patient to accept treatment, usually drugs and counseling, delivered at a community mental health center, rather than in a hospital. The patient has to report to the mental health center at frequent intervals to receive the treatment. Outpatient commitment is a new approach, and it is too early to tell whether is an acceptable solution to the problem of suffering among the untreated mentally ill.[41]

A primary problem is getting the public to provide money to establish community mental health centers and to staff them with people who are trained to supervise the treatment of psychiatric outpatients. Research is also needed to determine whether involuntary community treatment actually is beneficial to unwilling patients. Will the unwilling patients actually abide by the court orders to participate in the treatment? Do the patients get better? Do they become more capable of caring for themselves? After they have obtained treatment, are they glad they were forced to do so?[42]

Outpatient commitment also has potential civil liberties problems. In some states that have experimented with outpatient commitment, treatment has been imposed on unwilling patients in a more authoritarian and paternalistic manner than is allowed for hospital treatment. Outpatient treatment has been ordered without a hearing to establish incompetence, without right of appeal, and without representation for the patient. This achieves great bureaucratic efficiency, but it also restricts patients' rights. The imposition of outpatient treatment without a full hearing is allegedly justified on the grounds that it is vastly less restrictive than hospitalization. Patients, however, may refuse to comply with court-ordered treatments. They may refuse to take drugs or refuse to report for counseling and checkups. In response, the courts may commit them to the hospital as an enforcement measure. Thus, competent, nondangerous people may end up in the hospital against their will, deprived of liberty in the absence of due process.[43]

Practical Problems with the Legal Protections of Patient's Rights

The resolution of conflict by rational argument in the courts is a praiseworthy custom, but it carries a high price. The price is a lowering in the amount and quality of care. Psychologists and psychiatrists have to spend more hours with lawyers and judges and fewer with patients. More money is spent on court hearings, lawyers, legal guardians, patient advocates, and outside consultants. Treatment is delayed. Irwin Perr found that required legal procedures added $30,000 to the cost of treatment for two drug-refusing patients in a New Jersey private hospital. Most of the added expense was a consequence of the time required to obtain a court order for involuntary commitment. Waiting for the courts delayed the onset of drug treatment and prolonged hospitalization for several months. The nonmonetary costs of the delay were also substantial. When treatment is delayed, relief of suffering is delayed.[44]

The costs of litigation are a strong incentive for hospitals simply to release unwilling patients rather than support the expense of commitment for needed care. Some patients are lucky enough to have family who will try to provide for them. But a seriously ill patient will rapidly exhaust the emotional and financial resources of most families. Failing to treat the mentally ill does not save public money in the long run. Families of patients, incidently, typically oppose elaborate procedural safeguards of patients' rights to refuse treatment. The families want efficient methods of forcing their ill, refusing relatives into treatment.

Drugs are feared because they are perceived to be too powerful and to give psychiatrists too much authority. Judge Tauro said that drugs were a form of "mind control," a view also held by the radical psychiatrists. We believe, however, that this evaluation is incorrect. When used properly for the treatment of mental illness, there is no evidence that psychiatric drugs have the power to coerce conformist ideas or behavior. They do not suppress genius or other forms of nonill eccentricity. On the contrary, the drugs increase the variety of behaviors and mental activities that patients can perform. The drugs routinely reduce patients' dependence on others. They restore patients' capacity to think freely and to use the powers of thought to achieve their own objectives. A political revolutionary suffering from schizophrenia or depression would be more likely to overthrow the government after receiving drug treatment than before.

The legitimate scope of psychiatry is narrow. Only a limited number of well-defined illnesses can be treated effectively. Diagnosing mental illness to suit political needs, as occurred with General Grigorenko, is political repression, not medical care. We believe that normality should be given the broadest possible range of variation. Rigorous adherence to the concept that an illness involves the patient's suffering and disability will help check the tendency to treat nonill, nonconforming people as if they were ill. An objective method of diagnosis, as encouraged by the *DSM-III-R*, opens diagnostic decision making to public scrutiny and inhibits malicious mischief. Legal restraints on civil commitment, like those proposed by Stone and Roth, will restrict compulsory treatment to those who are genuinely benefited by it and are harmed without it. Providing treatment in the least restrictive environment that is consistent with treatment success will minimize abridgement of liberties that do not conflict with required treatment.

Unfair power relationships between psychiatrists and patients will never be fully prevented by judicial and procedural measures alone. In addition, treatment must be delivered by empathetic and benevolent caregivers who, out of respect for every person's dignity, strive to achieve an egalitarian relationship with each patient.

THE MEDICAL MODEL: A SUMMATION

We have explained and defended the medical model of mental illness, believing it a valid blueprint for understanding and coping with the problem of pathological irrationality of thought, perception, emotion, and behavior. According to the model, mental illnesses are biological phenomena having diverse genetic and environmental causes, not defects of character or lapses in morality; they are not an occasion for casting blame. Mental illnesses are not sane responses to an insane world or sets of bad habits acquired through unfortunate learning experiences. As Wilhelm Greisinger declared in the nineteenth century, "mental diseases are brain diseases."[45] They should be treated if effective treatment is available. The treatments may use both somatic and psychological techniques.

Advocates of the medical model invest faith in the scientific method of inquiry. Through research the causes of mental illness can be discovered and perhaps eliminated. Admittedly, scientists are still ignorant of many important aspects of mental illness. But during the past four decades, much has been learned about how the brain works, and new laboratory techniques have been developed for learning still more. Five important new scientific discoveries have been made: (1) there are genetically transmitted risk factors for severe mental illnesses; (2) antipsychotic drugs block dopamine receptors; (3) antidepressant drugs alter norepinephrine and serotonin synapses in several ways; (4) antianxiety drugs enhance inhibition at GABA synapses; and (5) abnormal activity in the frontal and temporal lobes is correlated with schizophrenia, depression, and anxiety disorders. These discoveries have led to a major advance in our ability to form hypotheses about possible causes and more effective treatments for severe mental illness.

According to the medical model, it is unethical to give treatments that are not based on the best available scientific knowledge or to give treatments that are not known to be effective. Proponents of the medical model are adamantly opposed to treatment cults or allegedly therapeutic procedures that are based on little more than superstition, especially when these treatments are accompanied by promises that cannot be kept. Caregivers must speak clearly and directly with patients about the goals and effectiveness of proposed treatments. It must be explained that currently available drugs can relieve many symptoms, but they are not cures, and they are not solutions to personal problems.[46] The solution of personal problems may often be an important part of effective therapy.

The role of the therapist is to relieve suffering, encourage good health, and prolong life through empathy with the patient and application of scientific knowledge. The therapist has no responsibility, and should assume none, for enforcing social conformity. Instead, the therapist should respect the individuality of each patient and strive to enhance the value of human life in all its diverse forms.

APPENDIX

—

GENERIC NAME	TRADE NAME	USUAL DAILY DOSE (MG)
D. Other		
Molindone hydrochloride	Moban	50 – 100
Loxapine hydrochloride	Loxitane	60 – 100
II. Drugs for Major Depression		
A. Tricyclic Antidepressants		
Imipramine hydrochloride	Janimine, Tofranil	50 – 200
Desipramine hydrochloride	Norpramin, Pertofrane	75 – 200
Amitriptyline hydrochloride	Elavil, Endep	75 – 150
Nortriptyline hydrochloride	Pamelor	75 – 100
Doxepin hydrochloride	Adapin, Sinequan	75 – 150
Protriptyline hydrochloride	Vivactil	15 – 40
Amoxapine	Asendin	200 – 300
B. Monoamine Oxidase Inhibitors		
Isocarboxazid	Marplan	10 – 30
Phenelzine sulfate	Nardil	15 – 30
Tranylcypromine sulfate	Parnate	20 – 30
C. Other Antidepressants		
Maprotiline hydrochloride	Ludiomil	75 – 150
Trazodone hydrochloride	Desyrel	150 – 600
Fluoxetine	Prozac	20 – 80
III. Drugs for Bipolar Disorder		
Lithium carbonate	Eskalith, Lithane, Lithobid	900 – 1,500
IV. Drugs for Anxiety		
A. Benzodiazepines		
Chlordiazepoxide hydrochloride	Librium	15 – 40

GENERIC NAME	TRADE NAME	USUAL DAILY DOSE (MG)
Clorazepate dipotassium	Tranxene	30
Diazepam	Valium	4–40
Lorazepam	Ativan	2–6
Halazepam	Paxipam	60–160
Alprazolam	Xanax	0.75–1.5
Oxazepam	Serax	30–60
Prazepam	Centrax	20–40
B. Barbiturates		
Aprobarbital	Alurate	120–240
Butabarbital sodium	Butisol	45–120
Pentobarbital sodium	Nembutal	60–80
Phenobarbital sodium	Generic	30–120
C. Other Antianxiety Drugs		
Buspirone hydrochloride	BuSpar	15–30
Meprobamate	Equanil, Miltown, and others	1,200–1,600
Glutethimide	Doriden	250–500
Methyprylon	Noludar	150–400
Ethchlorvynol	Placidyl	200–600
V. Drugs for OCD		
Clomipramine	Anafranil	100–250

Sources: R. J. Baldessarini, "Drugs and the Treatment of Psychiatric Disorders," in *The Pharmacological Basis of Therapeutics*, edited by A. G. Gilman, L. S. Goodman, and A. Gilman (New York: Macmillan, 1985), 387–445; S. C. Harvey, "Hypnotics and Sedatives," in *The Pharmacological Basis of Therapeutics*, edited by A. G. Gilman, L. S. Goodman, and A. Gilman (New York: Macmillan, 1985), 339–71; *Physician's Desk Reference*, 43rd ed. (Oradell, N.J.: Medical Economics, 1989); *Facts and Comparisons, Inc.* (St. Louis: Lippincott).

NOTES

—

CHAPTER 1

1. F. U. Ayd, and B. Blackwell, eds., *Discoveries in Biological Psychiatry* (Philadelphia: Lippincott, 1970).
2. P. A. Berger, "Medical Treatment of Mental Illness," *Science* 200:975, 1978; U.S. Department of Commerce, *Statistical Abstract of the United States*, 107th ed. (1987), 100; 108th ed., (1988), 104; 109th ed. (1989), 109.
3. Ellen L. Bassuk, "The Homelessness Problem," *Scientific American* July 1984, 40–45.
4. Berger, "Medical Treatment of Mental Illness." *Science* 200:974–975.
5. J. Harpole, "Right to Refuse Medical Treatment." *ACLU of Oregon Newsletter*, March 1988; Paul S. Appelbaum, "Is the Need for Treatment Constitutionally Acceptable as a Basis for Civil Commitment?" *Law Medicine and Health Care* 12(1984):144–49; Paul S. Appelbaum, "Civil Commitment." In Gerald L. Klerman, et al., eds., *Social, Epi-*

demiologic and Legal Psychiatry (Basic Books, Philadelphia, 1986), pp 383–99.

6. T. Szasz, Insanity, the Idea and Its Consequences (New York: John Wiley & Sons, 1987) pp 279–365; T. Szasz, Psychiatric Slavery (New York: The Free Press, 1977) pp 133–39; T. Szasz, The Myth of Mental Illness, rev. ed. (New York: Harper & Row, 1974) pp 1–103.

7. K. Kesey, One Flew over the Cuckoo's Nest (New York: Viking Press, 1962).

CHAPTER 2

1. More information about nerve cells and how drugs affect them can be found in neuroscience textbooks. Among our favorites are D. P. Kimble, Biological Psychology (Fort Worth, Tex.: Holt, Rinehart and Winston, 1988); S. W. Kuffler, et al., From Neuron to Brain, 2d ed. (Sunderland, Mass.: Sinauer Associates, 1984); J. R. Cooper and F. E. Bloom, The Biochemical Basis of Neuropharmacology (New York: Oxford University Press, 1986); E. R. Kandel and J. H. Schwartz, Principles of Neuroscience, 2d ed. (New York: Elsevier, 1985).

CHAPTER 3

1. R. L. Spitzer and P. Wilson, "Nosology and the Official Psychiatric Nomenclature," in H. I. Kaplan, A. M. Freedman, and B. J. Sadock, eds., Comprehensive Textbook of Psychiatry, 2d ed. (Baltimore: Williams & Wilkins, 1975), 826–45; R. L. Spitzer and J. B. W. Williams, "Classification of Mental Disorders and DSM-III," in H. I. Kaplan, A. M. Freedman, and B. J. Sadock, eds., Comprehensive Textbook of Psychiatry, 3d ed. (Baltimore: Williams & Wilkins, 1980), 1035–72.

2. "Reagan Wounded by Gunman," New York Times, 31 March 1981, 1.

3. "Jury Finds Hinkley Not Guilty, Accepting His Defense of Insanity," New York Times, 22 June 1982, 1; T. Wicker, "Verdict Hurt Psychiatry the Most," Eugene Register Guard, 28 June 1982, 7A.

4. D. Faust and J. Ziskin, "The Expert Witness in Psychology and Psychiatry," Science 241(1988):31–35.

5. G. Klerman, J. Endicott, et al., "Neurotic Depressions: A Systematic Analysis of Multiple Criteria and Meanings," American Journal of Psychiatry 136(1979):57–67.

6. R. E. Kendall, J. E. Cooper, et al., "Diagnostic Criteria of American and British Psychiatrists," Archives of General Psychiatry 25(1971):123–30.

7. J. Endicott and R. L. Spitzer," Use of the Research Diagnostic Criteria and Schedule for Affective Disorders and Schizophrenia to Study Affective Disorders," *American Journal of Psychiatry*, 136(1979):52–56.

8. Spitzer and Wilson, "Nosology and the Official Psychiatric Nomenclature."

9. T. Szasz, *The Myth of Mental Illness*, rev. ed. (New York: Harper & Row, 1974) pp 1–103; T. Szasz, *Insanity, The Idea and Its Consequences* (New York: John Wiley & Sons, 1987):9–26, 47–98.

10. Spitzer and Wilson, Nosology and the Official Psychiatric Nomenclature.

11. Ibid.; Spitzer and Williams, "Classification of Mental Disorders and DSM-III"; American Psychiatric Association, *Diagnostic and Statistical Manual of Mental Disorders*, 3d ed (Washington, D.C.: The Association, 1980).

12. B. J. Carroll et al., "A Specific Laboratory Test for the Diagnosis of Melancholia," *Archives of General Psychiatry* 38(1981):15–23; J. M. Davis, "Clinical Utility of Biochemical Assays in Psychiatry," *Annual Review of Medicine* 38(1987):149–56.

13. Spitzer and Wilson, "Nosology and the Official Psychiatric Nomenclature"; Spitzer and Williams, "Classification of Mental Disorders and DSM-III."

14. American Psychiatric Association, *Diagnostic and Statistical Manual of Mental Disorders,* 3d ed., rev. (Washington, D.C.: The Association, 1987).

15. R. L. Spitzer, J. B. W. Williams, et al., "DSM-III: The Major Achievement and an Overview," *American Journal of Psychiatry* 136(1980): 151–63.

16. American Psychiatric Association, *Diagnostic and Statistical Manual of Mental Disorders,* 2d ed. (Washington, D.C.: The Association, 1968).

17. Spitzer, et al., "DSM-III: The Major Achievement and an Overview"; 151–163. R. L. Spitzer, "Introduction," in American Psychiatric Association, *Diagnostic and Statistical Manual of Mental Disorders*, 3d ed., 1–12; Spitzer and Williams, "Classification of Mental Disorders and DSM-III."

18. J. P. Feighner, E. Robins, et al., "Diagnostic Criteria for Use in Psychiatric Research," *Archives of General Psychiatry* 26(1972):27–63.

19. G. Winokur and M. Zimmerman, "'Cause the Bible Tells Me So," *Archives of General Psychiatry* 45(1988):683–84.

20. J. Endicott and R. L. Spitzer, "A Diagnostic Interview: The Schedule for Affective Disorders and Schizophrenia, *Archives of General Psychiatry* 35(1978):837–44; L. N. Robins, J. E. Helzer, et al., "National Institute of Mental Health Diagnostic Interview Schedule," *Archives of General Psychiatry* 38(1981):381–89.

21. R. L. Spitzer and J. B. W. Williams, *"Introduction" DSM-III-R*, xvii.

CHAPTER 4

1. American Psychiatric Association, *Diagnostic and Statistical Manual of Mental Disorders,* 3d ed. (Washington, D.C.: The Association, 1980); American Psychiatric Association, *Diagnostic and Statistical Manual of Mental Disorders,* 3d ed., rev. (Washington, D.C.: The Association, 1987), 187–98; J. R. Bemporad and H. Pinsker, "Schizophrenia: The Manifest Symptomatology," in *American Handbook of Psychiatry,* 2d ed., edited by S. Arieti, and E. B. Brody (New York: Basic Books, 1974), 524–50; R. Cancro, "Overview of Schizophrenia," *Comprehensive Textbook of Psychiatry,* 3d ed., edited by H. I. Kaplan, A. M. Freedman, and B. J. Sadock (Baltimore: Williams & Wilkins, 1980), 1093–104; H. E. Lehmann, "Schizophrenia: Clinical Features," *Comprehensive Textbook of Psychiatry,* 3d ed., 1153–92; K. S. Kendler, R. L. Spitzer, et al., "Psychotic Disorders in DSM-III-R," *American Journal of Psychiatry* 146(1989):953–62.
2. Lehmann, "Schizophrenia: Clinical Features."
3. S. Sheehan, "A Reporter at Large (Creedmoor — Part II)," *The New Yorker,* 1 June 1981, 74; idem, "A Reporter at Large Creedmoor — Part IV)," *The New Yorker,* 15 June 1981, 121.
4. L. N. Robins, J. E. Helzer, et al., "Lifetime Prevalence of Specific Psychiatric Disorders in Three Sites," *Archives of General Psychiatry* 41(1984):949–58.
5. R. L. Spitzer, A. E. Skodol, et al., *DSM-III Case Book* (Washington, D.C.: American Psychiatric Association, 1981).
6. Z. J. Lipowski, "Organic Mental Disorders: Introduction and Review of Syndromes," in *Comprehensive Textbook of Psychiatry,* 3d ed., edited by H. I. Kaplan, A. M. Freedman, and B. J. Sadock (Baltimore: Williams & Wilkins, 1980), 1359–91; J. R. Bemporad, and H. Pinsker, "Schizophrenia: The Manifest Symptomatology," in *American Handbook of Psychiatry,* 2d ed., edited by S. Arieti, and E. B. Brody (New York: Basic Books, 1974), 524–50; Lehmann, "Schizophrenia: Clinical Features."

CHAPTER 5

1. R. C. Shelton and D. R. Weinberger, "Brain Morphology in Schizophrenia," in *Psychopharmacology: The Third Generation of Progress,* edited by H. Y. Meltzer (New York: Raven Press, 1987), 773–81; D. G. Pearlson et al., "Ventricle – Brain Ratio, Computed Tomographic Density, and Brain Area in 50 Schizophrenics," *Archives of General Psychiatry* 46(1989):690–97.
2. N. C. Andreason, "Brain Imaging: Applications in Psychiatry," *Science* 239(1988):1381–88.
3. Ibid., Shelton and Weinberger, "Brain Morphology in Schizophrenia."

4. P. Tyrer and A. MacKay, "Schizophrenia: No Longer a Functional Psychosis," *Trends in Neurosci* 9(1986):537–38; R. Brown, et al., "Postmortem Evidence of Structural Brain Changes in Schizophrenia," *Archives of General Psychiatry* 43(1986):36–42.

5. R. L. Suddath et al., "Temporal Lobe Pathology in Schizophrenia: A Quantitative Magnetic Resonance Imaging Study," *American Journal of Psychiatry* 146(1989):464–72.

6. D. R. Weinberger, K. F. Berman, and R. F. Zee, "Physiologic Dysfunction of Dorsolateral Prefrontal Cortex in Schizophrenia. I. Regional Cerebral Blood Flow Evidence." *Archives of General Psychiatry* 43(1986):114–24; K. F. Berman, R. F. Zee, and D. R. Weinberger, "Physiologic Dysfunction of Dorsolateral Prefrontal Cortex in Schizophrenia. II. Role of Neuroleptic Treatment, Attention, and Mental Effort," *Archives of General Psychiatry* 43(1986):126–35; D. R. Weinberger, K. F. Berman, and B. P. Illowsky, "Physiologic Dysfunction of Dorsolateral Prefrontal Cortex in Schizophrenia. III. A New Cohort and Evidence for a Monoaminergic Mechanism," *Archives of General Psychiatry* 45(1988):609–15; K. F. Berman, B. P. Illowsky, and D. R. Weinberger, "Physiologic Dysfunction of Dorsolateral Prefrontal Cortex in Schizophrenia. IV. Further Evidence for Regional and Behavioral Specificity," *Archives of General Psychiatry* 45(1988):616–22; K. F. Berman, "Cortical 'Stress Tests' in Schizophrenia: Regional Cerebral Blood Flow Studies," *Biological Psychiatry* 22(1987):1304–26.

7. R. M. Cohen, et al., "From Syndrome to Illness: Delineating the Pathophysiology of Schizophrenia with PET," *Schizophrenia Bulletin* 14 (1988):169–76.

8. T. S. Early, et al., "Left Globus Pallidus Abnormality in Never-Medicated Patients with Schizophrenia," *Proceedings of the National Academy of Sciences, USA* 84(1987):561–63.

9. H. S. Bracha, "Asymmetric Rotational (Circling) Behavior, a Dopamine-Related Asymmetry: Preliminary Findings in Unmedicated and Never-Medicated Schizophrenic Patients," *Biological Psychiatry* 22 (1987):995–1003; M. I. Posner et al., "Asymmetries in Hemispheric Control of Attention in Schizophrenia," *Archives of General Psychiatry* 45(1988):814–21.

10. S. S. Kety, "Disorders of the Human Brain," *Scientific American*, September 1979, 202–14.

11. L. I. Gardner, "Deprivation Dwarfism," *Scientific American*, July 1972, 76–82; G. F. Powell, J. A. Brasel, and R. M. Blizzard," Emotional Deprivation and Growth Retardation Simulating Idiopathic Hypopituitarism. I. Clinical Evaluation of the Syndrome," *New England Journal of Medicine* 276(1967):1271–78; G. F. Powell, J. A. Brasel, S. Raiti, and R. M. Blizzard, "Emotional Deprivation and Growth Retardation Simu-

lating Idiopathic Hypopituitarism. II. Endocrinologic Evaluation of the Syndrome," *New England Journal of Medicine* 276(1967):1279–83.

12. Kety, "Disorders of the Human Brain."

13. J. L. Fuller and W. R. Thompson, *Foundations of Behavior Genetics* (St. Louis: Mosby, 1978), 370.

14. I. I. Gottesman and A. Bertelsen, "Confirming Unexpressed Genotypes for Schizophrenia," *Archives of General Psychiatry* 46(1989):867–72; E. Kringlen and G. Cramer, "Offspring of Monozygotic Twins Discordant for Schizophrenia," *Archives of General Psychiatry* 46(1989): 873–77.

15. S. S. Kety, "The Biological Roots of Mental Illness: Their Ramifications Through Cerebral Metabolism, Synaptic Activity, Genetics and the Environment," in *Harvey Lectures 1975–76* (New York: Academic Press, 1978) 1–22; S. S. Kety, D. Rosenthal, P. H. Wender, F. Schulsinger, and B. Jacobsen, "Mental Illness in the Biological and Adoptive Families of Adopted Individuals Who Have Become Schizophrenic: A Preliminary Report Based on Psychiatric Interviews," in *Genetic Research in Psychiatry*, edited by R. R. Fieve, A. Rosenthal, and H. Brill (Baltimore, Johns Hopkins University Press, 1975), 147–66.

16. K. S. Kendler, A. M. Gruenberg, and J. S. Strauss, "An Independent Analysis of the Copenhagen Sample of the Danish Adoption Study of Schizophrenia. III. The Relationship Between Paranoid Psychosis (Delusional Disorder) and the Schizophrenia Spectrum Disorders," *Archives of General Psychiatry* 38(1981):985–87.

17. W. B. Byerly et al., "Mapping Genes for Manic-Depression and Schizophrenia with DNA Markers," *Trends in Neurosciences* 12(1989):46–48.

18. R. Sherington et al., "Localization of a Susceptibility Locus for Schizophrenia on Chromosome 5," *Nature* 336(1988):164–67; J. L. Kennedy et al., "Evidence Against Linkage of Schizophrenia to Markers on Chromosome 5 in a Northern Swedish Pedigree," *Nature* 336(1988):167–70; D. St. Clair et al., "No Linkage of Chromosome 5q11–q13 Markers to Schizophrenia in Scottish Families," *Nature* 339(1989):305–6.

19. R. D. Laing, *The Politics of Experience* (New York: Ballantine Books, 1967), 115.

20. S. S. Kety, "From Rationalization to Reason," *American Journal of Psychiatry* 131(1974):957–63.

21. I. I. Gottesman and J. Shields, *Schizophrenia the Epigenetic Puzzle* (Cambridge: Cambridge University Press, 1982); M. E. Paul, ed., *International Directory of Genetic Services* (White Plains, N.Y.: March of Dimes Birth Defects Foundation, 1986).

22. H. Pardes, "Genetics and Psychiatry: Past Discoveries, Current Dilemmas, and Future Directions," *American Journal of Psychiatry* 146 (1989):435–43.

23. Gottesman and Bertelsen, "Confirming Unrepressed Genotypes for Schizophrenia."
24. For a review of this subject, see S. R. Hirsch, "Do Parents Cause Schizophrenia?" *Trends in Neurosciences* 2(1979):49–52.
25. P. H. Wender, D. Rosenthal, S. S. Kety, F. Schulsinger, and J. Welner, "Cross Fostering, a Research Strategy for Clarifying the Role of Genetic and Experiential Factors in the Etiology of Schizophrenia," *Archives of General Psychiatry* 30(1974):121–28.
26. A. F. Mirsky, et al., "Adult Outcomes of High-Risk Children: Differential Effects of Town and Kibbutz Rearing," *Schizophrenia Bulletin* 11(1985):150–54.
27. K. S. Kendler, "The Genetics of Schizophrenia: A Current Perspective," in *Psychopharmacology: The Third Generation of Progress*, edited by H. Y. Meltzer (New York: Raven Press, 1987), 705–13.
28. D. Rosenhan, "On Being Sane in Insane Places," *Science* 179(1973): 250–58.
29. J. M. Murphy, "Psychiatric Labelling in Cross-Cultural Perspective," *Science* 191(1976):1019–28.
30. A. Jablensky and N. Sartorius, "Is schizophrenia universal?" *Acta Psychiatrica Scandinavica* 78(1988):65–70.
31. Murphy, "Psychiatric Labelling in Cross-cultural perspective."
32. H. M. Babigian, "Schizophrenia: Epidemiology," in *Comprehensive Textbook of Psychiatry/III*, edited by H. I. Kaplan, A. M. Freedman, and B. J. Sadock (Baltimore: Williams & Wilkins, 1980), 1113–21.
33. A. Jablensky and N. Sartorius, "Is Schizophrenia Universal?" *Acta Psychiatrica Scandinavica* 78(1988):65–70.
34. R. J. Turner, "Social Mobility and Schizophrenia," *Journal of Health and Social Behavior* 9(1968):194–203; E. H. Hare, J. S. Price, and E. Slater, "Parental Social Class in Psychiatric Patients," *British Journal of Psychiatry* 121(1972):515–24.

CHAPTER 6

1. J. P. Swazey, *Chlorpromazine in Psychiatry* (Cambridge, Mass.: MIT Press, 1974).
2. R. J. Baldessarini, "Drugs and the Treatment of Psychiatric Disorders," in *The Pharmacological Basis of Therapeutics*, edited by A. G. Gilman, L. S. Goodman, and A. Gilman (New York: MacMillan, 1980), 408–11.
3. D. Rosenhan, "On Being Sane in Insane Places," *Science* 179(1973): 250–58.
4. National Institute of Mental Health Pharmacology Service Center, Collaborative Study Group, "Phenothiazine Treatment in Acute Schizophrenia," *Archives of General Psychiatry* 10(1964):246–61; P. Hymo-

witz and H. Spohn, "The Effects of Antipsychotic Medication on the Linguistic Ability of Schizophrenics," *Journal of Nervous and Mental Disease* 168(1980):287–96.

5. Swazey, *Chlorpromazine in Psychiatry*, 209.
6. Ibid., 219.
7. M. Vonnegut, *Eden Express* (New York, Bantam, 1976).
8. Ibid., 164.
9. C. North and R. Cadoret, "Diagnostic Discrepancy in Personal Accounts of Patients with Schizophrenia," *Archives of General Psychiatry* 38(1981):133–37.
10. S. Sheehan, "Creedmoor," *The New Yorker*, 25 May, 1 June, 8 June, and 15 June 1981.
11. National Institute of Mental Health Pharmacology Service Center, Collaborative Study Group, "Phenothiazine Treatment in Acute Schizophrenia."
12. P. R. A. May, *Treatment of Schizophrenia* (New York: Science House, 1968), 151–54; P. R. A. May, A. H. Tuma, "A Followup Study of the Results of Schizophrenia Treatment," in *Evaluation of Psychological Therapies*, edited by R. L. Spitzer and D. F. Klein (Baltimore: Johns Hopkins University Press, 1979), 256–84.
13. J. M. Davis, "Antipsychotic Drugs," in *Comprehensive Textbook of Psychiatry/III*, edited by H. I. Kaplan, A. M. Freedman, and B. J. Sadock (Baltimore: Williams & Wilkins, 1980), 2257–89.
14. T. J. Crow, "Positive and Negative Schizophrenic Symptoms and the Role of Dopamine," *British Journal of Psychiatry* 137(1980):383–86; E. C. Johnstone et al., "Mechanism of the Antipsychotic Effect in the Treatment of Acute Schizophrenia," *Lancet* 1(1978):848–51.
15. A. Breier et al., "Neuroleptic Responsivity of Negative and Positive Symptoms in Schizophrenia," *American Journal of Psychiatry* 144 (1987):1549–55; S. C. Goldberg, "Negative and Deficit Symptoms in Schizophrenia Do Respond to Neuroleptics," *Schizophrenia Bulletin* 11(1985):453–56; S. R. Kay and M. M. Singh, "The Positive–Negative Distinction in Drug-Free Schizophrenic Patients," *Archives of General Psychiatry* 46(1989):711–18.
16. A. Rifkin and S. Siris, "Drug Treatment of Acute Schizophrenia," in *Psychopharmacology: The Third Generation of Progress*, edited by H. Y. Meltzer (New York: Raven Press, 1987), 1095–101.
17. J. K. Kane et al., "Clozapine for the Treatment-Resistant Schizophrenic," *Archives of General Psychiatry* 45(1988):789–96.
18. G. W. Hogarty and S. C. Goldberg, "Drug and Sociotherapy in the Aftercare of Schizophrenic Patients. I. One Year Relapse Rates," *Archives of General Psychiatry* 28(1973):54–64; G. W. Hogarty, S. C. Goldberg, N. R. Schooler, and R. F. Ulrich, "Drug and Sociotherapy in

the Aftercare of Schizophrenic Patients. II. Two Year Relapse Rates," *Archives of General Psychiatry* 31(1974):603–6.

19. G. E. Hogarty et al., "Fluphenazine and Social Therapy in the Aftercare of Schizophrenic Patients," *Archives of General Psychiatry* 36(1979): 1283–94; N. R. Schooler, et al., "Prevention of Relapse in Schizophrenia," *Archives of General Psychiatry* 37(1980):16–24.

20. G. Gardos, and J. O. Cole, "Maintenance Antipsychotic Therapy: For Whom and How Long?" in *Psychopharmacology: A Generation of Progress*, edited by M. A. Lipton, A. DiMascio, and K. F. Killam (New York: Raven Press, 1978), 1169–78.

21. J. A. Lieberman et al., "Methylphenidate Challenge as a Predictor of Relapse in Schizophrenia," *American Journal of Psychiatry* 141(1984): 633–38; M. Davidson et al., "L-Dopa Challenge and Relapse in Schizophrenia," *American Journal of Psychiatry* 144(1987):934–38; B. Angrist et al., "Amphetamine Response and Relapse Risk After Depot Neuroleptic Discontinuation," *Psychopharmacology* 85(1985):277–83.

22. J. M. Kane et al., "High-Dose vs Low-Dose Strategies in the Treatment of Schizophrenia," *Psychopharmacology Bulletin* 21(1985):533–37; S. R. Marder et al., "Low- and Conventional-Dose Maintenance Therapy with Fluphenazine Decanoate," *Archives of General Psychiatry* 44(1987):518–21; G. E. Hogarty et al., "Dose of Fluphenazine, Familiar Expressed Emotion, and Outcome in Schizophrenia," *Archives of General Psychiatry* 45:(1988):797–805; R. J. Baldessarini, B. M. Cohen, and M. H. Teicher, "Significance of Neuroleptic Dose and Plasma Level in the Pharmacological Treatment of Psychoses," *Archives of General Psychiatry* 45(1988):79–81; D. A. W. Johnson et al., "Double-Blind Comparison of Half-Dose and Standard Dose of Flupenthixol Decanoate in the Maintenance Treatment of Stabilized Out-patients with Schizophrenia," *British Journal of Psychiatry* 151(1987):634–38.

23. J. M. Kane and J. A. Lieberman, "Maintenance Pharmacotherapy in Schizophrenia," in *Psychopharmacology: The Third Generation of Progress*, edited by H. Y. Meltzer (New York: Raven Press, 1987), 1103–9.

24. H. E. Lehmann, "Schizophrenia, Clinical Features." In *Comprehensive Textbook of Psychiatry/III*, edited by H. I. Kaplan, A. M. Freedman, and B. J. Sadock (Baltimore: Williams & Wilkins, 1980), 1153–92; L. E. Hollister, "Antipsychotic Medications and the Treatment of Schizophrenia," in *Psychopharmacology*, edited by J. D. Barchas, P. A. Berger, R. D. Ciaranello, and G. R. Elliot (New York: Oxford University Press, 1977), 121–50; M. Harrow, R. R. Grinker, and M. L. Silvester, "Is Modern Day Schizophrenia Outcome Still Negative?" *American Journal of Psychiatry* 135(1978):1156–62; M. T. Tsuang, R. F. Woolson, and J. A. Flemming, "Long Term Outcome of Major Psychoses. I. Schizophrenia and Affective Disorders Compared with Psychiatrically Symptom

Free Surgical Conditions," *Archives of General Psychiatry* 36(1979):1295–301; R. C. Bland, R. C. Parker, and H. Orn, "Prognosis in Schizophrenia: A 10-Year Followup of First Admissions," *Archives of General Psychiatry* 33(1976):949–54.

25. Bland et al., "Prognosis in Schizophrenia."
26. Lehmann, "Schizophrenia, Clinical Features."
27. Harrow et al., "Is Modern Day Schizophrenia Outcome Still Negative?"
28. Lehmann, "Schizophrenia, Clinical Features," 918.
29. K. Kesey, *One Flew Over the Cuckoo's Nest* (New York: Viking Press, 1962).
30. Davis, "Antipsychotic Drugs."
31. Ibid.
32. Vonnegut, *Eden Express*, 253.
33. Kane and Lieberman, "Maintenance Pharmacotherapy in Schizophrenia."
34. M. E. Jarvik, "Drugs Used in the Treatment of Psychiatric Disorders," in *The Pharmacological Basis of Therapeutics*, 4th ed. edited by L. S. Goodman and A. Gilman (New York: Macmillan, 1970), 169.
35. Vonnegut, *Eden Express*, 248.
36. Ibid., 269.
37. W. T. Carpenter, T. H. McGlashan, and J. S. Strauss, "The Treatment of Acute Schizophrenia Without Drugs: An Investigation of Some Current Assumptions," *American Journal of Psychiatry* 134(1977):14–20.
38. May, *Treatment of Schizophrenia*.
39. P. R. A. May, A. H. Tuma, and W. J. Dixon, "Schizophrenia—A Followup Study of the Results of 5 Forms of Treatment," *Archives of General Psychiatry* 38(1981):776–84.
40. M. Greenblatt, "Foreword" to May, *Treatment of Schizophrenia*.
41. P. R. A. May and G. M. Simpson, "Evaluation of Treatment Methods," in *Comprehensive Textbook of Psychiatry/III*, edited by H. I. Kaplan, A. M. Freedman, and B. J. Sadock (Baltimore: Williams & Wilkins, 1980), 1240–74; D. B. Feinsilver, and J. G. Gunderson, "Psychotherapy for Schizophrenics—Is It Indicated? A Review of the Relevant Literature," *Schizophrenia Bulletin* Fall (1972):11–23.
42. Vonnegut, *Eden Express*, 249.
43. May, *Treatment of Schizophrenia*, 231–42.
44. Hogarty et al., "Drug and Sociotherapy in the Aftercare of Schizophrenic Patients"; Hogarty et al., "Fluphenazine and Social Therapy in the Aftercare of Schizophrenic Patients"; Schooler et al., "Prevention of Relapse in Schizophrenia."
45. J. G. Gunderson et al., "Effects of Psychotherapy in Schizophrenia. II. Comparative Outcome of Two Forms of Treatment," *Schizophrenia Bulletin* 10(1984):564–98.
48. G. W. Hogarty et al., "Family Psychoeducation, Social Skills Training,

and Maintenance Chemotherapy in the Aftercare Treatment of Schizophrenia," *Archives of General Psychiatry* 43(1986):633–42; I. R. Falloon et al., "Family Management in the Prevention of Exacerbations of Schizophrenia," *New England Journal of Medicine* 306(1982):1437–40.

CHAPTER 7

1. P. Seeman, "Dopamine Receptors and the Dopamine Hypothesis of Schizophrenia," *Synapse* 1(1987):133–152.
2. B. S. Bunney, S. R. Sesak, and N. Silva, "Midbrain Dopaminergic Systems: Neurophysiology and Electrophysiological Pharmacology," in *Psychopharmacology: The Third Generation of Progress*, edited by H. Y. Meltzer (New York: Raven Press, 1987), 113–26.
3. Seeman, "Dopamine Receptors and the Dopamine Hypothesis of Schizophrenia"; R. H. Roth, M. E. Wolf, and A. Y. Deutch, "Neurochemistry of Midbrain Dopamine Systems," in *Psychopharmacology: The Third Generation of Progress*, edited by H. Y. Meltzer (New York: Raven Press, 1987), 81–94; R. H. Roth, "CNS Dopamine Autoreceptors: Distribution, Pharmacology, and Function," *Annals of the New York Academy of Sciences* 430(1984):27–53; I. Helmreich et al., "Are Presynaptic Dopamine Autoreceptors and Postsynaptic Dopamine Receptors in the Rabbit Caudate Nucleus Pharmacologically Different?" *Neuroscience* 7(1982):1559–66.
4. D. R. Burt, I. Creese, and S. H. Snyder, "Dopamine Receptor Binding in the Corpus Striatum of Mammalian Brain," *Proceedings of the National Academy of Sciences USA* 72(1975):4655–59; P. Seeman, T. Lee, M. Chau-Wong, and K. Wong, "Antipsychotic Drug Classes and Neuroleptic/Dopamine Receptors," *Nature* 261(1976):717–19.
5. B. S. Bunney and G. K. Aghajanian, "Mesolimbic and Mesocortical Dopaminergic Systems: Physiology and Pharmacology," in *Psychopharmacology: A Generation of Progress*, edited by M. A. Lipton, A. DiMascio, and K. F. Killam (New York: Raven Press, 1978), 159–70.
6. D. R. Burt, I. Creese, and S. H. Synder, "Properties of ^{3}H Haloperidol and ^{3}H Dopamine Binding Associated with Dopamine Receptors in Calf Brain Membranes," *Molecular Pharmacology* 12(1976):800–12; S. H. Snyder, D. R. Burt, and I. Creese, "Dopamine Receptors of Mammalian Brain: Direct Demonstration of Binding to Agonist and Antagonist States," in *Neurotransmitters, Hormones and Receptors: Novel Approaches*, edited by A. J. Ferendelli, B. S. McEwen, and S. H. Snyder (Bethesda, Md.: Society for Neuroscience, 1976), 28–49; Seeman et al., "Antipsychotic Drug Classes and Neuroleptic/Dopamine Receptors."

7. Snyder, Burt, and Creese, "Dopamine Receptors of Mammalian Brain: Direct Demonstration of Binding to Agonist and Antagonist States."

8. J. W. Kebabian and D. B. Calne, "Multiple Receptors for Dopamine," *Nature* 277(1979):93–96.

9. S. H. Snyder, "Amphetamine Psychosis: A 'Model' Schizophrenia Mediated by Catecholamines," *American Journal of Psychiatry* 130(1973): 60–61; J. H. Biel and B. A. Bopp, "Amphetamines: Structure–Activity Relationships," in *Handbook of Psychopharmacology*, vol. 11, edited by L. L. Iversen, S. D. Iversen, and S. H. Snyder (New York: Plenum Press, 1978), 1–39.

10. B. Angrist and A. Sudilovsky, "Central Nervous System Stimulants: Historical Aspects and Clinical Effects," in *Handbook of Psychopharmacology*, vol. 11, edited by L. L. Iversen, S. D. Iversen, and S. H. Snyder 99–165.

11. D. S. Janowsky, M. F. El-Yousef, J. M. Davis, and H. S. Sererke, "Provocation of Schizophrenic Symptoms by Intravenous Injection of Methylphenidate," *Archives of General Psychiatry* 28(1973):185–91.

12. Ibid.; D. S. Janowsky and J. M. Davis, "Methylphenidate, Dextroamphetamine and Levamphetamine: Effects on Schizophrenic Symptoms," *American Journal of Psychiatry* 33(1976):304–8; S. H. Snyder, S. P. Banerjee, H. I. Yamamura, and D. Greenberg, "Drugs, Neurotransmitters, and Schizophrenia," *Science* 184(1974):1243–53.

13. Ibid.; L. E. Hollister, "Drug-Induced Psychoses and Schizophrenic Reactions: A Critical Comparison," *Annals of the New York Academy of Sciences* 96(1962):80–92.

14. Angrist and Sudilovsky, "Central Nervous System Stimulants"; Snyder et al., "Drugs, Neurotransmitters, and Schizophrenia"; B. Angrist, H. K. Lee, and S. Gershon, "The Antagonism of Amphetamine-Induced Symptomatology by a Neuroleptic," *American Journal of Psychiatry* 131(1974):817–19; R. J. Baldessarini, *Chemotherapy in Psychiatry* (Cambridge, Mass.: Harvard University Press, 1977), 124.

15. Snyder et al., "Dopamine Receptors of Mammalian Brain."

16. B. Angrist, G. Sathananthan, and S. Gershon, "Behavioral Effects of L-dopa in schizophrenic patients," *Psychopharmacologia* 31 (1973):1–12.

17. R. H. Roth, "CNS Dopamine Autoreceptors: Distribution, Pharmacology, and Function," *Annals of the New York Academy of Sciences* 430(1984):27–53.

18. Bunney et al., "Midbrain Dopaminergic Systems"; L. A. Chiodo, and B. S. Bunney, "Typical and Atypical Neuroleptics: Differential Effects of Chronic Administration on the Activity of A9 and A10 Midbrain Dopaminergic Neurons," *Journal of Neuroscience* 3(1983):1607–19; M. J. Bannon, et al., "The Electrophysiological and Biochemical Pharmacology of the Mesolimbic and Mesocortical Dopamine Neurons," in *Hand-*

book of Psychopharmacology, vol. 19, edited by L. L. Iversen, S. D. Iversen, and S. H. Snyder (New York: Plenum Press, 1987), 329–74; B. S. Bunney, "Antipsychotic Drug Effects on the Electrical Activity of Dopaminergic Neurons," *Trends in Neuroscience* 7(1984):212–15.

19. R. H. Roth, "CNS Dopamine Autoreceptors: Distribution, Pharmacology, and Function," *Annals of the New York Academy of Sciences* 430(1984):27–53.

20. M. J. Bannon et al., "Unique Response to Antipsychotic Drugs Is Due to Absence of Terminal Autoreceptors in Mesocortical Dopamine Neurones," *Nature* 296(1982):444–46.

21. M. B. Bowers, "Plasma Monoamine Metabolites in Psychotic Disorders," *Archives of General Psychiatry* 45(1988):595–96; R. Davila et al., "Plasma Homovanillic Acid as a Predictor of Response to Neuroleptics," *Archives of General Psychiatry* 45(1988):564–67; D. Pickar et al., "Longitudinal Measurement of Plasma Homovanillic Acid Levels in Schizophrenic Patients," *Archives of General Psychiatry* 43:(1986):669–76.

22. P. Muller and P. Seeman, "Dopaminergic Supersensitivity After Neuroleptics: Time Course and Specificity," *Psychopharmacology* 60(1978): 1–11; D. R. Burt, I. Creese, and S. H. Snyder, "Antischizophrenic Drugs: Chronic Treatment Elevates Dopamine Receptor Binding in Brain," *Science* 196(1977):326–28.

23. R. J. Baldessarini and D. Tarsy, "Dopamine and the Pathophysiology of Dyskinesias Induced by Antipsychotic Drugs," *Annual Review of Neurobiology* 3(1980):23–41; I. Creese and S. H. Snyder, "Behavioral and Biochemical Properties of the Dopamine Receptor," in *Psychopharmacology: A Generation of Progress*, edited by M. A. Lipton, A. DiMascio, and K. F. Killam (New York: Raven Press, 1978), 377–88.

24. M. F. Losonczy, M. Davidson, and K. L. Davis, "The Dopamine Hypothesis of Schizophrenia," in *Psychopharmacology: The Third Generation of Progress*, edited by H. Y. Meltzer (New York: Raven Press, 1987), 715–26.

25. D. F. Wong et al., "Positron Emission Tomography Reveals Elevated D_2 Dopamine Receptors in Drug-Naive Schizophrenics," *Science* 234(1986):1558–63.

26. G. Sedvall, L. Farde, and F.-A. Wiesel, "Quantitative Determination of D2 Dopamine Receptor Characteristics in Healthy Human Subjects and Psychiatric Patients," *Life Sciences* 41(1987):813–16; J-L. Martinot et al., "Striatal D_2 Dopaminergic Receptors Assessed with Positron Emission Tomography and [^{76}Br]Bromospiperone in Untreated Schizophrenic Patients," *American Journal of Psychiatry* 147(1990):44–50.

27. M. F. Losonczy, M. Davidson, and K. L. Davis, "The Dopamine Hypothesis of Schizophrenia," in *Psychopharmacology: The Third Genera-

tion of Progress, edited by H. Y. Meltzer (New York: Raven Press, 1987), 715–26; A. Wolkin et al., "Dopamine Blockade and Clinical Response: Evidence for Two Biological Subgroups of Schizophrenia," *American Journal of Psychiatry* 146(1989):905–8.

28. Losonczy et al., "The Dopamine Hypothesis of Schizophrenia."

CHAPTER 8

1. R. J. Baldessarini, "Drugs and the Treatment of Psychiatric Disorders," in *The Pharmacological Basis of Therapeutics* edited by A. G. Gilman, L. S. Goodman, and A. Gilman (New York: Macmillan, 1980), 391– 447; J. M. Davis, "Antipsychotic Drugs," in *Comprehensive Textbook of Psychiatry/III*, edited by H. I. Kaplan, A. M. Freedman, and B. J. Sadock (Baltimore: Williams & Wilkins, 1980), 2257–89.

2. Baldessarini, "Drugs and the Treatment of Psychiatric Disorders"; Davis, "Antipsychotic Drugs"; P. A. Berger, "Medical Treatment of Mental Illness," *Science* 200(1978):974–81.

3. L. E. Hollister, "Antipsychotic Medications and the Treatment of Schizophrenia," in *Psychopharmacology. From Theory to Practice*, edited by J. D. Barchas et al. (New York: Oxford University Press, 1977), 121–50.

4. R. J. Baldessarini and D. Tarsy, "Dopamine and the Pathophysiology of Dyskinesias Induced by Antipsychotic Drugs," *Annual Review of Neuroscience* 3(1980):23–41; R. J. Baldessarini and D. Tarsey, "Tardive Dyskinesia," in *Psychopharmacology: A Generation of Progress*, edited by M. A. Lipton, A. DiMascio, and K. F. Killam, (New York: Raven Press, 1978), 993–1004.

5. D. V. Jeste and R. J. Wyatt, *Understanding Tardive Dyskinesia* (New York: The Guilford Press, 1982), 10–38.

6. National Institute of Mental Health, "Abnormal Involuntary Movement Scale," in *Early Clinical Drug Evaluation Unit Assessment Manual* edited by W. Guy (Rockville, Md.: U.S. Department of Health and Human Services, 1976), 534–37.

7. P. A. Berger, "Medical Treatment of Mental Illness," *Science* 200(1978):974–81; D. E. Casey, "The Differential Diagnosis of Tardive Dyskinesia," *Acta Psychiatrica Scandinavica* 63(1981, Supp. 291):71–87; J. M. Smith and R. J. Baldessarini, "Changes in Prevalence, Severity and Recovery in Tardive Dyskinesia with Age," *Archives of General Psychiatry* 37(1980):1368–73; Baldessarini and Tarsy, "Tardive Dyskinesia"; J. M. Kane and J. M. Smith, "Tardive Dyskinesia," *Archives of General Psychiatry* 39(1982):473–82; D. V. Jeste and R. J. Wyatt, "Changing Epidemiology of Tardive Dyskinesia: An Overview," *American Journal of Psychiatry* 138(1981):297–309; D. E. Casey, "Tar-

dive Dyskinesia," in *Psychopharmacology: The Third Generation of Progress*, edited by H. Y. Meltzer (New York: Raven Press, 1987), 1411– 19; Jeste and Wyatt, *Understanding Tardive Dyskinesia.*

8. S. Mukherjee et al., "Persistent Tardive Dyskinesia in Bipolar Patients," *Archives of General Psychiatry* 43(1986):342–46.

9. Casey, "Tardive Dyskinesia."

10. Jeste and Wyatt, *Understanding Tardive Dyskinesia*; Smith and Baldessarini, "Changes in Prevalence, Severity, and Recovery in Tardive Dyskinesia with Age."

11. Casey, "Tardive Dyskinesia"; J. M. Kane et al., "Incidence of Tardive Dyskinesia: Five-Year Data from a Prospective Study," *Psychopharmacology Bulletin* 20(1984):387–89; L. M. Toenniessen, D. E. Casey, and B. H. McFarland, "Tardive Dyskinesia in the Aged," *Archives of General Psychiatry* 42(1985):278–84; R. Yassa, V. Nair, and G. Schwartz, "Early Versus Late Onset Psychosis and Tardive Dyskinesia," *Biological Psychiatry* 21(1986):1291–97.

12. J. L. Waddington et al., "Cognitive Dysfunction, Negative Symptoms, and Tardive Dyskinesia in Schizophrenia," *Archives of General Psychiatry* 44(1987):907–12; J. L. Waddington and H. A. Youssef, "Late Onset Involuntary Movements in Chronic Schizophrenia: Relationship of 'Tardive' Dyskinesia to Intellectual Impariment and Negative Symptoms," *British Journal of Psychiatry* 149(1986):616–20.

13. S. R. Marder and T. Van Putten, "Who Should Receive Clozapine?" *Archives of General Psychiatry* 45(1988):865–67.

14. Casey, "Tardive Dyskinesia"; Jeste and Wyatt, *Understanding Tardive Dyskinesia*; Yassa, et al., "Early Versus Late Onset Psychosis and Tardive Dyskinesia."

15. Baldessarini and Tarsy, "Dopamine and the Pathophysiology of Dyskinesias."

16. Ibid.

17. Baldessarini and Tarsy, "Dopamine and the Pathophysiology of Dyskinesia"; idem, "Tardive Dyskinesia."

18. Casey, "Tardive Dyskinesia."

19. Baldessarini and Tarsy, "Dopamine and the Pathophysiology of Dyskinesias"; idem, "Tardive Dyskinesia"; Smith and Baldessarini, "Changes in Prevalence, Severity, and Recovery in Tardive Dyskinesia."

20. Baldessarini and Tarsy, "Dopamine and the Pathophysiology of Dyskinesias."

21. Jeste and Wyatt, *Understanding Tardive Dyskinesia*; H. L. Klawans, C. M. Tanner, and C. G. Goetz, "Epidemiology and Pathophysiology of Tardive Dyskinesias," in *Advances in Neurology, Vol 49: Facial Dyskinesias*, edited by J. Jankovic and E. Tolosa (New York: Raven Press, 1988), 185–97.

22. T. R. E. Barnes, T. Kidger, and S. M. Gore, "Tardive Dyskinesia: A

3-Year Follow-up Study," *Psychological Medicine* 13(1983):17–81; Casey, "Tardive Dyskinesia."

23. R. L. Binder et al., "Tardive Dyskinesia and Neuroleptic-Induced Parkinsonism in Japan," *American Journal of Psychiatry* 144(1987): 1494–96.

24. H. Y. Meltzer, D. J. Goode, and V. S. Fang, "The Effects of Psychotropic Drugs on Endocrine Function. I. Neuroleptics, Precursors and Agonists," in *Psychopharmacology: A Generation of Progress*, edited by M. A. Lipton, A. DiMascio, and K. F. Killam (New York: Raven Press, 1978), 509–29.

25. Davis, "Antipsychotic Drugs."

26. I, Creese, D. R. Burt, and S. H. Snyder, "Biochemical Actions of Neuroleptic Drugs; Focus on Dopamine Receptor," in *Handbook of Psychopharmacology*, vol. 10, edited by L. L. Iversen, S. D. Iversen, and S. H. Snyder (New York: Plenum Press, 1978), 37–89; Davis, "Antipsychotic Drugs."

27. C. A. Kaufman and R. J. Wyatt, "Neuroleptic Malignant Syndrome," in *Psychopharmacology: The Third Generation of Progress*, edited by H. Y. Meltzer (New York: Raven Press, 1987), 1421–30; P. E. Keck et al., "Frequency and Presentation of Neuroleptic Malignant Syndrome: A Prospective Study," *American Journal of Psychiatry* 144(1987): 1344–46.

28. P. Rosenbush and T. Stewart, "A Prospective Analysis of 24 Episodes of Neuroleptic Malignant Syndrome," *American Journal of Psychiatry* 146(1989):717–25.

29. D. F. Levinson and G. M. Simpson, "Serious Nonextrapyramidal Adverse Effects of Neuroleptics: Sudden Death, Agranulocytosis, and Hepatotoxicity," in *Psychopharmacology: The Third Generation of Progress*, edited by H. Y. Meltzer (New York: Raven Press, 1987), 1431–36.

30. S. R. Marder and T. Van Putten, "Who Should Receive Clozapine?" *Archives of General Psychiatry* 45(1988):865–67.

31. Baldessarini, "Drugs and the Treatment of Psychiatric Disorders."

32. Davis, "Antipsychotic Drugs."

33. Baldessarini, "Drugs and Psychiatric Disorders."

34. Davis, "Antipsychotic Drugs."

35. R. J. Baldessarini, *Chemotherapy in Psychiatry* (Cambridge, Mass.: Harvard University Press, 1977), 20–21; Davis, "Antipsychotic Drugs."

36. S. Sheehan, "A reporter at Large (Creedmoor—Part II)," *The New Yorker*, June 1, 1981, 79.

CHAPTER 9

1. American Psychiatric Association (APA), *Diagnostic and Statistical Manual of Mental Disorders*, 3d ed. (Washington, D.C.: The Association,

1980); J. Nelson and D. C. Charney, "The Symptoms of Major Depressive Illness," *American Journal of Psychiatry* 138(1981):1–13; J. P. Feighner, E. Robins, S. B. Guze, R. A. Woodruff, et al., "Diagnostic Criteria for Use in Psychiatric Research," *Archives of General Psychiatry* 26(1972):27–63; G. Klerman, "Affective Disorders: Overview of Affective Disorders," in *Comprehensive Textbook of Psychiatry*, 3d ed., edited by H. I. Kaplan, A. M. Freedman, and B. J. Sadock (Baltimore: Williams & Wilkins, 1980), 1305–19; E. A. Wolpert, "Major Affective Disorders," in *Comprehensive Textbook of Psychiatry*, 3d ed., edited by H. I. Kaplan, A. M. Freedman, and B. J. Sadock (Baltimore: Williams & Wilkins, 1980), 1319–31; S. Arieti, "Affective Disorders, Manic Depressive Psychosis and Psychotic Depression. Manifest Symptomatology, Psychodynamics, Sociological Factors and Psychotherapy," in *American Handbook of Psychiatry*, 2d ed., edited by S. Arieti and E. B. Brody (New York: Basic Books, 1974), 449–90; Robert L. Spitzer, Andrew E. Skodol, Miriam Gibbon, et al., *DSM-III Case Book* (Washington, D.C.: American Psychiatric Association, 1981); idem, *Diagnostic and Statistical Manual of Mental Disorders*, 3d ed., rev. (Washington, D.C.: The Association, 1987), 213–33.

2. Spitzer et al., *DSM-III Case Book*, 98–99.

3. Wolpert, "Major Affective Disorders."

4. Jerome K. Myers, Myrna M. Weissman, et al., "Six-Month Prevalence of Psychiatric Disorders in Three Communities," *Archives of General Psychiatry* 41(1984):959; Lee N. Robins, John E. Helzer et al., "Lifetime prevalence of specific psychiatric disorders in three sites," *Archives of General Psychiatry* 41(1984):949–58.

5. G. L. Klerman, "Long Term Treatment of Affective Disorders," in *Psychopharmacology: A Generation of Progress*, edited by M. A. Lipton, A. DiMascio, and K. F. Killam (New York: Raven Press, 1978), 1303–12; P. M. Lewinsohn, A. Zeiss et al., "Probability of Relapse After Recovery from an Episode of Depression," *Abnormal Psychology* 98(1989): 107–16.

6. M. M. Weissman, Jerome K. Myers, and W. Douglas Thompson, "Depression and Its Treatment in a US Urban Community 1975–1976," *Archives of General Psychiatry* 38(1981):417–21.

7. M. M. Weissman and J. K. Myers, "Affective Disorders in a US Urban Community," *Archives of General Psychiatry* 35(1978):1304–11.

8. R. R. Fieve, *Moodswing* (New York: Bantam Books, 1975), 68.

9. Ibid., 42–44.

10. Ibid., 192–95.

11. Kenneth S. Kendler, Robert L. Spitzer, and Janet B. W. Williams, "Psychotic Disorders in DSM-III-R," *American Journal of Psychiatry* 146(1989):953–62.

12. M. M. Weissman et al., "Suicidal Ideation and Suicide Attempts in

Panic Disorder and Attacks," *New England Journal of Medicine* 321 (1989):1209–14.

13. Spitzer et al., *DSM-III Case Book*, 215–18.

14. Max Hamilton, "Development of a Rating Scale for Primary Depressive Illness," *British Journal of Clinical Psychology* 6(1967):278–96.

CHAPTER 10

1. S. Sheehan, "Creedmoor," *The New Yorker*, May 25, June 1, June 8, June 15, 1981.

2. G. L. Klerman, "Long Term Treatment of Affective Disorders," in *Psychopharmacology: A Generation of Progress*, edited by M. A. Lipton, A. DiMascio, K. F. Killam (New York: Raven Press, 1978), 1303–12; P. J. Clayton, "Prevalence and Course of Affective Disorders," in *Depression, Basic Mechanisms, Diagnosis and Treatment*, edited by A. J. Rush and K. Z. Altshuler (New York: Guilford Press, 1986), 32–44.

3. M. T. Tsuang, R. F. Woolson, and J. A. Fleming, "Premature Deaths in Schizophrenia and Affective Disorders," *Archives of General Psychiatry*, 37(1980):979–83.

4. M. T. Tsuang, "Suicide in Schizophrenics, Manics, Depressives, and Surgical Controls," *Archives of General Psychiatry* 35(1978):153–55; S. B. Guze and E. Robins, "Suicide and Primary Affective Disorder," *British Journal of Psychiatry* 17(1970):437–38.

5. U.S. Department of Commerce, Bureau of the Census, *Statistical Abstract of the United States* (Washington, D.C.: GPO, 1980), 78.

6. F. A. Whitlock, "Depression and Suicide," in *Handbook of Studies on Depression*, edited by G. H. Burrows (New York: Excerpta Medica, 1977), 379–404.

7. L. N. Robins, et al., "Lifetime Prevalence of Specific Psychiatric Disorders in Three Sites," *Archives of General Psychiatry* 41(1984):949–58; D. A. Regier, et al., "One-Month Prevalence of Mental Disorders in the United States," *Archives of General Psychiatry* 45(1986):977–86.

8. P. M. Lewinsohn, and M. Rosenbaum, "Recall of Parental Behavior by Acute Depressives, Remitted Depressives, and Nondepressives," *Journal of Personality and Social Psychology* 52(1987):611–19.

9. M. M. Weissman, and J. K. Myers, "Affective Disorders in a US Urban Community: The Use of Research Diagnostic Criteria in an Epidemiological Survey," *Archives of General Psychiatry* 35(1978):1304–11; Robins et al., "Lifetime Prevalence of Specific Psychiatric Disorders in Three Sites;" Regier et al., "One-Month Prevalence of Mental Disorders in the United States;" P. M. Lewinsohn et al., "Age at First Onset for Nonbipolar Depression," *Journal of Abnormal Psychology* 95 (1986):378–83.

10. J. H. Boyd and M. M. Weissman, "Epidemiology of Affective Disorders," *Archives of General Psychiatry* 38(1981):1039–46; Weissman and Myers, "Affective Disorders in a US Urban Community."

11. Robins et al., "Lifetime Prevalence of Specific Psychiatric Disorders in Three Sites;" Regier et al., "One-Month Prevalence of Mental Disorders in the United States."

12. A. Roy, "Five Risk Factors for Depression," *British Journal of Psychiatry* 150(1987):536–41; G. W. Brown and T. O. Harris, "*Social Origins of Depression—a Study of Psychiatric Disorder in Women* (London: Tavistock, 1978).

13. M. M. Weissman and G. L. Klerman, "Sex Differences and the Epidemiology of Depression," *Archives of General Psychiatry* 34(1977):98–111; C. S. Amenson and P. M. Lewinsohn, "An Investigation into the Observed Sex Difference in Prevalence of Unipolar Depression," *Journal of Abnormal Psychology* 90(1981):1–13; P. M. Lewinsohn, H. M. Hoberman and M. Rosenbaum, "A Prospective Study of Risk Factors for Unipolar Depression," *Journal of Abnormal Psychology* 97 (1988):251–64.

14. R. M. Hirschfeld and C. K. Cross, "Epidemiology of Affective Disorders," *Archives of General Psychiatry* 39(1982):35–46; Brown and Harris, *Social Origins of Depression*, 151; P. Bebbington, et al., "Epidemiology of Mental Disorders in Camberwell," *Psychological Medicine* 11(1981):561–79; Weissman and Myers, "Affective disorders in a US urban community"; Lewinsohn et al., "A Prospective Study of Risk Factors for Unipolar Depression"; Amenson and Lewinsohn, "An Investigation into the Observed Sex Difference in Prevalence of Unipolar Depression."

15. Weissman and Myers, "Affective Disorders in a US Urban Community."

16. Hirschfeld and Cross, "Epidemiology of Affective Disorders"; Robins et al., "Lifetime Prevalence of Specific Psychiatric Disorders in Three Sites."

17. Lewinsohn et al., "A Prospective Study of Risk Factors for Unipolar Depression"; S. M. Monroe, et al., "Social Support, Life Events, and Depressive Symptoms: A 1-Year Prospective Study," *Journal of Consulting and Clinical Psychology* 4(1986):424–31.

18. G. L. Klerman, "Overview of Affective Disorders," in *Comprehensive Textbook of Psychiatry/III*, edited by H. I. Kaplan, A. M. Freedman, and B. J. Sadock (Baltimore, Williams & Wilkins, 1980), 1305–18.

19. C. Lloyd, "Life Events and Depressive Disorder Reviewed. I. Events as Predisposing Factors," *Archives of General Psychiatry* 37(1980):529–535.

20. Lewinsohn et al., "A Prospective Study of Risk Factors for Unipolar Depression"; Monroe et al., "Social Support, Life Events, and Depressive Symptoms."

21. Lewinsohn et al., "A Prospective Study of Risk Factors for Unipolar Depression"; P. M. Lewinsohn et al., "Depression-Related Cognitions: Antecedent or Consequence?" *Journal of Abnormal Psychology* 90(1981):213–19.

22. Regier et al., "One-Month Prevalence of Mental Disorders in the United States."

23. A. J. Marsella et al., "Cross-Cultural Studies of Depressive Disorders: An Overview," In *Culture and Depression*, edited by A. Kleinman and B. Good (Berkeley: University of California Press, 1985), 299–324.

24. M. Beiser, "A Study of Depression Among Traditional Africans, Urban North Americans, and Southeast Asian Refugees," in *Culture and Depression* edited by A. Kleinman and B. Good (Berkeley: University of California Press, 1985), 273–98.

25. L. Baxter et al., "Reduction of Prefrontal Cortex Glucose Metabolism Common to 3 Types of Depression," *Archives of General Psychiatry* 46(1989):243–50.

26. M. S. Buchsbaum et al., "Brain Imaging in Affective Disorders," in *Depression, Basic Mechanisms, Diagnosis and Treatment*, edited by A. J. Rush and K. Z. Altshulzer (New York: Guilford Press, 1986), 126–42.

27. P. H. Wender et al., "Psychiatric Disorders in the Biological and Adoptive Families of Adopted Individuals with Affective Disorders," *Archives of General Psychiatry* 43(1986):923–29.

28. K. K. Kidd and M. M. Weissman, "Why We Do Not Yet Understand the Genetics of Affective Disorders," in *Depression: Biology, Psychodynamics, and Treatment*, edited by J. O. Cole, A. F. Schatzberg, and S. H. Frazier (New York: Plenum Press, 1978), 107–22; E. S. Gershon, et al., "Genetics of Affective Illness," in *Psychopharmacology: The Third Generation of Progress*, edited by H. Y. Meltzer (New York: Raven Press, 1987) 481–91.

29. J. Mendelwicz and J. D. Ranier, "Adoption Study Supporting Genetic Transmission in Manic-Depressive Illness," *Nature* 268(1977): 327–29.

30. Kidd and Weissman, "Why We Do Not Yet Understand the Genetics of Affective Disorders"; Gershon et al., "Genetics of Affective Illness."

31. J. A. Egeland et al., "Bipolar Affective Disorders Linked to DNA Markers on Chromosome 11," *Nature* 325(1987):783–87.

32. S. D. Detera-Wadleigh et al., "Close Linkage of c-Harvey-ras-1 and the Insulin Gene to Affective Disorder Is Ruled Out in Three North American Pedigrees," *Nature* 325(1987):806–8; S. Hodgkinson et al., "Molecular Genetic Evidence for Heterogeneity in Manic Depression," *Nature* 325(1987):805–6.

33. J. R. Kelsoe, "Re-evaluation of the Linkage Relationship Between Chromosome llp Loci and the Gene for Bipolar Affective Disorder in the Old Order Amish," *Nature* 342(1989):238–42.

CHAPTER 11

1. R. J. Baldessarini, "Drugs and the Treatment of Psychiatric Disorders," in *The Pharmacological Basis of Therapeutics*, edited by A. G. Gilman, L. S. Goodman and A. Gilman (New York: MacMillan, 1980), 391–447; I. Hindmarch, "A Pharmacological Profile of Fluoxetine and Other Antidepressants on Aspects of Skilled Performance and Car Handling Ability," *British Journal of Psychiatry* 153 (Suppl. 3) (1988):99–104.
2. J. M. Davis, "Antidepressant Drugs," in *Comprehensive Textbook of Psychiatry/III*, edited by H. I. Kaplan, A. M. Freedman, and B. J. Sadock (Baltimore: Williams & Wilkins, 1980), 2240–316.
3. K. A. Kessler, "Tricyclic Antidepressants: Mode of Action and Clinical Use," in *Psychopharmacology: A Generation of Progress*, edited by M. A. Lipton, A. DiMascio, and K. F. Killam (New York: Raven Press, 1978), 1289–1302; P. A. Berger, "Antidepressants and the Treatment of Depression," in *Psychopharmacology, from Theory to Practice*, edited by J. D. Barchas, P. A. Berger, R. D. Ciaranello, and G. R. Elliott (New York: Oxford University Press, 1977), 174–207.
4. M. Hamilton, "Development of a Rating Scale for Primary Depressive Illness," *British Journal of Social and Clinical Psychology* 6(1967): 278–96.
5. J. B. Morris and A. T. Beck, "The Efficacy of Antidepressant Drugs," *Archives of General Psychiatry* 30(1974):667–74.
6. A. Asberg-Wistedt, "A Double Blind Study of Zimelidine, a Serotonin Uptake Inhibitor, and Desipramine, a Noradrenaline Uptake Inhibitor, in Endogenous Depression," *Acta Psychiatrica Scandinavica* 66 (1982):50–65; C. L. Revaris et al., "Phenelzine and Amitryptiline in the Treatment of Depression," *Archives of General Psychiatry* 37(1980):1075–1080; R. J. Baldessarini, *Chemotherapy in Psychiatry, Principles and Practice* (Cambridge, Mass.: Harvard University Press, 1985); J. M. Davis "Antidepressant Drugs," in *Comprehensive Textbook of Psychiatry*, edited by H. I. Kaplan and B. J. Sadock (Baltimore: Williams & Wilkins, 1985), 1513–1537.
7. Kessler, "Tricyclic Antidepressants"; Berger, "Antidepressants and the Treatment of Depression."
8. M. Linnoila, T. Seppala, M. J. Mattille, R. Vihko, A. Pakarinen, and J. T. Skinner, "Clomipramine and Doxepin in Depressive Neurosis," *Archives of General Psychiatry* 37(1980):1295–99.
9. R. M. Glass, E. H. Uhlenhuth, F. W. Hartel, W. Matuzas, and M. W. Fischman, "Cognitive Dysfunction and Imipramine in Outpatient Depressives," *Archives of General Psychiatry* 38(1981):1048–51.
10. J. H. Kocsis et al., "Imipramine and Social-Vocational Adjustment in Chronic Depression," *American Journal of Psychiatry* 145 (1988):997–99.

11. G. L. Klerman, "Long Term Treatment of Affective Disorders," in *Psychopharmacology: A Generation of Progress*, edited by M. A. Lipton, A. DiMascio, and K. F. Killam (New York: Raven Press, 1978), 1303–12; M. W. Jann, A. H. Bitar, and A. Rao, "Lithium Prophylaxis of Tricyclic-Antidepressant-Induced Mania in Bipolar Patients," *American Journal of Psychiatry* 139(1982):683–84.

12. S. J. Kantor and A. H. Glassman, "Delusional Depression: Natural History and Response to Treatment," *British Journal of Psychiatry* 131(1977):351–60; Raskin A, et al., "Differential Response to Chlorpromazine, Imipramine and Placebo, *Archives of General Psychiatry* 23(1970):164–173.

13. Berger, "Antidepressants and the Treatment of Depression"; D. G. Spiker et al., "The Pharmacological Treatment of Delusional Depression," *American Journal of Psychiatry* 142(1985):430–36.

14. J. B. Morris and A. T. Beck, "The Efficacy of Antidepressant Drugs," *Archives of General Psychiatry* 30(1974):667–74; M. B. Keller et al., "Long-Term Outcome of Episodes of Major Depression," *Journal of the American Medical Association* 252(1984):788–92; P. J. Cowen, "Depression Resistant to Tricyclic Antidepressants," *British Medical Journal* 297(1988):435–36.

15. F. M. Quitkin et al., "Duration of Antidepressant Drug Treatment," *Archives of General Psychiatry* 41(1984):238–45.

16. Task Force on the Use of Laboratory Tests in Psychiatry, "Tricyclic Antidepressants — Blood Level Measurements and Clinical Outcome: An APA Task Force Report," *American Journal of Psychiatry* 142(1985):155–62.

17. A. H. Glassman, J. M. Perel, M. Shostak, S. J. Kantor, and J. L. Fleiss, "Clinical Implications of Imipramine Plasma Levels for Depressive Illness," *Archives of General Psychiatry* 34(1977):197–204.

18. J. C. Nelson et al., "Desipramine Plasma Concentration and Antidepressant Response," *Archives of General Psychiatry* 39(1982):1419–22.

19. M. Asberg et al., "Relationship Between Plasma Level and Therapeutic Effect of Nortriptyline," *British Medical Journal* 3(1971):331–34.

20. Task Force on the Use of Laboratory Tests in Psychiatry, "Tricyclic Antidepressants — Blood Level Measurements and Clinical Outcome."

21. F. M. Quitkin, "The Importance of Dosage in Prescribing Antidepressants," *British Journal of Psychiatry* 147(1985):593–97.

22. S. P. Roose et al., "Tricyclic Nonresponders: Phenomenology and Treatment," *American Journal of Psychiatry* 143(1986):345–48; L. H. Price et al., "Variability of Response to Lithium Augmentation in Refractory Depression," *American Journal of Psychiatry* 143(1986): 1387–92.

23. P. R. Joyce and E. S. Paykel, "Predictors of Drug Response in Depression," *Archives of General Psychiatry* 46(1989):89–99.

24. S. P. Roose et al., "Tricyclic Nonresponders: Phenomenology and Treatment," *American Journal of Psychiatry* 143(1986):345–48.
25. L. H. Price et al., "Variability of Response to Lithium Augmentation in Refractory Depression," *American Journal of Psychiatry* 143(1986): 1387–92; P. J. Cowen, "Depression Resistant to Tricyclic Antidepressants," *British Medical Journal* 297(1988):435–36.
26. Roose et al., "Tricyclic Nonresponders."
27. E. Frank et al., "Early Recurrence in Unipolar Depression," *Archives of General Psychiatry* 46(1989):397–400.
28. A. Coppen and M. Peet, "The Long-Term Management of Patients with Affective Disorders," in *Psychopharmacology of Affective Disorders*, edited by E. S. Paykel and A. Coppen (New York: Oxford University Press, 1979), 249–56; R. F. Prien et al., "Drug Therapy in the Prevention of Recurrences in Unipolar and Bipolar Affective Disorders," *Archives of General Psychiatry* 41(1984):1096–104; R. H. S. Mindham et al., "Continuation Therapy with Tricyclic Antidepressants in Depressive Illness," *Lancet* 2(1972):854–55.
29. G. L. Klerman, A. DiMascio, M. M. Weissman, B. Prusoff, and E. S. Paykel, "Treatment of Depression by Drugs and Psychotherapy," *American Journal of Psychiatry* 131(1974):186–91.
30. Coppen and Peet, "The Long-Term Management of Patients with Affective Disorders."
31. Prien et al., "Drug Therapy in the Prevention of Recurrences in Unipolar and Bipolar Affective Disorders."
32. M. M. Weissman and G. L. Klerman, "The Chronic Depressive in the Community: Unrecognized and Poorly Treated," *Comprehensive Psychiatry* 18(1977):523–32.
33. R. F. Prien and D. J. Kupfer, "Continuation Drug Therapy for Major Depressive Episodes: How Long Should It Be Maintained?" *American Journal of Psychiatry* 143(1986):18–23.
34. Weissman and Klerman, "The Chronic Depressive in the Community"; M. B. Keller et al., "The Persistent Risk of Chronicity in Recurrent Episodes of Nonbipolar Major Depressive Disorder: A Prospective Follow-up," *American Journal of Psychiatry* 143(1986):24–28.
35. D. Bialos, E. Giller, P. Jatlow, J. Doeherty, and L. Harkness, "Recurrence of Depression After Discontinuation of Long-Term Amitriptyline Treatment," *American Journal of Psychiatry* 139(1982):325–29.
36. Kessler, "Tricyclic Antidepressants"; T. A. Wehr and F. K. Goodwin, "Can Antidepressants Cause Mania and Worsen the Course of Affective Illness?" *American Journal of Psychiatry* 144(1987):1403–1411.
37. Baldessarini, "Drugs and the Treatment of Psychiatric Disorders."
38. D. A. W. Johnson, "Treatment Compliance in General Practice," *Acta Psychiatrica Scandinavica* 63 (Suppl. 290) (1981):447–53.
39. M. M. Weissman, J. K. Myers, and D. Thompson, "Depression and Its

Treatment in a US Urban Community 1975–1976," *Archives of General Psychiatry* 38(1981):417–21.

40. D. A. Regier, "The NIMH Depression Awareness, Recognition, and Treatment Program: Structure, Aims and Scientific Basis," *American Journal of Psychiatry*, 145(1988):1351–57; C. V. R. Blacker and A. W. Clare, "Depressive Disorder in Primary Care," *British Journal of Psychiatry* 150(1987):737–51; S. Shapiro et al., "Utilization of Health and Mental Health Services: Three Epidemiological Catchment Area Sites," *Archives of General Psychiatry* 41(1984):971–78.

41. M. B. Keller et al., "Treatment Received by Depressed Patients," *Journal of the American Medical Association* 248(1982):1848–55.

42. M. B. Keller et al., "Low Levels and Lack of Predictors of Somatotherapy and Psychotherapy Received by Depressed Patients," *Archives of General Psychiatry* 43(1986):458–66.

43. J. H. Barbar, "Depressive illness in general practice," *Acta Psychiatrica Scandinavica* 63 (Suppl. 290) (1981):441–46.

44. D. A. W. Johnson, "Treatment Compliance in General Practice," *Acta Psychiatrica Scandinavica* 63 (Suppl. 290) (1981):447–53.

45. M. A. Fauman, "Tricyclic Antidepressant Prescription by General Hospital Physicians," *American Journal of Psychiatry* 137(1980):490–91.

46. J. R. Hankin, D. M. Steinwachs, D. A. Regier, B. J. Burns, I. D. Goldberg, and E. W. Hoeper, "Use of General Medical Care Services by Persons with Mental Disorders," *Archives of General Psychiatry* 39(1982):225–31.

47. Regier, "The NIMH Depression Awareness, Recognition, and Treatment Program."

48. Baldessarini, "Drugs and the Treatment of Psychiatric Disorders."

49. Ibid.

CHAPTER 12

1. W. S. Appleton and J. M. Davis, *Practical Clinical Psychopharmacology* (Baltimore: Williams & Wilkins, 1980), 117–20; P.A. Berger, "Antidepressant Medications and the Treatment of Depression," in *Psychopharmacology, from Theory to Practice*, edited by J. D. Barchas, P. A. Berger, R. D. Ciaranello, and G. R. Elliott (New York: Oxford University Press, 1977), 174–207; C. L. Revaris, D. S. Robinson, J. O. Ives, N. Alexander, and D. Bartlett, "Phenelzine and Amitriptyline in the Treatment of Depression," *Archives of General Psychiatry* 37(1980):1075–80; J. M. Davis, "Antidepressant Drugs," in *Comprehensive Textbook of Psychiatry/III*, edited by H. I. Kaplan, A. M. Freed-

man, and B. J. Sadock (Baltimore: Williams & Wilkins, 1980), 2290–316.

2. Appleton and Davis, *Practical Clinical Psychopharmacology*, 117–120; Berger, "Antidepressant Medications and the Treatment of Depression"; Davis, "Antidepressant Drugs."

3. D. S. Robinson and N. M. Kurtz, "Monoamine Oxidase Inhibiting Drugs: Pharmacologic and Therapeutic Issues," in *Psychopharmacology: The Third Generation of Progress*, edited by H. Y. Meltzer (New York: Raven Press, 1987), 1297–304.

4. M. R. Liebowitz et al., "Antidepressant Specificity in Atypical Depression," *Archives of General Psychiatry* 45(1988):129–37; F. M. Quitkin et al., "Phenylzine Versus Imipramine in the Treatment of Probable Atypical Depression: Defining Syndrome Boundaries of Selective MAOI Responders," *American Journal of Psychiatry* 145(1988):306–311.

5. Davis, "Antidepressant Drugs."

6. M. Lader, "Fluoxetine Efficacy vs Comparative Drugs: An Overview," *British Journal of Psychiatry* 153 (Suppl. 3) (1988):51–58.

7. S. A. Montgomery, "The Prophylactic Efficacy of Fluoxetine in Unipolar Depression," *British Journal of Psychiatry* 153 (Suppl. 3) (1988):69–76.

8. K. Kesey, *One Flew Over the Cuckoo's Nest* (New York: Viking Press, 1962).

9. Ibid., 236.

10. Ibid., 242.

11. R. D. Weiner, "The Psychiatric Use of Electrically Induced Seizures," *American Journal of Psychiatry* 131(1979):1507–17; I. S. Turek and T. P. Hanlon, "The Effectiveness and Safety of Electroconvulsive Therapy (ECT)," *Journal of Nervous and Mental Disease* 164(1977):419–31.

12. A. Glassman, S. J. Kantor, M. Shostak, "Depression, Delusions and Drug Response," *American Journal of Psychiatry* 132(1975):716–19; M. Fink, "Efficacy and Safety of Induced Seizures (EST) in Man," *Comprehensive Psychiatry* 19(1978):1–18; D. Avery and A. Lubrano, "Depression Treated with Imipramine and ECT: The DeCarolis Study Reconsidered," *American Journal of Psychiatry* 136(1979):559–62; M. Fink, "Convulsive Therapy in Affective Disorder: A Decade of Understanding and Acceptance," in *Psychopharmacology: The Third Generation of Progress*, edited by H. Y. Meltzer (New York: Raven Press, 1987), 1071–76.

13. D. G. Spiker, "The Pharmacological Treatment of Delusional Depression," *American Journal of Psychiatry* 142(1985):430–36.

14. Glassman et al., "Depression, Delusions and Drug Response"; Fink, "Efficacy and Safety of Induced Seizures"; Avery and Lubrano, "Depression Treated with Imipramine and ECT."

15. D. Kay, T. Fahy, and R. Garside, "A Seven Month Double-Blind Trial of Amitriptyline and Diazepam in ECT-Treated Patients," *British Journal of Psychiatry* 117(1970):667–71; P. Perry and M. T. Tsuang, "Treatment of Unipolar Depression Following Electroconvulsive Therapy," *Journal of Affective Disorders* 1(1979):123–29; A. Coppen and M. Peet, "The Long-Term Management of Patients with Affective Disorders," in *Psychopharmacology of Affective Disorders*, edited by E. S. Paykel and A. Coppen (New York: Oxford University Press, 1979), 248–56.

16. A. Coppen, M. T. Abou-Saleh, P. Milln, J. Bailey, M. Metcalfe, B. H. Burns, and A. Armond, "Lithium Continuation Following Electroconvulsive Therapy," *British Journal of Psychiatry* 139(1981):284–87.

17. E. A. Wolpert, "Major Affective Disorders," in *Comprehensive Textbook of Psychiatry/III*, edited by H. I. Kaplan, A. M. Freedman, and B. J. Sadock (Baltimore: Williams & Wilkins, 1980), 1319–31.

18. D. Avery and G. Winokur, "Mortality in Depressed Patients Treated with Electroconvulsive Therapy and Antidepressants," *Archives of General Psychiatry* 33(1976):1029–37.

19. L. B. Kalinowsky, "Convulsive Therapies," in *Comprehensive Textbook of Psychiatry/III*, edited by H. I. Kaplan, A. M. Freedman, and B. J. Sadock (Baltimore: Williams & Wilkins, 1980), 2335–2342; Fink, "Efficacy and Safety of Induced Seizures (EST) in man."

20. Avery and Winokur, "Mortality in Depressed Patients Treated with Electroconvulsive Therapy and Antidepressants."

21. F. H. Frankel, "Current Perspectives on ECT: A Discussion," *American Journal of Psychiatry* 134(1977):1014–19.

22. M. Fink, "Myths of Shock Therapy," *American Journal of Psychiatry* 134(1977):991–96.

23. Frankel, "Current Perspectives on ECT."

24. C. E. Coffey, "Effects of ECT on Brain Structure: A Pilot Prospective Magnetic Resonance Imaging Study," *American Journal of Psychiatry* 145(1988):701–06.

25. L. R. Squire, "Neurological Effects of ECT," in *Electroconvulsive Therapy, Biological Foundations and Clinical Applications*, edited by R. Abrams (New York: SP Medical and Scientific Books, 1982), 169–86.

26. L. R. Squire, "ECT and Memory Loss," *American Journal of Psychiatry* 134(1977):997–1001; L. R. Squire, P. C. Slater, and P. L. Miller, "Retrograde Amnesia and Bilateral Electroconvulsive Therapy," *Archives of General Psychiatry* 38(1981):89–95; L. R. Squire, "Memory Functions as Affected by Electroconvulsive Therapy," in *Electroconvulsive Therapy: Clinical and Basic Research Issues*, edited by S. Malitz and H. A. Sackeim (New York: The New York Academy of Sciences, 1986), 307–14.

27. R. D. Weiner et al., "Effects of Stimulus Parameters on Cognitive Side Effects," In *Electroconvulsive Therapy: Clinical and Basic Research Issues*, edited by S. Malitz and H. A. Sackeim (New York: The New York Academy of Sciences, 1986) 315–25.

28. G. D'Elia and H. Raotma, "Is Unilateral ECT Less Effective Than Bilateral ECT?" *British Journal of Psychiatry* 126(1975):83–89; Davis, "Antidepressant drugs"; Squire, "ECT and Memory Loss"; Kalinowsky, "Convulsive Therapies"; Fink, "Efficacy and Safety of Induced Seizures (EST) in Man"; M. Greenblatt, "Efficacy of ECT in Affective and Schizophrenic Illness," *American Journal of Psychiatry* 134(1977): 1001–5; Glassman et al., "Depression, Delusions and Drug Response"; W. W. K. Zung, "Evaluating Treatment Methods for Depressive Disorders," *American Journal of Psychiatry* 124(1968):40–48; R. Abrams, "Is Unilateral Electroconvulsive Therapy Really the Treatment of Choice in Endogenous Depression?" in *Electroconvulsive Therapy: Clinical and Basic Research Issues*, edited by S. Malitz and H. A. Sackeim (New York: The New York Academy of Sciences, 1986), 50–55.

29. R. L. Horne et al., "Comparing Bilateral to Unilateral Electroconvulsive Therapy in a Randomized Study with EEG Monitoring," *Archives of General Psychiatry* 42(1985):1087–92; Fink, "Convulsive Therapy in Affective Disorder"; Weiner et al., "Effects of Stimulus Parameters on Cognitive Side Effects."

30. H. A. Sackeim, "Effects of Electrode Placement on the Efficacy in Titrated, Low-Dose ECT," *American Journal of Psychiatry* 144(1987):1449–55.

31. Weiner et al., "Effects of Stimulus Parameters on Cognitive Side Effects."

32. M. M. Weissman, "Psychotherapy and Its Relevance to the Pharmacotherapy of Affective Disorders: From Ideology to Evidence," in *Psychopharmacology: A Generation of Progress*, edited by M. A. Lipton, A. DiMascio, and K. F. Killam (New York: Raven Press, 1978), 1313–21.

33. M. M. Weissman, G. L. Klerman, E. D. Paykel, B. Prusoff, and B. Hanson, "Treatment Effects on the Social Adjustment of Depressed Patients," *Archives of General Psychiatry* 30(1974):771–78.

34. A. T. Beck, A. J. Rush, B. F. Shaw, and G. Emery, *Cognitive Therapy of Depression* (New York: Guilford Press, 1979); M. Kovacs, J. Rush, A. T. Beck, and S. D. Hollon, "Depressed Outpatients Treated with Cognitive Therapy or Pharmacotherapy," *Archives of General Psychiatry* 38(1981):33–39.

35. P. M. Lewinsohn, J. M. Sullivan, and S. J. Grosscup, "Changing Reinforcing Events: An Approach to the Treatment of Depression," *Psychotherapy: Theory, Research and Practice* 17(1980):322–34.

36. A. Zeiss et al., "Nonspecific Improvement Effects in Depression Using Interpersonal Skills Training, Pleasant Activities Schedules or Cognitive Training," *Journal of Consulting and Clinical Psychology* 47(1979): 427–39.

37. G. E. Murphy et al. "Cognitive Therapy and Pharmacotherapy," *Archives of General Psychiatry* 41(1984):33–41.

38. L. Covi, R. S. Lipman, L. R. Derogatis, J. E. Smith, and J. H. Pattison, "Drugs and Group Psychotherapy in Neurotic Depression," *American Journal of Psychiatry* 131(1974):191–98.

39. M. Kovacs, J. Rush, A. T. Beck, and S. D. Hollon, "Depressed Outpatients Treated with Cognitive Therapy or Pharmacotherapy," *Archives of General Psychiatry* 38(1981):33–39.

40. M. M. Weissman et al., "Psychotherapy and Its Relevance to the Pharmacotherapy of Major Depression: A Decade Later (1976–1985)," in *Psychopharmacology: The Third Generation of Progress*, edited by H. Y. Meltzer (New York: Raven Press, 1987), 1059–69; I. Elkin et al., "National Institute of Mental Health Treatment of Depression Collaborative Research Program: 1. General Effectiveness of Treatments," *Archives of General Psychiatry* 46(1989):971–82.

41. Elkin et al., "National Institute of Mental Health Treatment of Depression Collaborative Research Program."

42. M. Kovacs, J. Rush, A. T. Beck, and S. D. Hollon, "Depressed Outpatients Treated with Cognitive Therapy or Pharmacotherapy," *Archives of General Psychiatry* 38(1981):33–39; R. Herceg-Baron, B. Prusoff, M. Weissman, A. DiMascio, C. Neu, and G. L. Klerman, "Pharmacotherapy and Psychotherapy in Acute Depressed Patients: A Study of Attrition Patterns in a Clinical Trial," *Comprehensive Psychiatry* 20(1979):315–25; C. G. Last et al., "Patterns of Attrition for Psychosocial and Pharmacologic Treatments of Depression," *Journal of Clinical Psychiatry* 46(1985):361–66.

43. Herceg-Baron et al., "Pharmacotherapy and Psychotherapy in Acute Depressed Patients."

44. Ibid.

45. A. Freedman, "Interaction of Drug Therapy with Marital Therapy in Depressed Patients," *Archives of General Psychiatry* 32(1975):619–37; A. S. Bellack, M. Hersen, and J. Himmelhoch, "Social Skills Training Compared with Pharmacotherapy and Psychotherapy in the Treatment of Unipolar Depression," *American Journal of Psychiatry* 138 (1981):1562–67; M. M. Weissman, B. A. Prusoff, and A. DiMascio, "The Efficacy of Drugs and Psychotherapy in the Treatment of Acute Depressive Episodes," *American Journal of Psychiatry* 136(1979):555–58; Weissman et al., "Psychotherapy and Its Relevance to the Pharmacotherapy of Major Depression"; I. M. Blackburn, S. Bishop, A. I. M. Glen, L. J. Whalley, J. E. Christie, "The Efficacy of Cognitive Therapy in Depression—a Treatment Trial Using Cognitive Therapy and Phar-

macotherapy, Each Alone and in Combination," *British Journal of Psychiatry* 139(1981):181–89.

46. H. R. Conte, "Combined Psychotherapy and Pharmacotherapy for Depression," *Archives of General Psychiatry* 43(1986):471–79.

47. M. M. Weissman, G. L. Klerman, B. A. Prusoff, D. Sholomskas, and M. S. Padian, "Depressed Outpatients: Results One Year After Treatment with Drugs and/or Interpersonal Psychotherapy," *Archives of General Psychiatry* 38(1981):51–55.

48. A. J. Rush, M. Kovacs, A. T. Beck, J. Weissenburger and S. D. Hollon, "Differential Effects of Cognitive Therapy and Pharmacotherapy on Depressive Symptoms," *Journal of Affective Disorders* 3(1981):221–29; A. J. Rush et al., "Comparison of the Effects of Cognitive Therapy and Pharmacotherapy on Hopelessness and Self-Concept," *American Journal of Psychiatry* 139(1982):862–66.

49. A. D. Simons et al., "The Process of Change in Cognitive Therapy and Pharmacotherapy for Depression," *American Journal of Psychiatry* 41(1984):45–51.

50. B. A. Prusoff, M. M. Weissman, and G. L. Klerman, "Research Diagnostic Criteria Subtypes of Depression: Their Role as Predictors of Differential Response to Psychotherapy and Drug Treatment," *Archives of General Psychiatry* 37(1980):796–801.

51. Last et al., "Patterns of Attrition for Psychosocial and Pharmacologic Treatments of Depression."

52. Blackburn et al., "The Efficacy of Cognitive Therapy in Depression."

53. Ibid.; Rush et al., "Differential Effects of Cognitive Therapy and Pharmacotherapy on Depressive Symptoms."

54. Weissman et al., "Depressed Outpatients: Results One Year After Treatment with Drugs and/or Interpersonal Psychotherapy."

55. Rush et al., "Differential Effects of Cognitive Therapy and Pharmacotherapy on Depressive Symptoms."

56. Murphy et al., "Cognitive Therapy and Pharmacotherapy"; A. D. Simons et al., "Cognitive Therapy and Pharmacotherapy for Depression: Sustained Improvement Over One Year," *Archives of General Psychiatry* 43(1986):43–48.

57. G. L. Klerman et al., "Treatment of Depression by Drugs and Psychotherapy," *American Journal of Psychiatry* 131(1974):186–91.

58. E. Frank et al., "Early Recurrence in Unipolar Depression," *Archives of General Psychiatry* 46(1989):397–400.

59. Herceg-Baron et al., "Pharmacotherapy and Psychotherapy in Acute Depressed Patients."

60. B. Blackwell, "Newer Antidepressant Drugs," in *Psychopharmacology: The Third Generation of Progress*, edited by H. Y. Meltzer (New York: Raven Press, 1987), 1041–49; B. Shopsin, "Second Generation Antidepressants," *Journal of Clinical Psychiatry* 41(1980):45–56; M. M. Al-Yassiri, S. F. Ankier, and P. K. Bridges, "Trazodone—a New Anti-

depressant," *Life Sciences* 28(1981):2449–58; L. E. Hollister, "Current Antidepressant Drugs: Their Clinical Use," *Drugs* 22(1981):129–52.

CHAPTER 13

1. N. Weiner, "Drugs That Inhibit Adrenergic Nerves and Block Adrenergic Receptors," in *The Pharmacological Basis of Therapeutics*, edited by A. G. Gilman, L. S. Goodman, and A. Gilman (New York: MacMillan, 1980), 176–210; W. W. Douglas, "Histamine and 5-hydroxytryptamine (Serotonin) and Their Antagonists," in *The Pharmacological Basis of Therapeutics*, edited by A. G. Gilman, L. S. Goodman, and A. Gilman (New York: MacMillan, 1980), 609–46.

2. R. J. Baldessarini, "Drugs and the Treatment of Psychiatric Disorders," in *The Pharmacological Basis of Therapeutics*, edited by A. G. Gilman, L. S. Goodman, and A. Gilman (New York: MacMillan, 1980), 391–447.

3. J. Glowinski and J. Axelrod, "Inhibition of Uptake of Tritiated Noradrenaline in the Intact Rat Brain by Imipramine and Structurally Related Compounds," *Nature* 204(1964):1318–19.

4. F. K. Goodwin, R. W. Cowdry, and M. H. Webster, "Predictors of Drug Response in the Affective Disorders: Toward an Integrated Approach," in *Psychopharmacology: A Generation of Progress*, edited by M. A. Lipton, A. DiMascio, and K. F. Killam (New York: Raven Press, 1978), 1277–88; F. K. Goodwin, and W. Z. Potter, "The Biology of Affective Illness: Amine Neurotransmitters and Drug Response," in *Depression: Biology, Psychodynamics and Treatment*, edited by J. O. Cole, A. F. Schatzberg, and F. H. Frazier (New York: Plenum Press, 1978), 41–73.

5. Goodwin et al., "Predictions of Drug Response in the Affective Disorders"; P. Lindbrink, G. Jonsson, and K. Fuxe, "The Effect of Imipramine-like Drugs and Antihistamine Drugs on Uptake Mechanisms in the Central Noradrenaline and 5-Hydroxytryptamine Neurons," *Neuropharmacology* 10(1971):521–36; J. J. Schildkraut, "The Catecholamine Hypothesis of Affective Disorders: A Review of the Supporting Evidence," *American Journal of Psychiatry* 122(1965):509–522; W. E. Bunney, Jr., and J. M. Davis, "Norepinephrine in Depressive Reactions," *Archives of General Psychiatry* 13(1965):483–94; K. A. Kessler, "Tricyclic Antidepressants: Mode of Action and Clinical Use," in *Psychopharmacology: A Generation of Progress*, edited by M. A. Lipton, A. DiMascio, and K. F. Killam (New York: Raven Press, 1978), 1289–1302; P. A. Berger and J. D. Barchas, "Biochemical Hypotheses of Affective Disorders," in *Psychopharmacology, from Theory to Practice*, edited by J. D. Barchas, P. A. Berger, R. D. Ciaranello, and G. R. Elliott (New York: Oxford University Press, 1977), 151–73.

6. W. Z. Potter, F. Karoum, and M. Linnoila, "Common Mechanism of Action of Biochemically 'Specific' Antidepressants," *Progress in Neuro-*

psychopharmacology and Biological Psychiatry 8(1984):153–61; W. Z. Potter et al., "Selective Antidepressants and Cerebrospinal Fluid," *Archives of General Psychiatry* 42(1985):1171–77; M. Linnoila et al., "Alteration of Norepinephrine Metabolism with Desipramine and Zimelidine in Depressed Patients," *Archives of General Psychiatry* 39(1982):1025–028; R. N. Golden et al., "Antidepressants Reduce Whole-Body Norepinephrine Turnover While Enhancing 6-Hydroxymelatonin Output," *Archives of General Psychiatry* 45(1988):150–54. (1988):150–54.

7. G. R. Henninger and D. S. Charney, "Mechanism of Action of Antidepressant Treatments: Implications for the Etiology and Treatment of Depressive Disorders," in *Psychopharmacology: The Third Generation of Progress*, edited by H. Y. Meltzer (New York: Raven Press, 1987), 535–45.

8. Ibid.; J. E. Rosenblatt, C. B. Pert, J. F. Tallman, A. Pert, and E. W. Bunney, Jr., "The Effect of Imipramine and Lithium on Alpha and Beta Receptors Binding in Rat Brain," *Brain Research* 160(1979):186–91; F. Sulser, J. Vetulani, and P. L. Mobley, "Mode of Action of Antidepressant Drugs," *Biochemical Pharmacology* 27(1978):257–61; D. S. Charney, D. B. Menkes, and G. R. Heninger, "Receptor Sensitivity and the Mechanism of Action of Antidepressant Treatment," *Archives of General Psychiatry* 38(1981):1160–80.

9. H. Y. Meltzer and M. T. Lowy, "The Serotonin Hypothesis of Depression," in *Psychopharmacology: The Third Generation of Progress*, edited by H. Y. Meltzer (New York: Raven Press, 1987), 513–26; J. Hyttel et al., "Biochemical Effects and Drug Levels in Rats After Long-Term Treatment with the Specific 5-HT Uptake Inhibitor, Citalopram," *Psychopharmacology* 83(1984):20–27; R. Mishra et al., "Subsensitivity of the Norepinephrine Receptor—Coupled Adenylate Cyclase System in Brain: Effects of Nisoxetine Versus Fluoxetine," *European Journal of Pharmacology* 60(1979):379–82; B. M. Baron et al., "Rapid Down Regulation of Beta-Adrenoceptors by Co-administration of Desipramine and Fluoxetine," *European Journal of Pharmacology* 154(1988):125–34; W. F. Byerley et al., "Decreased Beta-Adrenergic Receptors in Rat Brain After Chronic Administration of the Selective Serotonin Uptake Inhibitor Fluoxetine," *Psychopharmacology* 94(1988):141–43; A. A. Alhaider, "Desensitization of Beta-Adrenoceptors Following Repeated Injections of 2-Substituted 4-Phenylquinolines," *Journal of Pharmacy and Pharmacology* 39(1987):746–47.

10. G. R. Heninger and D. S. Charney; Mechanism of Action of Antidepressant Treatments: Implication for the Etiology and Treatment of Depression Disorders," in *Psychopharmacology: The Third Generation of Progress*, edited by H. Y. Meltzer (New York: Raven Press, 1987), 535–44.

11. P. W. Gold, F. K. Goodwin, and G. P. Chrousos, "Clinical and Bio-

chemical Manifestations of Depression: Relation to the Neurobiology of Stress," *New England Journal of Medicine* 319(1988):348–53; A. Roy et al., "Plasma Norepinephrine Level in Affective Disorders," *Archives of General Psychiatry* 42(1985):1181–85; J. M. Davis et al., "Cerebrospinal Fluid and Urinary Biogenic Amines in Depressed Patients and Healthy Controls," *Archives of General Psychiatry* 45(1988):705–17; J. W. Maas et al., "Catecholamine Metabolism and Disposition in Healthy and Depressed Subjects," *Archives of General Psychiatry* 44(1987):337–44.

12. L. J. Siever, "Role of Noradrenergic Mechanism in the Etiology of the Affective Disorders," in *Psychopharmacology: The Third Generation of Progress*, edited by H. Y. Meltzer (New York: Raven Press, 1987), 493–504.

13. J. P. Halper, "Blunted Beta-Adrenergic Responsivity of Peripheral Blood Mononuclear Cells in Endogenous Depression," *Archives of General Psychiatry* 45(1988):241–44.

14. M. V. Rudorfer et al., "Exaggerated Orthostatic Responsivity of Plasma Norepinephrine in Depression," *Archives of General Psychiatry* 42(1985):1186–92.

15. C. B. Nemeroff, "Clinical Significance of Psychoneuroendocrinology in Psychiatry: Focus on the Thyroid and Adrenal," *Journal of Clinical Psychiatry* 50 (May Suppl) (1989):13–20.

16. C. B. Nemeroff, "The Role of Corticotropin-Releasing Factor in the Pathogenesis of Major Depression," *Pharmacopsychiatry* 21(1988): 76–82.

17. Ibid.

18. E. Widerlow et al., "Monoamine Metabolites, Corticotropin Releasing Factor and Somatostatin as CSF Markers in Depressed Patients," *Journal of Affective Disorders* 14(1988):99–107.

19. Baldessarini, "Drugs and the Treatment of Psychiatric Disorders"; idem, *Chemotherapy in Psychiatry* (Cambridge, Mass.: Harvard University Press, 1977), 101–14; Kessler, "Tricyclic Antidepressants"; P. A. Berger, "Antidepressant Medications and the Treatment of Depression," in *Psychopharmacology, from Theory to Practice*, edited by J. D. Barchas, P. A. Berger, R. D. Ciaranello, and G. R. Elliott (New York: Oxford University Press, 1977), 174–207.

20. Baldessarini, "Drugs and the Treatment of Psychiatric Disorders."

21. Ibid.

22. A. H. Glassman, "Cardiovascular Effects of Tricyclic Antidepressants," in *Psychopharmacology: The Third Generation of Progress*, edited by H. Y. Meltzer (New York: Raven Press, 1987), 1437–42; J. P. Halper and J. J. Mann, "Cardiovascular Effects of Antidepressant Medications," *British Journal of Psychiatry* 153 (Suppl. 3) (1988) 153:87–98.

23. A. Georgotas, "Affective Disorders: Pharmacotherapy," in *Comprehensive Textbook of Psychiatry*, 4th ed., edited by H. I. Kaplan and B. J. Saddock (Baltimore: Williams & Wilkins, 1985), 821–31; R. J. Baldessarini, *Chemotherapy in Psychiatry: Principles and Practice* (Cambridge, Mass.: Harvard University Press, 1985); J. Racy and E. A. Ward-Racy, "Tinnitus in Imipramine Therapy," *American Journal of Psychiatry* 137(1980):854–55.

24. L. L. Judd et al., "Effects of Psychotropic Drugs on Cognition and Memory in Normal Humans and Animals," in *Psychopharmacology: The Third Generation of Progress*, edited by H. Y. Meltzer (New York: Raven Press, 1987), 1467–75; I. Hindmarch, "A Pharmacological Profile of Fluoxetine and Other Antidepressants on Aspects of Skilled Performance and Car Handling Ability," *British Journal of Psychiatry* 153 (Suppl. 3) (1988) 153:99–104; H. V. Curran et al., "Antidepressants and Human Memory: An Investigation of Four Drugs with Different Sedative and Anticholinergic Properties," *Psychopharmacology* 95(1988):520–27.

25. Hindmarch, "A Pharmacological Profile of Fluoxetine and Other Antidepressants"; Curran et al., "Antidepressants and Human Memory"; K. R. Siegfried et al., "Cognitive Dysfunction in Depression: Difference Between Depressed and Nondepressed Elderly Patients and Differential Cognitive Effects of Nomifensine," *Drug Development Research* 4(1984):533–53; R. Liljequist et al., "Amitriptyline- and Mianserin-Induced Changes in Acquisition of Pair-Association Learning Task," *British Journal of Clinical Pharmacology* 5(1978):149–53.

26. J. P. Feighner et al., "Comparison of alprazolam, imipramine, and placebo in the treatment of depression," *Journal of the American Medical Association*, 249(1983):3057–64; Siegfried et al., "Cognitive Dysfunction in Depression"; D. E. Sternberg and M. E. Jarvik, "Memory Functions in Depression," *Archives of General Psychiatry* 33 (1976):219–24; R. M. Glass et al., "Cognitive Dysfunction and Imipramine in Outpatient Depressives," *Archives of General Psychiatry* 38(1981):1048–51.

27. M. Linnoila, "Clomipramine and Doxepin in Depressive Neurosis," *Archives of General Psychiatry* 37(1980):1295–99; T. Seppala et al., "Psychomotor Skills in Depressed Out-patients Treated with l-Tryptophan, Doxepin, or Clomipramine," *Annals of Clinical Research* 10(1978):214–21; Siegfried et al., "Cognitive Dysfunction in Depression."

28. R. T. Seagraves, "Sexual Side-Effects of Psychiatric Drugs," *International Journal of Psychiatry in Medicine* 18(1988):243–52.

29. W. M. Harrison et al., "A Controlled Study of the Effects of Antidepressants on Sexual Function," *Psychopharmacology Bulletin*

21(1985):85–88; W. O. Monteiro et al., "Anorgasmia from Clomipramine in Obsessive-Compulsive Disorder, a Controlled Trial." *British Journal of Psychiatry* 151(1987):102–12.

30. A. Kowalski et al., "The Sexual Side-Effects of Antidepressant Medication: A Double-Blind Comparison of Two Antidepressants in a Nonpsychiatric Population," *British Journal of Psychiatry* 147(1985): 413–18.

31. C. A. Pedersen and A. J. Prange, Jr., "Effects of Drugs and Neuropeptides on Sexual and Maternal Behavior in Mammals," in *Psychopharmacology: The Third Generation of Progress*, edited by H. Y. Meltzer (New York: Raven Press, 1987), 1477–83.

32. Seagraves, "Sexual Side-Effects of Psychiatric Drugs."

33. Berger, "Antidepressant Medications and the Treatment of Depression"; Baldessarini, "Drugs and the Treatment of Psychiatric Disorders"; idem, *Chemotherapy in Psychiatry*.

34. Berger, "Antidepressant Medications and the Treatment of Depression"; Baldessarini, "Drugs and the Treatment of Psychiatric Disorders"; idem, *Chemotherapy in Psychiatry*.

35. J. P. Halper and J. J. Mann, "Cardiovascular Effects of Antidepressant Medications," *British Journal of Psychiatry* 153 (Suppl. 3) (1988): 87–98.

36. G. L. Cooper, "The Safety of Fluoxetine—an Update," *British Journal of Psychiatry* 153 (Suppl. 3) (1988):77–86.

CHAPTER 14

1. C. Krauthammer and G. L. Klerman, "The Epidemiology of Mania," in *Manic Illness*, edited by B. Shopsin (New York: Raven Press, 1979), 11–28; M. M. Weissman, J. K. Myers, and D. Thompson, "Depression and Its Treatment in a US Urban Community 1975–1976," *Archives of General Psychiatry* 38(1981):417–21.

2. American Psychiatric Association, *Diagnostic and Statistical Manual of Mental Disorders*, 3rd ed. (Washington, D.C.: The Association, 1980), 217.

3. Krauthammer and Klerman, "The Epidemiology of Mania."

4. J. Mendelwicz and J. D. Ranier, "Adoption Study Supporting Genetic Transmission in Manic-Depressive Illness," *Nature* 268(1977): 327–29.

5. Krauthammer and Klerman, "The Epidemiology of Mania."

6. N. S. Kline, "A Narrative Account of Lithium Usage in Psychiatry," in *Lithium, Its Role in Psychiatric Research and Treatment*, edited by S. Gershon and B. Shopsin (New York: Plenum Press, 1973), 5–14;

L. Gerbino, M. Oleshansky, and M. Gershon, "Clinical Use and Mode of Action of Lithium," in *Psychopharmacology: A Generation of Progress*, edited by M. A. Lipton, A. DiMascio, and K. F. Killam (New York: Raven Press, 1978), 1261–75.

7. Kline, "A Narrative Account of Lithium Usage in Psychiatry"; R. J. Baldessarini, "Drugs and the Treatment of Psychiatric Disorders," in *The Pharmacological Basis of Therapeutics*, edited by A. G. Goodman, L. S. Goodman, and A. Gilman (New York: Macmillan, 1980), 391–447.

8. Kline, "A Narrative Account of Lithium Usage in Psychiatry."

9. M. Schou, "Lithium as Prophylactic Agent in Unipolar Affective Illness," *Archives of General Psychiatry* 36(1979):849–51.

10. W. E. Bunney, Jr., F. K. Goodwin, J. M. Davis, J. A. Fawcett, "A Behavioral-Biochemical Study of Lithium Treatment," *American Journal of Psychiatry* 125(1968):499–512.

11. F. M. Quitkin, A. Rifkin, D. F. Klein, "Lithium in Other Psychiatric Disorders," in *Lithium, Its Role in Psychiatric Research and Treatment*, edited by S. Gershon and B. Shopsin (New York: Plenum Press, 1973), 295–315.

12. F. K. Goodwin and M. E. Ebert, "Lithium in Mania: Clinical Trials and Controlled Studies," in *Lithium, Its Role in Psychiatric Research and Treatment*, edited by S. Gershon and B. Shopsin (New York: Plenum Press, 1973), 237–52; B. Shopsin, A. Georgotas, and S. Kane, "Psychopharmacology of Mania," in *Manic Illness*, edited by B. Shopsin (New York: Raven Press, 1979), 177–218.

13. J. Mendlewicz, R. R. Fieve, and F. Stallone, "Relationship Between the Effectiveness of Lithium Therapy and Family History," *American Journal of Psychiatry* 130(1973):1011–13.

14. M. Schou, "Prophylactic Lithium Maintenance Treatment in Recurrent Endogenous Affective Disorders," in *Lithium, Its Role in Psychiatric Research and Treatment*, edited by S. Gershon and B. Shopsin (New York: Plenum Press, 1973), 269–94.

15. J. M. Davis, "Overview: Maintenance Therapy in Psychiatry. II. Affective disorders," *American Journal of Psychiatry* 133(1976):1–13; F. Stallone, E. Shelley, J. Mendlewicz, and R. R. Fieve, "The Use of Lithium in Affective disorders. III. A Double-Blind Study of Prophylaxis in Bipolar Illness," *American Journal of Psychiatry* 130(1973):1006–10.

16. A. Reifman and R. J. Wyatt, "Lithium: A Brake in the Rising Cost of Mental Illness," *Archives of General Psychiatry* 37(1980):385–88.

17. R. R. Fieve, *Moodswing* (New York: Bantam Books, 1978), 47–53.

18. Gerbino et al., "Clinical Use and Mode of Action of Lithium"; R. R. Fieve, S. R. Platman, and R. R. Plutchik, "The Use of Lithium in Affective Disorders. I. Acute Endogenous Depression," *American Journal of Psychiatry* 125(1968):482–91; R. R. Fieve, "Overview of Thera-

peutic and Prophylactic Trials with Lithium in Psychiatric Patients," in *Lithium, Its Role in Psychiatric Research and Treatment*, edited by S. Gershon and B. Shopsin (New York: Plenum Press, 1973), 317–50.

19. Shopsin et al, "Psychopharmacology of Mania"; W. E. Bunney, Jr., "Psychopharmacology of the Switch Process in Affective Illness," in *Psychopharmacology: A Generation of Progress*, edited by M. A. Lipton, A. DiMascio, and K. F. Killam (New York: Raven Press, 1978), 1249–59; M. W. Jann, A. H. Bitar, A. Rao, "Lithium Prophylaxis of Tricyclic-Antidepressant-Induced Mania in Bipolar Patients," *American Journal of Psychiatry* 139(1982):683–84; T. A. Wehr and F. K. Goodwin, "Can Antidepressants Cause Mania and Worsen the Course of Affective Illness?" *American Journal of Psychiatry* 144(1987):1403–11.

20. Schou, "Lithium as Prophylactic Agent in Unipolar Affective Illness."

21. G. L. Klerman, "Long-Term Treatment of Affective Disorders," in *Psychopharmacology: A Generation of Progress*, edited by M. A. Lipton, A. DiMascio, and K. F. Killam (New York: Raven Press, 1978), 1303–11.

22. D. R. Shapiro et al., "Response to Maintenance Therapy in Bipolar Illness," *Archives of General Psychiatry* 46(1989):401–5.

23. M. E. Lickey and B. Gordon, *Drugs for Mental Illness* (New York: W. H. Freeman, 1983).

24. R. J. Miller, "Protein Kinase C: A Key Regulator of Neuronal Excitability," *Trends in Neurosciences* 9(1986):538–41; P. F. Worley et al., "Lithium Blocks a Phosphoinositide-Mediated Cholinergic Response in Hippocampal Slices," *Science* 239(1988):1428–29.

25. S. H. Snyder, "Molecular Strategies in Neuropsychopharmacology: Old and New," in *Psychopharmacology: The Third Generation of Progress*, edited by H. Y. Meltzer (New York: Raven Press, 1987), 17–21; A. H. Drummond, "Lithium and Inositol Lipid-Linked Signalling Mechanisms," *Trends in Pharmacological Sciences* 8(1987):129–33.

26. S. Avissar and G. Schreiber, "Muscarinic Receptor Subclassification and G-Proteins: Significance for Lithium Action in Affective Disorders and for the Treatment of the Extrapyramidal Side Effects of Neuroleptics," *Biological Psychiatry* 26(1989):113–30; Snyder, "Molecular Strategies in Neuropsychopharmacology"; Drummond, "Lithium and Inositol Lipid-Linked Signalling Mechanisms."

27. Avissar and Schreiber, "Muscarinic Receptor Subclassification and G-Proteins"; Snyder, "Molecular Strategies in Neuropsychopharmacology"; Drummond, "Lithium and Inositol Lipid-Linked Signalling Mechanisms."

28. Worley et al., "Lithium Blocks a Phosphoinositide-Mediated Cholinergic Response in Hippocampal Slices."

29. B. Shopsin and S. Gershon, "Pharmacology-Toxicology of the Lithium Ion," in *Lithium, Its Role in Psychiatric Research and Treatment*, edited by S. Gershon and B. Shopsin (New York: Plenum Press, 1973), 107–46;

E. A. Walpert, "Major Affective Disorders," in *Comprehensive Textbook of Psychiatry/III*, edited by H. I. Kaplan, A. M. Freedman, and B. J. Sadock (Baltimore: Williams & Wilkins, 1980), 1319–31; R. R. Fieve, "Lithium Therapy," in *Comprehensive Textbook of Psychiatry/III*, edited by H. I. Kaplan, A. M. Freedman, and B. J. Sadock (Baltimore: Williams & Wilkins, 1980), 2348–52; A. Georgotas, "Affective Disorders: Pharmacotherapy," in *Comprehensive Textbook of Psychiatry*, 4th ed., edited by H. I. Kaplan and B. J. Saddock (Baltimore: Williams & Wilkins, 1985), 821–33.

30. Fieve, "Lithium Therapy."

31. R. L. Sack and E. De Fraites, "Lithium and the Treatment of Mania, in *Psychopharmacology: From Theory to Practice*, edited by J. D. Barchas, et al. (New York: Oxford University Press, 1977), 208–25.

32. Shopsin and Gershon, "Pharmacology-Toxicology of the Lithium Ion."

33. Ibid.; Baldessarini, "Drugs and the Treatment of Psychiatric Disorders"; Fieve, "Lithium Therapy."

34. L. L. Judd, "The Effect of Lithium Carbonate on the Cognitive Functions of Normal Subjects," *Archives of General Psychiatry* 34(1977): 355–57; V. I. Reus, et al., "Effect of Lithium Carbonate on Memory Processes of Bipolar Affectively Ill Patients," *Psychopharmacology* 63(1979):39–42; E. D. Shaw et al., "Effects of Lithium Carbonate on Associative Productivity and Idiosyncracy in Bipolar Outpatients," *American Journal of Psychiatry* 143(1986): 1166–69.

35. Judd, "The Effect of Lithium Carbonate on the Cognitive Functions of Normal Subjects"; Shaw et al., "Effects of Lithium Carbonate on Associative Productivity and Idiosyncrasy in Bipolar Outpatients."

36. Baldessarini, "Drugs and the Treatment of Psychiatric Disorders"; E. A. Jenner, "Lithium and the Question of Kidney Damage," *Archives of General Psychiatry* 36(1979):888–90.

37. Ibid.; T. A. Ramsey and M. Cox, "Lithium and the Kidney: A Review," *American Journal of Psychiatry* 139(1982):443–49; J. R. DePaulo, et al., "Renal Function and Lithium: A Longitudinal Study," *American Journal of Psychiatry* 143(1986):892–95; G. F. S. Johnson et al., "Renal Function and Lithium Treatment: Initial and Follow-up Tests in Manic-Depressive Patients," *Journal of Affective Disorders* 6(1984):249–63; M. Schou, "Lithium Prophylaxis: Myths and Realities," *American Journal of Psychiatry* 146(1989):573–76.

38. Ramsey and Cox, "Lithium and the Kidney"; R. G. Walker and P. Kincaid-Smith, "Kidneys and the Fluid Regulatory System," in *Depression and Mania*, edited by F. N. Johnson (Oxford, IRL Press, 1987), 206–13.

39. Schou, "Lithium Prophylaxis"; idem, "Effects of Long-Term Lithium Treatment on Kidney Function: An Overview," *Journal of Psychiatric Research* 22(1988):287–96.

40. Gerbino et al., "Clinical Use and Mode of Action of Lithium"; F. K. Goodwin and A. P. Zis, "Lithium in the Treatment of Mania," *Archives of General Psychiatry* 36(1979):835–44; Shopsin et al., "Psychopharmacology of Mania."

41. R. F. Prien and A. J. Gelenberg, "Alternatives to Lithium for Preventive Treatment of Bipolar Disorder," *American Journal of Psychiatry* 146(1989):840–48; S. P. Tyer, "Lithium in the Treatment of Mania," *Journal of Affective Disorders*, 8(1985):251–57.

42. Prien and Gelenberg, "Alternatives to Lithium for Preventive Treatment of Bipolar Disorder."

43. S. E. Watkins et al., "The Effect of Carbamazepine and Lithium on Remission from Affective Illness," *British Journal of Psychiatry* 150(1987):180–82; T. Okuma et al., "A Preliminary Double-Blind Study on the Efficacy of Carbamazepine in Prophylaxis of Manic-Depressive Illness," *Psychopharmacology* 73(1981):95–96.

44. B. Lerer et al., "Carbamazepine and Lithium: Different Profiles in Affective Disorder?" *Psychopharmacology Bulletin* 21(1985): 18–22; Watkins et al., "The Effect of Carbamazepine and Lithium on Remission from Affective Illness.

45. R. M. Post and T. W. Uhde, "Carbamazepine in Psychiatric Disorders," *Psychopharmacology Bulletin* 21(1985):10–17; J. C. Ballenger and R. M. Post, "Carbamazepine in Manic-Depressive Illness: A New Treatment," *American Journal of Psychiatry* 137(1980):782–90; R. M. Post et al., "Prophylactic Efficacy of Carbamazepine in Manic-Depressive Illness," *American Journal of Psychiatry* 140(1983):1602–04; J. M. Post et al., "Efficacy of Carbamazepine in Manic-Depressive Illness: Implications for Underlying Mechanisms," In *Neurobiology of Mood Disorders*, edited by R. M. Post and J. C. Ballenger (Baltimore: Williams & Wilkins, 1984).

46. K. G. Kramlinger and R. M. Post, "Adding Lithium Carbonate to Carbamazepine: Antimanic Efficacy in Treatment-Resistant Mania," *Acta Psychiatrica Scandinavica* 79(1989):378–85.

47. H. M. Emrich and D. von Zerssen, "The Use of Sodium Valproate, Carbamazepine and Oxcarbazepine in Patients with Affective Disorders," *Journal of Affective Disorders* 8(1985):243–50; J. Fawcett, "Valproate Use in Acute Mania and Bipolar Disorder: An International Perspective," *Journal of Clinical Psychiatry* 50 (March Suppl) (1989):10–12.

48. Fawcett, "Valproate Use in Acute Mania and Bipolar Disorder"; R. Brown, "U.S. Experience with Valproate in Manic Depressive Illness: A Multicenter Trial," *Journal of Clinical Psychiatry* 50 (March Suppl)(1989):13–16.

49. S. G. Hayes, "Long-Term Use of Valproate in Primary Psychiatric Disorders," *Journal of Clinical Psychiatry* 50 (March Suppl)(1989): 35–39; Emrich and von Zerssen, "The Use of Sodium Valproate,

Carbamazepine and Oxcarbazepine in Patients with Affective Disorders."

50. Fieve, *Moodswing*, 47–53.

CHAPTER 15

1. American Psychiatric Association, "Anxiety Disorders (or Anxiety and Phobic Neuroses)," *Diagnostic and Statistical Manual of Mental Disorders*, 3rd ed., rev. [APA, *DSM-III-R*] (Washington, D.C.: The Association, 1987), 235–53; D. J. Greenblatt, R. I. Shader, *Benzodiazepines and Clinical Practice* (New York: Raven Press, 1974), 63; J. C. Nemiah, "Anxiety State," in *Comprehensive Textbook of Psychiatry*, 3rd ed., edited by H. I. Kaplan, A. M. Freedman, and B. J. Sadock (Baltimore: Williams & Wilkins, 1980), 1483–93; K. Rickels, "Use of Antianxiety Agents in Anxious Outpatients," *Psychopharmacology* 58(1978):1–17.

2. APA, *DSM-III-R*, 235–52.

3. Ibid., 241–43.

4. Ibid., 243–45.

5. Ibid., 247–51.

6. D. F. Klein, "Delineation of Two Drug Responsive Anxiety Syndromes," *Psychopharmacology* 5(1964):397–408.

7. C. M. Zitrin, D. F. Klein, M. G. Woerner, and D. C. Ross, "Treatment of Phobias. I. Comparison of Imipramine Hydrochloride and Placebo," *Archives of General Psychiatry* 40(1983):125–38.

8. P. L. Amies, M. G. Gelder, and P. M. Shaw, "Social Phobia: A Comparative Clinical Study," *British Journal of Psychiatry* 142(1983):174–79.

9. T. A. Mellman and T. W. Uhde, "Electroencephalographic Sleep in Panic Disorder," *Archives of General Psychiatry* 46(1989):178–84.

10. J. K. Myers, M. M. Weissman, et al., "Six-Month Prevalence of Psychiatric Disorders in Three Communities," *Archives of General Psychiatry* 41(1984):959–67.

11. L. N. Robins, J. E. Helzer, M. M. Weissman, et al., "Lifetime Prevalence of Specific Psychiatric Disorders in Three Sites," *Archives of General Psychiatry* 41(1984):949–58.

12. M. A. Lee, P. Flegel, J. F. Greden, and O. G. Cameron, "Anxiogenic Effects of Caffeine on Panic and Depressed Patients," *American Journal of Psychiatry* 145(1988):632–35; A. Breier, D. S. Charney, and G. R. Heninger, "Agoraphobia with Panic Attacks: Development, Diagnostic Stability, and Course of Illness," *Archives of General Psychiatry* 43(1986):1029–36; J. M. Gorman, M. R. Fyer, M. R. Liebowitz, and D. F. Klein, "Pharmacologic Provocation of Panic Attacks," in *Psychopharmacology: The Third Generation of Progress*, edited by H. Y. Meltzer (New York: Raven Press, 1987), 985–93; D. S. Charney, G. R. Heninger, and P. I. Jatlow, "Increased Anxiogenic Effects of Caffeine in Panic Disorders," *Archives of General Psychiatry* 42(1985):233–43.

13. Klein, "Delineation of Two Drug Responsive Anxiety Syndromes"; Zitrin et al., "Treatment of Phobias."
14. Breier et al., "Agoraphobia with Panic Attacks."
15. APA, *DSM-III-R*, 235–53; A. J. Fyer, "Differential Diagnosis and Assessment of Anxiety: Recent Developments," in *Psychopharmacology: The Third Generation of Progress*, edited by H. Y. Meltzer (New York: Raven Press, 1987), 1177–91; M. Humble, "Aetiology and Mechanisms of Anxiety Disorders," *Acta Psychiatrica Scandinavica* 76 (Suppl 335)(1987):15–30; I. M. Marks, *Fears, Phobias and Rituals* (New York: Oxford: Oxford University Press, 1987); C. A. Pollard, S. S. Bronson, and M. R. Kenny, "Prevalence of Agoraphobia Without Panic in Clinical Settings," *American Journal of Psychiatry* 146(1989):559.
16. APA, *DSM-III-R*, 235–53.
17. M. M. Weissman, P. J. Leaf, C. E. Holzer III, and K. R. Merikangas, "The Epidemiology of Anxiety Disorders: A Highlight of Recent Evidence," *Psychopharmacology Bulletin* 21(1985):538–41.
18. Ibid.
19. J. L. Rapoport, *The Boy Who Couldn't Stop Washing* (New York: Dutton, 1989).
20. R. L. Spitzer, A. E. Skodol, M. Gibbon, and J. B. W. Williams, *DSM-III Case Book* (Washington, D.C.: American Psychiatric Association, 1981).
21. S. M. Turner, D. C. Beidel, and R. S. Nathan, "Biological Factors in Obsessive-Compulsive Disorders," *Psychological Bulletin* 97(1985): 430–50.
22. J. L. Rapoport, "The Biology of Obsessions and Compulsions," *Scientific American* (March 1989), 83–89.
23. APA, *DSM-III-R*, 235–53.
24. Robins et al., "Lifetime Prevalence of Specific Psychiatric Disorders in Three Sites"; Myers et al., "Six-Month Prevalence of Psychiatric Disorders in Three Communities."
25. S. E. Swedo, J. L. Rapoport, H. Leonard, J. Lenane, and D. Cheslow, "Obsessive-Compulsive Disorder in Children and Adolescents," *Archives of General Psychiatry* 46(1989):335–41.
26. Fyer, "Differential Diagnosis and Assessment of Anxiety"; E. H. Uhlenhuth, M. B. Balter, G. D. Mellinger, I. H. Cisin, and J. Clinthorne, "Symptom Checklist Syndromes in the General Population," *Archives of General Psychiatry* 40(1983):1167–73; N. Breslau and G. C. Davis, "DSM-III Generalized Anxiety Disorder: An Empirical Investigation of More Stringent Criteria," *Psychiatric Research* 14(1985):231–38.
27. Fyer, "Differential Diagnosis and Assessment of Anxiety."
28. Ibid.
29. Breier et al., "Agoraphobia with Panic Attacks"; Breslau and Davis, "DSM-III Generalized Anxiety Disorder."
30. J. F. Leckman, M. M. Weissman, K. R. Merikangas, D. L. Pauls, and

B. A. Prusoff, "Panic Disorder and Major Depression: Increased Risk of Depression, Alcoholism, Panic, and Phobic Disorders in Families of Depressed Probands with Panic Disorder," *Archives of General Psychiatry* 40(1983):1055–60.

31. Turner et al., "Biological Factors in Obsessive-Compulsive Disorders."
32. Breier et al., "Agoraphobia with Panic Attacks."
33. Turner et al., "Biological Factors in Obsessive-Compulsive Disorders"; J. Zohar and T. R. Insel, "Obsessive-Compulsive Disorder: Psychobiological Approaches to Diagnosis, Treatment, and Pathophysiology," *Biological Psychiatry* 22(1987):667–87; W. Coryell, R. Noyes, and J. Schlechte, "The Significance of the HPA Axis in Panic Disorder," *Biological Psychiatry* 25(1989):989–1002.
34. Amies et al., "Social phobia"; Breier et al., "Agoraphobia with Panic Attacks"; Myers and Weissman, "Six-Month Prevalence of Psychiatric Disorders in Three Communities"; Robins et al., "Lifetime Prevalence of Specific Psychiatric Disorders in Three Sites."
35. K. J. Weiss and D. J. Rosenberg, "Prevalence of Anxiety Disorder Among Alcoholics," *Journal of Clinical Psychiatry* 46(1985):3–5.
36. F. M. Quitkin, A. Rifkin, J. Kaplan, and D. F. Klein, "Phobic Anxiety Syndrome Complicated by Drug Dependence and Addiction," *Archives of General Psychiatry* 27(1972):159–62; Amies et al., "Social phobia"; K. Rickels and E. E. Schweizer, "Current Pharmacotherapy of Anxiety and Panic," in *Psychopharmacology: The Third Generation of Progress*, edited by H. Y. Meltzer (New York: Raven Press, 1987), 1193–203.
37. P. Smail, T. Stockwell, S. Canter, and R. Hodgson, "Alcohol Dependence and Phobic Anxiety States. I. A Prevalence Study," *British Journal of Psychiatry* 144(1984):53–57.

CHAPTER 16

1. U.S. Food and Drug Administration (FDA) *Drug Utilization in the United States, 1985, 7th Annual Review* (Washington, D.C.: U.S. Department of Health and Human Services, 1986), 35.
2. S. Shapiro, E. A. Skinner, et al., "Utilization of Health and Mental Health Services," *Archives of General Psychiatry* 41(1984):971–78; K. Rickels and E. E. Schweizer, "Current Pharmacotherapy of Anxiety and Panic," in *Psychopharmacology: Third Generation of Progress*, edited by H. Y. Meltzer (New York: Raven Press, 1987), 1193–203.
3. D. J. Greenblatt, R. I. Shader, and D. R. Abernethy, "Clinical Use of Benzodiazepines" (second of two parts), *New England Journal of Medicine* 309(1983):410–16; J. D. Hasday, and F. E. Karch, "Benzodiazepine Prescribing in a Family Medicine Center," *Journal of the American Medical Association* 246(1981):1321–25; R. J. Baldessarini, *Chemother-*

apy in Psychiatry (Cambridge, Mass.: Harvard University Press, 1977), 136; J. M. Davis, "Minor Tranquilizers, Sedatives, and Hypnotics," In *Comprehensive Textbook of Psychiatry*, 3d ed., edited by H. I. Kaplan, A. M. Freedman, and B. J. Sadock (Baltimore: Williams & Wilkins, 1980), 2316–33; H. J. Parry, M. B. Balter, G. D. Mellinger, I. H. Cisin, and D. I. Manheimer, "National Patterns of Psychotherapeutic Drug Use," *Archives of General Psychiatry* 28(1973):769–83.

4. U.S. Department of Health and Human Services, *Alcohol and Health*, USDHHS Publ. No. (ADM) 87–1519 (1987): 60–79; J. M. Ritchie, "The Aliphatic Alcohols," in *Goodman and Gilman's Pharmacological Basis of Therapeutics*, edited by A. G. Gillman, A. Goodman, T. W. Rall, and F. Murad (New York: Macmillan, 1985), 372–86.

5. S. Sharpless, "Hypnotics and Sedatives, I. The Barbiturates," in *The Pharmacological Basis of Therapeutics*, 3d ed., edited by L. S. Goodman and A. Gilman (New York: Macmillan, 1965), 105–28.

6. C. Allgulander, "Dependence on Sedative and Hypnotic Drugs, a Comparative Clinical and Social Study," *Acta Psychiatrica Scandinavica* (Suppl. 270) 1978.

7. S. Sharpless, "Hypnotics and Sedatives. I. The Barbiturates," in *The Pharmacological Basis of Therapeutics*, 3d ed., edited by L. S. Goodman and A. Gilman (New York: Macmillan, 1965), 105–28.

8. S. C. Harvey, "Hypnotics and Sedatives," in *The Pharmacological Basis of Therapeutics*, 6th ed., edited by A. G. Gilman, L. S. Goodman and A. Gilman (New York: Macmillan, 1980), 339–75; S. E. Mayer, K. L. Melmon, and A. G. Gilman, "Introduction; the Dynamics of Drug Absorption, Distribution, and Elimination," in *The Pharmacological Basis of Therapeutics*, 6th ed., edited by A. G. Gilman, L. S. Goodman and A. Gilman (New York: Macmillan, 1980), 1–27.

9. R. J. Baldessarini, "Drugs and the Treatment of Psychiatric Disorders," in *The Pharmacological Basis of Therapeutics*, 6th ed., edited by A. G. Gilman, L. S. Goodman and A. Gilman (New York: Macmillan, 1980), 391–447; Allgulander, "Dependence on Sedative and Hypnotic Drugs."

10. Wallace Laboratories, Advertisement for Miltown, *American Journal of Psychiatry* 112(1955): xxv.

11. Allgulander, "Dependence on Sedative and Hypnotic Drugs; M. Sittig, *Pharmacological Manufacturing Encyclopedia*, 2nd ed., (Park Ridge, New Jersey: Noyes Publications, 1988), 585–6, 733–4, 969–71, 1001–2.

12. Allgulander, "Dependence on Sedative and Hypnotic Drugs"; Harvey, "Hypnotics and Sedatives"; J. Jaffe, "Drug Addiction and Drug Abuse," in *The Pharmacological Basis of Therapeutics*, 6th ed., edited by A. G. Gilman, A. Goodman and A. Gilman (New York: Macmillan, 1980), 535–84.

13. Allgulander, "Dependence on Sedative and Hypnotic Drugs."

14. FDA, *Drug Utilization in the United States* (1985):21.

15. K. Rickels, "Use of Antianxiety Agents in Anxious Outpatients," *Psychopharmacology* 58(1978):1–17.
16. Baldessarini, "Drugs and the Treatment of Psychiatric Disorders."
17. D. J. Greenblatt and R. I. Shader, "Pharmacotherapy of Anxiety with Benzodiazepines and Beta-Adrenergic Blockers," in *Psychopharmacology: A Generation of Progress*, edited by A. Lipton, S. DiMascio, and K. F. Killam (New York: Raven Press, 1978), 1381–90.
18. Allgulander, "Dependence on Sedative and Hypnotic Drugs"; D. J. Greenblatt and R. I. Shader, "Dependence, Tolerance and Addiction to Benzodiazepines: Clinical and Pharmacokinetic Considerations," *Drug Metabolism Reviews* 8(1978):13–28.
19. R. L. Katz, "Drug Therapy: Sedatives and Tranquilizers," *New England Journal of Medicine* 286(1972):757–60; K. Rickels, "Benzodiazepines: Clinical Use Patterns," in *Benzodiazepines: A Review of Research Results*. NIDA Research Monograph 33, edited by S. I. Szara and J. P. Ludford (Washington, D.C.: Department of Health and Human Services, 1980), 43–60.
20. Rickels, "Use of Antianxiety Agents in Anxious Outpatients."
21. FDA, *Drug Utilization in the United States, 1988, 10th Annual Review* (Washington, D.C.: U.S. Department of Health and Human Services, 1989), 8.
22. "The Top 200," *American Druggist*, February, 1990, 28.
23. Greenblatt and Shader, "Dependence, Tolerance and Addiction to Benzodiazepines"; J. Marks, *The Benzodiazepines: Use, Overuse, Misuse, Abuse* (Baltimore: University Park Press, 1978); Rickels, "Benzodiazepines"; A. Nagy, "Long-Term Treatment with Benzodiazepines: Theoretical, Ideological and Practical Aspects," *Acta Psychiatrica Scandinavica* 76 (Suppl. 335)(1987):47–55.
24. Greenblatt and Shader, "Pharmacotherapy of Anxiety with Benzodiazepines and Beta-Adrenergic Blockers."
25. Parry et al., "National Patterns of Psychotherapeutic Drug Use."
26. M. B. Balter, J. Levine, and D. I. Manheimer, "Cross National Study of the Extent of Antianxiety/Sedative Drug Use," *New England Journal of Medicine* 290(1974):769–74.
27. Ibid.; D. J. Greenblatt, R. I. Shader, and J. Koch-Wesser, "Psychotropic Drug Use in the Boston Area," *Archives of General Psychiatry* 32(1975):518–21; Hasday and Karch, "Benzodiazepine Prescribing in a Family Medicine Center"; Parry et al., "National Patterns of Psychotherapeutic Drug Use."
28. Davis, "Minor Tranquilizers, Sedatives, and Hypnotics."
29. D. J. Greenblatt and R. I. Shader, *Benzodiazepines and Clinical Practice* (New York: Raven Press, 1974), 231–35, 250–52; Harvey, "Hypnotics and Sedatives"; *Physicians' Desk Reference*, 30th ed. (Oradell, N.J.: Medical Economics, 1976), 543, 571–72, 1173, 1324, 1549–50.
30. M. M. Weissman, G. L. Klerman, J. S. Markowitz, and R. Ouellette,

"Suicidal Ideation and Suicide Attempts in Panic Disorder and Attacks," *New England Journal of Medicine* 321(1989):1209–14.

31. S. C. Harvey, "Hypnotics and Sedatives," in *Goodman and Gilman's Pharmacological Basis of Therapeutics*, 7th ed., edited by A. G. Gilman, A. Goodman, T. W. Rall, and F. Murad, (New York: Macmillan, 1985), 339–71.

32. Greenblatt and Shader, *Benzodiazepines and Clinical Practice*, 43–59; S. D. Iversen, and L. L. Iversen, *Behavioral Pharmacology*, 2d ed. (New York: Oxford University Press, 1981).

33. P. T. Hesbacher, K. Rickels, et al., "Setting, Patient, and Doctor Effects on Drug Response in Neurotic Patients. I. Differential Attrition, Dosage Deviation, and Side Reaction Responses to Treatment," *Psychopharmacologia* 18(1970):180–208; idem, "Setting, Patient, and Doctor Effects on Drug Response in Neurotic Patients. II. Differential Improvement," *Psychopharmacologia* 18(1970):209–26.

34. Davis, "Minor Tranquilizers, Sedatives, and Hypnotics"; Greenblatt and Shader, *Benzodiazepines and Clinical Practice*, 65–79; Greenblatt, Shader, "Pharmacotherapy of Anxiety with Benzodiazepines and Beta-Adrenergic Blockers."

35. Davis, "Minor Tranquilizers, Sedatives, and Hypnotics"; Rickels and Schweizer, "Current Pharmacotherapy of Anxiety and Panic"; Greenblatt et al., "Clinical Use of Benzodiazepines"; S. C. Harvey, "Hypnotics and Sedatives," in *The Pharmacological Basis of Therapeutics*, sixth ed., edited by A. G. Gilman, L. S. Goodman, and A. Gilman (New York: Macmillan, 1980), 339–75; J. L. Taylor and J. R. Tinkelberg, "Cognitive Impairment and Benzodiazepines," in *Psychopharmacology: Third Generation of Progress*, edited by H. Y. Meltzer (New York: Raven Press, 1987), 1449–56.

36. D. J. Greenblatt and R. I. Shader, "Pharmacokinetics of Antianxiety Agents," in *Psychopharmacology: Third Generation of Progress*, edited by H. Y. Meltzer (New York: Raven Press, 1987), 1377–86; Taylor and Tinkelberg, "Cognitive Impairment and Benzodiazepines."

37. Baldessarini, "Drugs and the Treatment of Psychiatric Disorders"; Harvey, "Hypnotics and Sedatives"; M. Lader, "Clinical Pharmacology of Benzodiazepines," *Annual Review of Medicine* 38(1987):19–28.

38. I. Lucki, K. Rickels, and A. M. Geller, "Chronic Use of Benzodiazepines and Psychomotor and Cognitive Test Performance," *Psychopharmacology Bulletin* 22(1986):426–33.

39. R. Hoehn-Saric and D. R. McLeod, "Physiologic and Performance Responses to Diazepam: Two Types of Effects," *Psychopharmacology* 22(1986):439–43; Taylor and Tinkelberg, "Cognitive Impairment and Benzodiazepines."

40. K. Rickels, W. G. Case, et al., "Long-Term Diazepam Therapy and Clinical Outcome," *Journal of the American Medical Association* 250(1983):767–71.

41. Greenblatt et al., "Current Status of Benzodiazepines."
42. G. C. Aden and S. G. Thein, "Alprazolam Compared to Diazepam and Placebo in the Treatment of Anxiety," *Journal of Clinical Psychiatry* 41(1980):245–48.
43. Rickels and Schweizer, "Current Pharmacotherapy of Anxiety and Panic."
44. K. Rickels, I. Csanalosi, et al., "A Controlled Clinical Trial of Alprazolam for the Treatment of Anxiety," *American Journal of Psychiatry* 140(1983):82–85.
45. B. Soderpalm, "Pharmacology of the Benzodiazepines; with Special Emphasis on Alprazolam," *Acta Psychiatrica Scandinavica* 76 (Suppl. 335)(1987):39–46.
46. Baldessarini, "Drugs and the Treatment of Psychiatric Disorders"; Davis, "Minor Tranquilizers, Sedatives, and Hypnotics"; Greenblatt and Shader, *Benzodiazepines and Clinical Practice*, 83–86.
47. Greenblatt and Shader, *Benzodiazepines and Clinical Practice*, 83–4.
48. C. Salzman, G. E. Kochansky, et al., "Chlordiazepoxide-Induced Hostility in a Small Group Setting," *Archives of General Psychiatry* 31(1974):401–5.
49. Baldessarini, "Drugs and the Treatment of Psychiatric Disorders"; Greenblatt and Shader, *Benzodiazepines and Clinical Practice*, 231, 235–50; Harvey, "Hypnotics and Sedatives."
50. J. R. Cooper, F. E. Bloom, and R. H. Roth, *The Biochemical Basis of Neuropharmacology* (New York: Oxford University Press, 1986); S. W. Kuffler, J. D. Nichols, and A. R. Martin, *From Neuron to Brain*, 2d ed. (Sunderland, Mass.: Sinauer, 1984).
51. R. W. Olsen, "Drug Interactions at the GABA Receptor–Ionophore Complex," *Annual Review of Pharmacology and Toxicology* 22 (1982):245–77; J. F. Tallman, P. Skolnik, and D. W. Gallagher, "Receptors for the Age of Anxiety: Pharmacology of the Benzodiazepines," *Science* 207(1980):274–81.
52. W. P. Stratten and C. D. Barnes, "Diazepam and Presynaptic Inhibition, *Neuropharmacology* 10(1971):685–96.
53. R. E. Study and J. L. Barker, "Diazepam and (−)-Pentobarbital: Fluctuation Analysis Reveals Different Mechanisms for Potentiation of Gamma-Aminobutyric Acid Responses in Cultured Central Neurons," *Proceedings of the National Academy of Science (USA)* 78(1981):7180.
54. J. L. Barker and D. G. Owen, "Electrophysiological Pharmacology of GABA and Diazepam in Cultured CNS Neurons," in *Benzodiazepine/ GABA Receptors and Chloride Channels: Structural and Functional Properties*, edited by R. W. Olsen and J. C. Venter (New York: Alan R. Liss, 1986), 135–65.
55. R. F. Squires and C. Braestrup, "Benzodiazepine Receptors in Rat Brain," *Nature* 266(1977):732–34; H. Mohler and T. Okada, "Benzo-

diazepine Receptor: Demonstration in the Central Nervous System," *Science* 198(1977):849–51.

56. E. Siegel and E. A. Barnard, "A Gamma-Aminobutyric Acid/Benzodiazepine Receptor Complex from Bovine Cerebral Cortex: Improved Purification with Preservation of Regulatory Sites and Their Interactions," *Journal of Biological Chemistry* 259(1984):7219–23; F. A. Stephenson and E. A. Barnard, "Purification and Characterization of the Brain GABA/Benzodiazepine Receptor," in *Benzodiazepine/GABA Receptors and Chloride Channels: Structural and Functional Properties*, edited by R. W. Olsen and C. J. Venter (New York: Alan R. Liss, 1986), 261–274.

57. S. J. Enna and H. Mohler, "Gamma-Aminobutyric Acid (GABA) Receptors and Their Association with Benzodiazepine Recognition Sites," in *Psychopharmacology: The Third Generation of Progress*, edited by H. Y. Meltzer (New York: Raven Press, 1987), 265–72.

58. Ibid.; W. Haefely and P. Polc, "Physiology of GABA Enhancement by Benzodiazepines and Barbiturates," in *Benzodiazepine/GABA Receptors and Chloride Channels: Structural and Functional Properties*, edited by R. W. Olsen and J. C. Venter (New York: Alan R. Liss, 1986), 97–133; Olsen, "Drug Interactions at the GABA Receptor–Ionophore Complex"; P. R. Schofield, M. G. Darlison, et al., "Sequence and Functional Expression of the GABA Receptor Shows a Ligand-Gated Receptor Super-family, *Nature* 328(1987):221–27; Study and Barker, "Diazepam and (–)-Pentobarbital."

59. I. R. Ho and R. A. Harris, "Mechanism of Action of Barbiturates," *Annual Review of Pharmacology* 21(1981):83–111; R. Nicoll, "Selective Actions of Barbiturates on Synaptic Transmission," in *Psychopharmacology: A Generation of Progress*, edited by A. Lipton, S. DiMascio, and K. F. Killam (New York: Raven Press, 1978), 1337–48.

60. P. D. Suzdak, R. D. Schwartz, et al., "Ethanol Stimulates Gama-Aminobutyric Acid Receptor-Mediated Chloride Transport in Rat Brain Synaptoneurosomes," *Proceedings of the National Academy of Science (USA)* 83(1986):4071–75.

61. T. R. Insel, P. T. Ninan, et al., "A Benzodiazepine Receptor-Mediated Model of Anxiety," *Archives of General Psychiatry* 41(1984):741–50; Mohler and Okada, "Benzodiazepine Receptor"; Squires and Braestrup, "Benzodiazepine Receptors in Rat Brain."

62. J. M. Gorman, D. Battista, et al., "A Comparison of Sodium Bicarbonate and Sodium Lactate Infusion in the Induction of Panic Attacks," *Archives of General Psychiatry* 46(1989):145–50; D. E. Redmond, "Studies of the Nucleus Locus Coeruleus in Monkeys and Hypotheses for Neuropsychopharmacology," in *Psychopharmacology: The Third Generation of Progress*, edited by H. Y. Meltzer (New York: Raven Press, 1987), 967–75; E. M. Reiman, M. J. Fusselman, P. T. Fox, and M. E. Raichle,

"Neuroanatomical Correlates of Anticipatory Anxiety," *Science* 243(1989):1071–74; E. M. Reiman, M. E. Raichle, et al., "Neuroanatomical Correlates of a Lactate-Induced Anxiety Attack," *Archives of General Psychiatry* 46(1989):493–500.

63. A. Guidotti, C. M. Forchetti, et al., "Isolation, Characterization and Purification to Homogeneity of an Endogenous Polypeptide with Agonist Action on Benzodiazepine Receptors," *Proceedings of the National Academy of Science (USA)* 80(1983):3531–35.

64. M. L. Barbaccia, E. Costa, and A. Guidotti, "Endogenous Ligands for High-Affinity Recognition Sites of Psychotropic Drugs," *Annual Review of Pharmacology* 28(1988):451–76.

65. C. Braestrup, R. Schmiechen, et al., "Interaction of Convulsive Ligands with Benzodiazepine Receptors," *Science* 216(1982):1241–43.

66. Insel et al., "A Benzodiazepine Receptor-Mediated Model of Anxiety."

67. R. Darrow, R. Horowski, et al., "Severe Anxiety Induced by FG 7142, a Beta-Carboline Ligand for Benzodiazepine Receptors," *Lancet* 2(1983):98–99.

68. D. L. Temple, J. P. Yevich, and J. S. New, "Buspirone: Chemical Profile of a New Class of Anxioselective Agent," *Journal of Clinical Psychiatry* 43 (12, sec. 2) (1982):4–9.

69. L. A. Riblet, D. P. Taylor, et al., "Pharmacology and Neurochemistry of Buspirone," *Journal of Clinical Psychiatry* 43 (12, sec. 2) (1982):11–16.

70. J. P. Feighner, C. H. Merideth, and G. A. Hendrickson, "A Double-Blind Comparison of Buspirone and Diazepam in Outpatients with Generalized Anxiety Disorder," *Journal of Clinical Psychiatry* 43 (12, sec. 2) (1982):103–7; H. L. Goldberg and R. Finnerty, "Comparison of Buspirone in Two Separate Studies," *Journal of Clinical Psychiatry* 43 (12, sec. 2) (1982):87–91; K. Rickels, K. Weisman, et al., "Buspirone and Diazepam in Anxiety: A Controlled Study," *Journal of Clinical Psychiatry* 43 (12, sec. 2) (1982):81–6; J. B. Cohn, C. L. Bowden, et al., "Double-Blind Comparison of Buspirone and Clorazepate in Anxious Outpatients," *American Journal of Medicine* 80 (Suppl. 3B) (1986):10–16.

71. K. Rickels, E. Schweizer, et al., "Long-Term Treatment of Anxiety and Risk of Withdrawal," *Archives of General Psychiatry* 45(1988):444–50.

72. J. P. Feighner, "Buspirone in the Long-Term Treatment of Generalized Anxiety Disorder," *Journal of Clinical Psychiatry* 48 (12, Suppl.) (1987):3–6.

73. R. E. Newton, J. D. Marunycx, et al., "Review of the Side-Effect Profile of Buspirone," *American Journal of Medicine* 80 (Suppl. 3B) (1986): 17–21.

74. M. J. Mattila, K. Aranko, and T. Seppala, "Acute Effects of Buspirone and Alcohol on Psychomotor Skills," *Journal of Clinical Psychiatry* 43 (12, sec. 2) (1982):56–60; H. Moskowitz and A. Smiley, "Effects of

Chronically Administered Buspirone and Diazepam in Driving-Related Skills Performance," *Journal of Clinical Psychiatry* 43 (12, sec. 2) (1982):45–55; M. Lader, "Psychological Effects of Buspirone," *Journal of Clinical Psychiatry* 43 (12, sec. 2) (1982):62–67.

75. Lader, "Psychological Effects of Buspirone"; Mattila et al., "Acute Effects of Buspirone and Alcohol on Psychomotor Skills."

76. Redmond, "Studies of the Nucleus Locus Coeruleus in Monkeys and Hypotheses for Neuropsychopharmacology"; A. Basbaum, and H. L. Fields, "Endogenous Pain Control Systems: Brainstem Pathways and Endorphin Circuitry," *Annual Review of Neuroscience* 7(1984):309–38.

77. A. S. Eison, and D. L. Temple, "Buspirone: Review of Its Pharmacology and Current Perspectives on Its Mechanism of Action," *American Journal of Medicine* 80 (Suppl. 3B) (1986):1–9.

78. Riblet et al., "Pharmacology and Neurochemistry of Buspirone."

79. D. P. Taylor, "Buspirone, A New Approach to the Treatment of Anxiety," *The FASEB Journal* 2(1988):2445–52.

80. Feighner, "Buspirone in the Long-Term Treatment of Generalized Anxiety Disorder."

CHAPTER 17

1. J. G. Hubbell, "Danger! Prescription Drug Abuse," *Readers Digest*, April 1980, 100–4; R. Hughes and R. Brewin, *The Tranquilizing of America* (New York: Harcourt Brace Jovanovich, 1979).

2. S. I. Szara, "Introduction," in *Benzodiazepines: A Review of Research Results. NIDA Research Monograph 33*, edited by S. I. Szara and J. P. Ludford (Washington, D.C.: Department of Health and Human Services, 1980), 1–3.

3. E. M. Brecher, *Licit and Illicit Drugs* (Boston: Little Brown, 1972).

4. American Psychiatric Association, *Diagnostic and Statistical Manual of Mental Disorders*, 3d ed. rev. (Washington, D.C.: The Association, 1987).

5. J. H. Jaffe, "Drug Addiction and Drug Abuse," in *The Pharmacological Basis of Therapeutics*, 6th ed., edited by A. G. Gilman, A. Goodman, and A. Gilman (New York: Macmillan, 1980), 535–84.

6. P. L. Amies, M. G. Gelder, and P. M. Shaw, "Social Phobia: A Comparative Clinical Study," *British Journal of Psychiatry* 142(1983):174–79; P. Smail, T. Stockwell, S. Canter, and R. Hodgson, "Alcohol Dependence and Phobic Anxiety States," *British Journal of Psychiatry* 144 (1984):53–57.

7. K. J. Weiss and D. J. Rosenberg, "Prevalence of Anxiety Disorder Among Alcoholics," *Journal of Clinical Psychiatry* 46(1985):3–5; K. Rickels and E. E. Schweizer, "Current Pharmacotherapy of Anxiety

and Panic," in *Psychopharmacology: Third Generation of Progress*, edited by H. Y. Meltzer (New York: Raven Press, 1987), 1193–203.

8. U.S. Department of Health and Human Services, *Alcohol and Health*, US DHHS Publ. No. (ADM) 87–1519 1987; N. K. Mello and R. R. Griffiths, "Alcoholism and Drug Abuse: An Overview," in *Psychopharmacology: The Third Generation of Progress*, edited by H. Y. Meltzer (New York: Raven Press, 1987), 1511–14.

9. Hubbell, "Danger! Prescription Drug Abuse;" K. Dukakis, with J. Skovell, "The True Story," *Good Housekeeping*, September 1990, 202–13.

10. B. Ford, with C. Chase. *The Times of My Life* (New York: Harper & Row, 1978); Dukakis, "The True Story."

11. C. Allgulander, "Dependence on Sedative and Hypnotic Drugs, a Comparative Clinical and Social Study," *Acta Psychiatrica Scandinavica* (Suppl. 270) 1978.

12. R. R. Griffiths, S. E. Lukas, D. Bradford, J. V. Brady, and J. D. Snell, "Self-Injection of Barbiturates and Benzodiazepines in Baboons," in *Psychopharmacology* 75(1981):101–9; M. W. Fischman, "Cocaine and the Amphetamines," in *Psychopharmacology: The Third Generation of Progress*, edited by H. Y. Meltzer (New York: Raven Press, 1987), 1543–53.

13. R. L. Balster and W. L. Woolverton, "Intravenous Buspirone Self-Administration in Rhesus Monkeys," *Journal of Clinical Psychiatry* 43 (12, sec. 2) (1982):34–37; R. R. Griffiths, and N. A. Ator, "Benzodiazepine Self-Administration in Animals and Humans: A Comprehensive Review," in *Benzodiazepines: A Review of Research Results. NIDA Research Monograph 33*, edited by S. I. Szara and J. P. Ludford (Washington, D.C.: Department of Health and Human Services, 1980), 22–36.

14. R. R. Griffiths, and C. A. Sannerud, "Abuse of and Dependence on Benzodiazepines and Other Anxiolytic/Sedative Drugs," In *Psychopharmacology: The Third Generation of Progress*, edited by H. Y. Meltzer (New York: Raven Press, 1987), 1535–41.

15. Griffiths et al., "Self-Injection of Barbiturates and Benzodiazepines in Baboons."

16. Balster and Woolverton, "Intravenous Buspirone Self-Administration in Rhesus Monkeys."

17. Griffiths and Ator, "Benzodiazepine Self-Administration in Animals and Humans."

18. J. D. Griffith, D. R. Jasinski, G. P. Casten, and G. R. McKinney, "Investigation of the Abuse Liability of Buspirone in Alcohol-Dependent Patients," *American Journal of Medicine* 80 (Suppl. 3B) (1986): 30–35.

19. J. O. Cole, M. H. Orzack, B. Beaker, M. Bird, and Y. Bar-Tal, "Assessment of the Abuse Liability of Buspirone in Recreational Sedative Users," *Journal of Clinical Psychiatry* 43(1982):69–74.

20. J. M. Ritchie, "The Aliphatic Alcohols," in *The Pharmacological Basis of Therapeutics*, 3d ed., edited by L. S. Goodman and A. Gilman (New York: Macmillan, 1965), 143–158.

21. D. J. Greenblatt, and R. I. Shader, "Pharmacokinetics of Antianxiety Agents," In *Psychopharmacology: Third Generation of Progress*, edited by H. Y. Meltzer (New York: Raven Press, 1987), 1377–86.

22. S. Sharpless, "Hypnotics and Sedatives. I. The Barbiturates," in *The Pharmacological Basis of Therapeutics*, 3d ed., edited by L. S. Goodman and A. Gilman (New York: Macmillan, 1965), 105–28.

23. K. Rickels, E. Schweizer, I. Csanalosi, W. G. Case, and H. Chung, "Long-Term Treatment of Anxiety and Risk of Withdrawal," *Archives of General Psychiatry* 45(1988):444–50.

24. Cole et al., "Assessment of the Abuse Liability of Buspirone in Recreational Sedative Users"; R. E. Gammans, R. F. Mayol, and J. A. Labudde, "Metabolism and Disposition of Buspirone," *American Journal of Medicine* 80 (suppl. 3B) (1986):41.

25. Griffiths and Sannerud, "Abuse of and Dependence on Benzodiazepines and Other Anxiolytic/Sedative Drugs."

26. Ritchie, "The Aliphatic Alcohols"; Sharpless, "Hypnotics and Sedatives"; Greenblatt and Shader, Pharmacokinetics of Antianxiety Agents.

27. Jaffe, Drug Addiction and Drug Abuse.

28. D. Margules and L. Stein, "Increase of 'Antianxiety' Activity and Tolerance of Behavioral Depression During Chronic Administration of Oxazepam," *Psychopharmacology* 13(1968):74–80.

29. Rickels and Schweizer, "Current Pharmacotherapy of Anxiety and Panic"; D. J. Greenblatt, R. I. Shader, and D. R. Abernethy, "Current Status of Benzodiazepines" (first of two parts), *New England Journal of Medicine* 309(1983):354–58.

30. M. E. Jarvik, "Drugs Used in the Treatment of Psychiatric Disorders," in *The Pharmacological Basis of Therapeutics*, 4th ed., edited by L. S. Goodman and A. Gilman (New York: Macmillan, 1970), 151–203.

31. R. J. Baldessarini, *Chemotherapy in Psychiatry* (Cambridge, Mass.: Harvard University Press, 1977), 133.

32. L. E. Hollister, F. K. Conley, et al., "Long-Term Use of Diazepam," *Journal of the American Medical Association* 246(1981):1568–70.

33. K. Rickels, W. G. Case, R. W. Downing, and A. Winokur, "Long-Term Diazepam Therapy and Clinical Outcome," *Journal of the American Medical Association* 250(1983):767–71; K. Rickels, I. Csanalosi, P. Greisman, D. Dohen, J. Werblowsky, H. A. Ross, and H. Harris, "A Controlled Clinical Trial of Alprazolam for the Treatment of Anxiety," *American Journal of Psychiatry* 140(1983): 82–85.

34. I. Lucki, K. Rickels, and A. M. Geller, "Chronic Use of Benzodiazepines and Psychomotor and Cognitive Test Performance," *Psychopharmacology Bulletin* 22(1986):426–33.

35. C. Hallstrom and M. Lader, "The Incidence of Benzodiazepine Dependence in Long-Term Users," *Journal of Psychiatric Treatment and Evaluation* 4(1982):293–96.
36. D. Haskell, J. O. Cole, S. Schniebolk, and B. Lieberman, "A Survey of Diazepam Patients," *Psychopharmacology Bulletin* 22(1986):432–38.
37. Rickels and Schweizer, "Current Pharmacotherapy of Anxiety and Panic"; Greenblatt et al., "Current Status of Benzodiazepines."
38. R. Hoehn-Saric, and D. R. McLeod, "Physiologic and Performance Responses to Diazepam: Two Types of Effects," *Psychopharmacology* 22(1986):439–43.
39. D. J. Greenblatt, and R. I. Shader, "Long-Term Administration of Benzodiazepines. Pharmacokinetic Versus Pharmacodynamic Tolerance," *Psychopharmacology Bulletin* 22(1984):416–23.
40. B. Soderpalm, "Pharmacology of the Benzodiazepines; with Special Emphasis on Alprazolam," *Acta Psychiatria Scandinavica* 76 (Suppl. 335) (1987):39–46.
41. J. P. Feighner, "Buspirone in the Long-Term Treatment of Generalized Anxiety Disorders," *Journal of Clinical Psychiatry* 48 (12, Suppl.) (1987):3–6.
42. Jaffe, "Drug Addiction and Drug Abuse."
43. J. S. Pevnick, D. R. Jasinski, and C. A. Haertzen, "Abrupt Withdrawal from Therapeutically Administered Diazepam," *Archives of General Psychiatry* 35(1978):995–98; Griffiths and Sannerud, "Abuse of and Dependence on Benzodiazepines and Other Anxiolytic/Sedative Drugs"; M. Lader, "Assessing the Potential for Buspirone Dependence or Abuse and Effects of its Withdrawal." *American Journal of Medicine* 82 (Suppl. 5A) (1987):20–26; H. Ashton, "Benzodiazepine Withdrawal: An Unfinished Story," *British Medical Journal* 288(1983):1135–40.
44. L. E. Hollister, F. P. Motzenbecker, and R. O. Dagan, "Withdrawal Reactions to Chlordiazepoxide (Librium)," *Psychopharmacologia* 2(1961):63–68.
45. A. Winokur, K. Rickels, et al., "Withdrawal reaction from long term, low dosage administration of diazepam. A double blind, placebo controlled study", *Archives of General Psychiatry* 37(1980):101–105.
46. G. D. Mellinger, M. B. Balter, and E. H . Uhlenhuth, "Prevalence and Correlates of the Long-Term Regular Use of Anxiolytics," *Journal of the American Medical Association* 251(1984):375–79.
47. Griffiths and Sannerud, "Abuse of and Dependence on Benzodiazepines and Other Anxiolytic/Sedative Drugs."
48. P. Tyrer, R. Owen, and S. Dawling, "Gradual Withdrawal of Diazepam After Long-Term Therapy," *Lancet* 1(1983):1402–6.
49. Rickels et al., "Long-Term Treatment of Anxiety and Risk of Withdrawal."
50. K. Rickels, "Benzodiazepines: Clinical Use Patterns," in *Benzodiaze-*

pines: A Review of Research Results. NIDA Research Monograph 33, edited by S. I. Szara and J. P. Ludford (Washington, D.C.: Department of Health and Human Services, 1980), 43–60; Rickels et al., "Long-Term Diazepam Therapy and Clinical Outcome."

51. Griffiths and Sannerud, "Abuse of and Dependence on Benzodiazepines and Other Anxiolytic/Sedative Drugs."
52. Rickels et al., "Long-Term Treatment of Anxiety and Risk of Withdrawal."
53. Jaffe, "Drug Addiction and Drug Abuse."
54. H. Moskowitz and A. Smiley, "Effects of Chronically Administered Buspirone and Diazepam in Driving-Related Skills Performance," *Journal of Clinical Psychiatry* 43 (12, sec. 2) (1982):45–55.
55. L. A. Riblet, D. P. Taylor, M. S. Eison, and H. C. Stanton, "Pharmacology and Neurochemistry of Buspirone," *Journal of Clinical Psychiatry* 43 (12, sec. 2) (1982):11–16.
56. E. Schweizer and K. Rickels, "Failure of Buspirone to Manage Benzodiazepine Withdrawal," *American Journal of Psychiatry* 143(1986): 1590–92.
57. M. Lader and D. Olajide, "A Comparison of Buspirone and Placebo in Relieving Benzodiazepine Withdrawal Symptoms," *Journal of Clinical Psychopharmacology* 7(1987):11–15.
58. J. P. Feighner, "Impact of Anxiety Therapy on Patients' Quality of Life," *American Journal of Medicine* 82 (Suppl. 5A) (1987):14–19.
59. Feighner, "Buspirone in the Long-Term Treatment of Generalized Anxiety Disorder"; Rickels et al., "Long-Term Treatment of Anxiety and Risk of Withdrawal"; M. Lader, "Clinical Pharmacology of Benzodiazepines," *Annual Review of Medicine* 38(1987):19–28.
60. A. Nagy, "Long-Term Treatment with Benzodiazepines: Theoretical, Ideological and Practical Aspects," *Acta Psychiatrica Scandinavica* 76 (Suppl. 335) (1987):47–55.

CHAPTER 18

1. I. M. Marks, *Fears, Phobias and Rituals,* (New York, Oxford: Oxford University Press, 1987), 457–523.
2. D. F. Klein, "Delineation of Two Drug Responsive Anxiety Syndromes," *Psychopharmacology* 5(1964):397–408.
3. C. M. Zitrin, D. F. Klein, M. G. Woerner, and D. C. Ross, "Treatment of Phobias, I. Comparison of Imipramine Hydrochloride and Placebo," *Archives of General Psychiatry* 40(1983):125–38; D. V. Sheehan, J. Ballenger, and G. Jacobsen, "Treatment of Endogenous Anxiety with Phobic, Hysterical and Hypochondriacal Symptoms," *Archives of General Psychiatry* 37(1980):51–59; G. Chouinard, L. Annable, R. Ron-

taine, and L. Solyom, "Alprazolam in the Treatment of Generalized Anxiety and Panic Disorders: A Double-Blind Placebo-Controlled Study. *Psychopharmacology* 77(1982):229–33.

4. K. Rickels and E. E. Schweizer, "Current Pharmacotherapy of Anxiety and Panic," in *Psychopharmacology: Third Generation of Progress*, edited by H. Y. Meltzer (New York: Raven Press, 1987), 1193–203; M. Lader, "Clinical Pharmacology of Benzodiazepines," *Annual Review of Medicine* 38(1987):19–28.

5. D. V. Sheehan, J. Ballenger, and G. Jacobsen, "Treatment of Endogenous Anxiety with Phobic, Hysterical, and Hypochondriacal Symptoms," *Archives of General Psychiatry* 37(1980):51–59.

6. Zitrin et al., "Treatment of Phobias, I."

7. Ibid.

8. Ibid.

9. C. A. Pollard, S. S. Bronson, and M. R. Kenny, "Prevalence of Agoraphobia Without Panic in Clinical Settings," *American Journal of Psychiatry* 146(1989):559; M. M. Weissman, P. I. Leaf, C. E. Holzer III, and K. R. Merikangas, "The Epidemiology of Anxiety Disorders: A Highlight of Recent Evidence," *Psychopharmacology Bulletin* 21(1985):538–41.

10. M. R. Mavissakalian and J. M. Perel, "Imipramine Dose–Response Relationship in Panic Disorder with Agoraphobia; Preliminary Findings," *Archives of General Psychiatry* 46(1989):127.

11. Marks *Fears and Phobias and Rituals*, 457–494; D. F. Klein, C. M. Zitrin, M. G. Woerner, and D. C. Ross, "Treatment of Phobias, II. Behavior Therapy and Supportive Psychotherapy: Are There Any Specific Ingredients?" *Archives of General Psychiatry* 40(1983):139–45.

12. Marks, *Fears, Phobias and Rituals*, 457–78, 496–97, 505–06.

13. Ibid. 505.

14. J. M. Gorman, M. R. Liebowitz, A. J. Fyer, and J. Stein, "A Neuroanatomical Hypothesis for Panic Disorder," *American Journal of Psychiatry* 146(1989):148–61.

15. J. M. Gorman, M. R. Fyer et al., "Pharmacologic Provocation of Panic Attacks," in *Psychopharmacology: The Third Generation of Progress*, edited by H. Y. Meltzer (New York: Raven Press, 1987), 985–93.

16. Ibid.; J. M. Gorman, D. Battista, R. R. Goetz, D. J. Dillon, M. R. Liebowitz, A. J. Fyer, J. P. Kahn, D. Sandberg, and D. F. Klein, "A Comparison of Sodium Bicarbonate and Sodium Lactate Infusion in the Induction of Panic Attacks," *Archives of General Psychiatry* 46 (1989):145–50; Gorman et al., "A Neuroanatomical Hypothesis for Panic Disorder;" D. E. Redmond, "Studies of the Nucleus Locus Coeruleus in Monkeys and Hypotheses for Neuropsychopharmacology," in *Psychopharmacology: The Third Generation of Progress*, edited by H. Y. Meltzer (New York: Raven Press, 1987), 967–75.

17. Redmond, "Studies of the Nucleus Locus Coeruleus in Monkeys and Hypotheses for Neuropsychopharmacology."

18. E. M. Reiman, M. E. Raichle, E. Robins, F. K. Butler, P. Herscovitch, P. Fox, and J. Perlmutter, "The Application of Positron Emission Tomography to the Study of Panic Disorder," *American Journal of Psychiatry* 143(1986):469–77; E. M. Reiman, M. E. Raichle, E. Robins, M. A. Mintun, M. J. Fusselman, P. T. Fox, J. L. Price, and K. A. Hackman, "Neuroanatomical Correlates of a Lactate-Induced Anxiety Attack," *Archives of General Psychiatry* 46(1989):493–500.

19. P. Thoren, M. Asberg, B. Cronholm, L. Jornestedt, and L. Traskman, "Clomipramine Treatment of Obsessive-Compulsive Disorder," *Archives of General Psychiatry* 37(1980):1281–85.

20. I. M. Marks, R. S. Stern, D. Mawson, J. Cobb, and R. McDonald, "Clomipramine and Exposure for Obsessive-Compulsive Rituals: I," *British Journal of Psychiatry* 136(1980):1–25.

21. Ibid.

22. T. R. Insel, D. L. Murphy, R. M. Cohen, I. Alterman, C. Kilts, and M. Linnoila, "Obsessive-Compulsive Disorder: A Double Blind Trial of Clomipramine and Clorgyline," *Archives of General Psychiatry* 40 (1983):605–12; M. F. Flament, J. L. Rapoport, C. J. Berg, W. Sceery, C. Kilts, B. Mellstrom, and M. Linnoila, "Clomipramine Treatment of Childhood Obsessive-Compulsive Disorder: A Double Blind Study," *Archives of General Psychiatry* 42(1985):977–983.

23. Ibid.

24. Ibid.; J. Zohar, and T. R. Insel, "Obsessive-Compulsive Disorder: Psychobiological Approaches to Diagnosis, Treatment, and Pathophysiology," *Biological Psychiatry* 22(1987):667–87.

25. Marks, *Fears, Phobias and Rituals*, 457–467, 472–73, 484–86, 513–16; Marks et al., "Clomipramine and Exposure for Obsessive-Compulsive Rituals: I.," 4.

26. E. B. Foa, "Failure in Treating Obsessive-Compulsives," *Behavioral Research and Therapy* 17(1979):169–76; Marks, *Fears, Phobias and Rituals*, 497–98.

27. Marks et al., "Clomipramine and Exposure for Obsessive-Compulsive Rituals: I."

28. I. M. Marks, M. Basoglu, H. Noshirvani, W. Monteiro, D. Cohen, and Y. Kasvikis, "Clomipramine, Self-Exposure and Therapist-Aided Exposure for Obsessive-Compulsive Rituals," *British Journal of Psychiatry* 152(1988):522–34.

29. Marks, *Fears, Phobias and Rituals*, 498, 516–18.

30. Ibid. 537–38, 554. Foa, "Failure in Treating Obsessive-Compulsives."

31. Insel et al., "Obsessive-Compulsive Disorder"; M. T. Pato, R. Zohar-Kadouch, J. Zohar, and D. L. Murphey, "Return of Symptoms After Discontinuation of Clomipramine in Patients with Obsessive-Compul-

sive Disorder," *American Journal of Psychiatry* 145(1988):1521–25; Thoren et al., "Clomipramine Treatment of Obsessive-Compulsive Disorder."

32. Marks et al., "Clomipramine, Self-Exposure and Therapist-Aided Exposure for Obsessive-Compulsive Rituals"; Marks, *Fears, Phobias and Rituals*, 497–98; D. Mawson, I. M. Marks, and L. Ramm, "Clomipramine and Exposure for Chronic Obsessive-Compulsive Rituals: III. Two Year Follow-up and Further Findings," *British Journal of Psychiatry* 140(1982):11–18.

33. Flament et al., "Clomipramine Treatment of Childhood Obsessive-Compulsive Disorder."

34. W. K. Goodman, L. H. Price, S. A. Rasmussen, P. L. Delgado, G. R. Heninger, and D. S. Charney, "Efficacy of Fluvoxamine in Obsessive-Compulsive Disorder: A Double Blind Comparison," *Archives of General Psychiatry* 46(1989):36–44.

35. Thoren et al., "Clomipramine Treatment of Obsessive-Compulsive Disorder."

36. J. Volavka, F. Neziroglu, and J. A. Yaryura-Tobias, "Clomipramine and Imipramine in Obsessive-Compulsive Disorder," *Psychiatric Research* 14(1985):85–91; J. Anath and J. C. Pecknold et al., "Double Blind Comparative Study of Clomipramine and Amitriptyline in Obsessive Compulsive Disorder," *Progress in Neuropsychopharmacology and Biological Psychiatry* 5(1981):257–64; Zohar and Insel, "Obsessive-Compulsive Disorder"; J. L. Rapoport, "The Biology of Obsessions and Compulsions," *Scientific American*, March 1989, 83–89.

37. Insel et al., "Obsessive-Compulsive Disorder."

38. Zohar and Insel, "Obsessive-Compulsive Disorder"; Rapoport, "The Biology of Obsessions and Compulsions."

39. Goodman et al., "Efficacy of Fluvoxamine in Obsessive-Compulsive Disorder"; A. Prasad, "A Double Blind Study of Imipramine Versus Zimelidine in Treatment of Obsessive-Compulsive Neurosis," *Pharmacopsychiatry* 17(1984):61–62.

40. T. R. Insel, E. A. Mueller, I. Alterman, M. Linnoila, and D. L. Murphy, "Obsessive-Compulsive Disorder and Serotonin: Is There a Connection?" *Biological Psychiatry* 20(1985):1174–88.

41. M. A. Jenike, L. Buttolph, L. Baer, J. Ricciardi, and A. Holland, "Open Trial of Fluoxetine in Obsessive-Compulsive Disorder," *American Journal of Psychiatry* 146(1989):909–11; R. Fontaine and G. Chouinard, "Antiobsessive Effect of Fluoxetine," *American Journal of Psychiatry* 142(1985):989; S. M. Turner, D. C. Beidel, and R. S. Nathan, "Biological Factors in Obsessive-Compulsive Disorders," *Psychological Bulletin* 97(1985):430–50.

42. P. Thoren, M. Asberg, L. Bertilsson, B. Mellstrom, F. Sjoqvist, and L. Traskman, "Clomipramine Treatment of Obsessive-Compulsive Dis-

order, II. Biochemical Aspects," *Archives of General Psychiatry* 37(1980):1289–94.

43. M. F. Flament, J. L. Rapoport, D. L. Murphy, C. J. Berg and R. Lake, "Biochemical Changes During Clomipramine Treatment of Childhood Obsessive-Compulsive Disorder," *Archives of General Psychiatry* 44(1987):219–25.

44. J. Zohar, E. A. Mueller, T. R. Insel, R. C. Zohar-Kadouch, and D. L. Murphy, "Serotonergic Responsivity in Obsessive-Compulsive Disorder," *Archives of General Psychiatry* 44(1987):946–51.

45. E. Hollander, M. Fay, B. Cohen, R. Campeas, J. M. Gorman and M. R. Liebowitz, "Serotonergic and Noradrenergic Sensitivity in Obsessive-Compulsive Disorder: Behavioral Findings," *American Journal of Psychiatry* 145(1988):1015–17.

46. D. S. Charney, W. K. Goodman, L. H. Price, S. W. Woods, S. A. Rasmussen, and G. R. Heninger, "Serotonin Function in Obsessive-Compulsive Disorder," *Archives of General Psychiatry* 45(1988): 177–85.

47. J. Zohar, T. R. Insel, R. C. Zohar-Kadouch, J. L. Hill, and D. L. Murphy, "Serotonergic Responsivity in Obsessive-Compulsive Disorder," *Archives of General Psychiatry* 45(1988):167–72.

48. C. Benkelfat, D. L. Murphy et al., "Clomipramine in Obsessive-Compulsive Disorder: Further Evidence for a Serotonergic Mechanism," *Archives of General Psychiatry* 46(1989):23–28.

49. D. L. Pauls and J. F. Leckman, "The inheritance of Gilles de la Tourette's Syndrome and Associated Behaviors," *New England Journal of Medicine* 315(1986):993–97; J. L. Rapoport and S. P. Wise, Obsessive-Compulsive Disorder: Evidence for Basal Ganglia Dysfunction," *Psychopharmacology Bulletin* 24(1988):380–84; J. L. Cummings, "Psychosomatic Aspects of Movement Disorders," *Advances in Psychosomatic Medicine* 13(1985):111–32; Turner et al., "Biological Factors in Obsessive-Compulsive Disorders."

50. S. E. Swedo, J. L. Rapoport, D. L. Cheslow, H. L. Leonard, E. M. Ayoub, D. M. Hosier, and E. R. Wald, "High Prevalence of Obsessive-Compulsive Symptoms in Patients with Sydenham's Chorea," *American Journal of Psychiatry* 146(1989):246–49.

51. J. L. Cummings and M. Frankel, "Gilles de la Tourette Syndrome and the Neurological Basis of Obsessions and Compulsions," *Biological Psychiatry* 20(1985):1117–26.

52. L. R. Baxter, M. E. Phelps, J. C. Mazziotta, B. H. Guze, J. M. Schwartz, and C. E. Selin, "Local Cerebral Glucose Metabolic Rates in Obsessive-Compulsive Disorder: A Comparison with rates in Unipolar Depression and in Normal Controls," *Archives of General Psychiatry* 44(1987): 211–18; L. R. Baxter, J. M. Schwartz, J. C. Mazziotta, M. E. Phelps, J. J. Pahl, B. H. Guze, and L. Fairbanks, "Cerebral Glucose Metabolic

Rates in Nondepressed Patients with Obsessive-Compulsive Disorder," *American Journal of Psychiatry* 145(1988):1560–63.

53. S. E. Swedo, M. B. Schapiro, C. L. Grady, D. L. Cheslow, H. L. Leonard, A. Kumar, R. Friedland, S. I. Rapoport, and J. L. Rapoport, "Cerebral Glucose Metabolism in Childhood-Onset Obsessive-Compulsive Disorder," *Archives of General Psychiatry* 46(1989):518–23.

CHAPTER 19

1. J. Leo, "Danger Is Found in Some Remedies," *New York Times*, 9 February 1969, 92.

2. A. Frances and J. F. Clarkin, "No Treatment as the Prescription of Choice," *Archives of General Psychiatry* 38(1981):542–45; T. B. Karasu, "The Ethics of Psychotherapy," *American Journal of Psychiatry* 137(1980):1502–15.

3. M. Roth, "Psychiatry and Its Critics," *Canadian Psychiatric Association Journal* 17(1972):343–50; J. A. Talbot, "Radical Psychiatry: An Appreciation of the Issues," *American Journal of Psychiatry* 131(1972): 121–28.

4. T. Szasz, *The Myth of Mental Illness*, rev. ed. (New York: Harper & Row, 1974), 1–103; R. D. Laing, *The Politics of Experience* (New York: Ballantine, 1967), 100–130; R. D. Laing, *Wisdom, Madness and Folly* (New York: McGraw-Hill Book Company, 1985), 1–30; M. Cerrolaza, The Nebulous Scope of Current Psychiatry, *Comprehensive Psychiatry* 14 (1973):299–309.

5. T. Szasz, "Psychiatric Justice," *British Journal of Psychiatry* 154 (1989):864–69.

6. A. A. Stone, *Mental Health and Law: A System in Transition*, (New York: Jason Aronson, Inc, 1976), 1–8; P. S. Appelbaum and T. G. Guthein, "The Boston State Hospital Case: 'Involuntary Mind Control,' the Constitution, and the 'Right to Rot'" *American Journal of Psychiatry* 137(1980):720–723.

7. Szasz, *The Myth of Mental Illness*; idem, "Schizophrenia: The Sacred Symbol of Psychiatry," *British Journal of Psychiatry* 129(1976):308–16.

8. R. L. Spitzer and P. Wilson, "Nosology and the Official Psychiatric Nomenclature," in *Comprehensive Textbook of Psychiatry*, 2d ed., edited by H. K. Kaplan, A. M. Freedman, B. J. Sadock (Baltimore: Williams & Wilkins, 1975), 826–45.

9. S. Kety, "From Rationalization to Reason," *American Journal of Psychiatry* 137(1974):332–39; M. Ford, "The Psychiatrist's Double Bind: The Right to Refuse Medication," *American Journal of Psychiatry* 137 (1980):332–39; M. S. Moore, "Some Myths About 'Mental Illness,'" *Archives of General Psychiatry* 32(1975):1483–97; M. Cerrolaza, "The

Nebulous Scope of Current Psychiatry;" M. Roth, J. Kroll, *The Reality of Mental Illness* (Cambridge: Cambridge University Press, 1986).

10. S. Bloch and P. Reddaway, *Psychiatric Terror: How Soviet Psychiatry Is Used to Suppress Dissent* (New York: Basic Books, 1977), 107.

11. Ibid., 105–127; W. Reich, "The Case of General Grigorenko: A Psychiatric Reexamination of a Soviet Dissident," *Psychiatry* 43(1980): 303–23.

12. Ibid.; Bloch and Reddaway, *Psychiatric Terror*, 114–116.

13. W. Reich, "Soviet Psychiatry on Trial," *Commentary* 65(1978):40–48; A. Koryagin, "The Involvement of Soviet Psychiatry in Persecution of Dissenters," *British Journal of Psychiatry* 154(1989):336–40; V. Rich, "Soviet Psychiatry," *Nature* 301(1983):559.

14. Koryagin, "The Involvement of Soviet Psychiatry in Persecution of Dissenters"; W. J. Eaton, "Russians Enact Rules Limiting Commitment to Mental Hospitals," *Portland Oregonian*, 5 January 1987; C. Holden, "Politics and Soviet Psychiatry," *Science* 239(1988):551–53; idem, "Is Soviet Psychiatry Changing Its Ways?" *Science* 242(1988):505–6.

15. C. Holden, "Psychiatrists Examine Soviet System," *Science* 243(1989):1547; idem, "Soviet psychiatry: Real Progress or Just PR?" *Science* 245(1989):348; idem, "Soviets Back in World Psychiatric Body," *Science* 246(1989):450; Associated Press, "US Group Finishes Probe of Soviet Mental Hospitals," *Register Guard*, March 12, 1989.

16. P. S. Appelbaum, "Tarasoff and the Clinician: Problems in Fulfilling the Duty to Protect," *American Journal of Psychiatry* 142(1985):425–29; idem, "The New Preventive Detention: Psychiatry's Problematic Responsibility for the Control of Violence," *American Journal of Psychiatry* 145(1988):779–85; C. W. Lidz, E. P. Mulvey, P. S. Appelbaum, and S. Cleveland, "Commitment: The Consistency of Clinicians and the Use of Legal Standards," *American Journal of Psychiatry* 146(1989):176–81.

17. S. K. Hoge, G. Sachs, P. S. Appelbaum, A. Greer, and C. Gordon, "Limitations on Psychiatrists' Discretionary Civil Commitment Authority by the Stone and Dangerousness Criteria," *Archives of General Psychiatry* 45(1988):764–69.

18. P. Appelbaum, "Can Mental Patients Say No to Drugs?" *New York Times Magazine*, March 21, 1982, 51–59; idem, "Is the Need for Treatment Constitutionally Acceptable as a Basis for Civil Commitment?" *Law, Medicine and Health Care* 12(1984):144–49; A. A. Stone, "The Right to Refuse Treatment: Why Psychiatrists Should and Can Make It Work," *Archives of General Psychiatry* 38(1981):358–62; idem, *Mental Health and Law*, 1–4, 51–64.

19. Stone, "The Right to Refuse Treatment"; M. Ford, "The Psychiatrist's Double Bind: The Right to Refuse Medication," *American Journal of Psychiatry* 137(1980):332–39.

20. Appelbaum, "Is the Need for Treatment Constitutionally Acceptable as a Basis for Civil Commitment?"; T. G. Gutheil, "In Search of True Freedom: Drug Refusal, Involuntary Medication, and 'Rotting with Your Rights On,'" *American Journal of Psychiatry* 137(1980):327–28; S. J. Reiser, "Refusing Treatment for Mental Illness: Historical and Ethical Dimensions," *American Journal of Psychiatry* 137(1980):329–31; Stone, "The Right to Refuse Treatment"; R. K. Schwitzgebel, "Survey of State Civil Commitment Statutes," in *Civil Commitment and Social Policy*, USDHHS Publ. No. (ADM) 81–1011 (Washington, D.C.: U.S. Department of Health and Human Services, 1981), 47–83.

21. P. S. Appelbaum and L. H. Roth, "Assessing the NCSC Guidelines for Involuntary Civil Commitment from the Clinician's Point of View," *Hospital and Community Psychiatry* 39(1988):406–10; Ford, "The Psychiatrist's Double Bind"; J. Monahan, *The Clinical Prediction of Violent Behavior* (Washington, D.C.: U.S. Department of Health and Human Services, National Institute of Mental Health, 1981); Stone, *Mental Health and Law.*

22. J. S. Mill, "On Liberty," in *Collected Works of John Stuart Mill*, vol. 18, edited by J. M. Robson (Toronto: University of Toronto Press, 1977), 223–24.

23. Ford, "The Psychiatrist's Double Bind"; S. Schultz, "The Boston State Hospital Case: A Conflict of Civil Liberties and True Liberalism," *American Journal of Psychiatry* 139(1982):183–88; Appelbaum, "Can Mental Patients Say No to Drugs?"; Appelbaum and Gutheil, "The Boston State Hospital Case;" W. J. Curran, "The Management of Psychiatric Patients: Courts, Patients' Representatives, and the Refusal of Treatment," *New England Journal of Medicine* 302(1980):1297–99.

24. Appelbaum, "Can Mental Patients Say No to Drugs?"

25. A. Meisel, L. H. Roth, and C. W. Lidz, "Toward a Model of the Legal Doctrine of Informed Consent," *American Journal of Psychiatry* 134(1977):285–89.

26. Ford, "The Psychiatrist's Double Bind"; Appelbaum and Gutheil, "The Boston State Hospital Case."

27. Stone, "The Right to Refuse Treatment."

28. Quoted in Gutheil, "In search of true freedom," 327.

29. Ford, "The Psychiatrist's Double Bind"; Appelbaum and Gutheil, "The Boston State Hospital Case"; Stone, "The Right to Refuse Treatment."

30. Appelbaum and Roth "Assessing the NCSC Guidelines for Involuntary Civil Commitment . . ."; Appelbaum, "Is the Need for Treatment Constitutionally Acceptable as a Basis for Civil Commitment?"

31. Ford, "The Psychiatrist's Double Bind"; S. P. Segal, "Civil Commitment Standards and Patient Mix in England/Wales, Italy, and the United States," *American Journal of Psychiatry* 146(1989):187–93; A. A. Stone, "Recent Mental Health Litigation: A Critical Perspective,"

American Journal of Psychiatry 134(1977):273–79; Schultz, "The Boston State Hospital Case."

32. Reiser, "Refusing Treatment for Mental Illness"; Stone, *Mental Health and Law*, 46, 66–79, 102–106; Meisel et al., "Toward a Model of the Legal Doctrine of Informed Consent."

33. L. H. Roth, "A Commitment Law for Patients, Doctors, and Lawyers," *American Journal of Psychiatry* 136(1979):1121–27; T. G. Gutheil, R. Shapiro, and L. St. Clair, "Legal Guardianship in Drug Refusal: An Illusory Solution," *American Journal of Psychiatry* 137(1980):347–52.

34. P. S. Appelbaum, S. A. Mirkin, and A. L. Bateman, "Empirical Assessment of Competency to Consent to Psychiatric Hospitalization," *American Journal of Psychiatry* 138(1981):1170–76; Appelbaum and Gutheil, "The Boston State Hospital Case"; H. Owens, "When Is a Voluntary Commitment Really Voluntary?" *American Journal of Orthopsychiatry* 47(1977):104–10; Stone, *Mental Health and Law*, 46, 97–106, 199–215.

35. Stone, "The Right to Refuse Treatment"; Appelbaum, "Can Mental Patients Say No to Drugs?"; Curran, "The Management of Psychiatric Patients"; Appelbaum and Gutheil, "The Boston State Hospital Case."

36. Roth, "A Commitment Law for Patients, Doctors, and Lawyers."

37. Ibid.; Stone, *Mental Health and Law*, 65–79, 102–106.

38. American Psychiatric Association, "Guidelines for Legislation on the Psychiatric Hospitalization of Adults," *American Journal of Psychiatry* 140(1983):672–79.

39. Segal, "Civil Commitment Standards and Patient Mix in England/ Wales, Italy, and the United States."

40. R. J. Wilk, "Implications of Involuntary Outpatient Commitment for Community Mental Health Agencies," *American Journal of Orthoppsychiatry* 58(1988):580–91; Appelbaum, "Is the Need for Treatment Constitutionally Acceptable . . . ?"; A. A. Arce and M. J. Vergare, "Identifying and Characterizing the Mentally Ill Among the Homeless," in *The Homeless Mentally Ill* edited by R. C. Lamb (Washington, D.C.: American Psychiatric Association, 1984), 75–89.

41. Wilk, "Implications of Involuntary Outpatient Commitment for Community Mental Health Agencies."

42. J. L. Geller, "Rights, Wrongs, and the Dilemma of Coerced Community Treatment," *American Journal of Psychiatry* 143(1986):1259–64; V. A. Hiday and T. L. Scheid-Cook, "A Follow-up of Chronic Patients Committed to Outpatient Treatment," *Hospital and Community Psychiatry* 40(1989):52–59; Appelbaum and Roth "Assessing the NCSC Guidelines for Involuntary Civil Commitment. . . ."

43. Wilk, "Implications of Involuntary Outpatient Commitment for Community Mental Health Agencies."

44. I. Perr, "Effect of the Rennie Decision on Private Hospitalization in New Jersey: Two Case Reports," *American Journal of Psychiatry* 138(1981):774–78; A. A. Stone, "Overview: The Right to Treatment," *American Journal of Psychiatry* 132(1975):1125–34.
45. Spitzer and Wilson, "Nosology and the Official Psychiatric Nomenclature," 832.
46. T. B. Karasu, "The Ethics of Psychotherapy," *American Journal of Psychiatry* 137(1980):1502–15; B. Wooton, "Psychiatry, Ethics, and the Criminal Law," *British Journal of Psychiatry* 136(1980):525–32.

INDEX

—

mitochondrion, 27
monoamine oxidase inhibitors, *see* MAOIs
Monroe, S., 174
mood disorders, diagnosis, 147–167, 350
  prevalence of, 149–150
morning sickness, 103
morning worsening, 165
morphine, physiological dependence, 300
Moscowitz, H., 294
motor tasks, lithium effects on, 245
MRI, 70

National Institute of Mental Health study of antipsychotics, 91–94
nausea, 232, 244, 261, 263, 270, 315
Nemeroff, C. B., 227
nerve cells (neurons), 18, 20–22
nerve impulse, 22–23, 26, 28, 31
nervousness, 232, 294
neuroleptic malignant syndrome, 138–139
neurons, *see* nerve cells
neurosis, 39, 48
Newton, R., 294
niacin, 365
nicotine, 308
NIMH, educational program on depression, 199
Noludar, *see* methyprylon
nonconformity, 41, 43, 363–364
norepinephrine, 26, 28, 30, 32
  buspirone and, 295–296
  OCD, 344
  panic disorder, 334
norepinephrine/serotonin theory of depression, 221–225
norepinephrine synapses, 33
  depression and, 221–228
nortryptyline, efficacy for OCD, 337
  plasma level, 192
nose drops, 232
nuclei (group of brain cells), 29
nucleus (of single cell), 27
numbness, 261
nursing homes, 359–360

obsessions, 66, 265–268
  depressive, 162, 267–268
  different than delusions, 268
  drug, 267
  eating, 267
  guilt, 267–268
obsessive-compulsive disorder, *see* OCD
OCD, 30, 265–268, 270
  age at onset, 268
  biological causes of, 344–349
  coexistent depression, 339
  course, 268
  diagnosis, 263–273
  drug therapy, 336–343
  gender, 268
  hallucinations, 61
  prevalence of, 268
  psychotherapy, 336, 339–343
  treatment of, 327, 336–350
oculogyric crisis, 131
Olajide, D., 323
orbital cortex (orbital frontal cortex), 15, 333
  OCD, 347, 349
orgasmic impairment, 342
orthostatic hypotension, 137, 229
overactivity, 152, 154
overconfidence, 152–153
overdosage, 359–360
overvalued ideas, 268
Owen, R., 320
oxazepam, 310

pain, 30
palpitations, 233, 261, 263, 270, 315
panic, 315
panic attacks, lactate induction, 334–336
panic disorder, 256–263, 270, 275, 312, 321–322
  age at onset, 259
  alcoholism and, 301
  biological causes, 333–336
  case study, 255
  course, 259
  diagnosis, 258–262, 332
  gender, 259

ISBN 0-7167-2195-3

90000>

EAN

9 780716 721956